little addictions

little addictions

catherine gray

ASTER*

First published in Great Britain in 2026 by Aster, an imprint of
Octopus Publishing Group Ltd
Carmelite House
50 Victoria Embankment
London EC4Y 0DZ
www.octopusbooks.co.uk

An Hachette UK Company
www.hachette.co.uk

The authorized representative in the EEA is Hachette Ireland,
8 Castlecourt Centre, Dublin 15, D15 XTP3, Ireland (email: info@hbgi.ie)

Distributed in the US by Hachette Book Group
1290 Avenue of the Americas, 4th and 5th Floors
New York, NY 10104

Distributed in Canada by Canadian Manda Group
664 Annette St., Toronto, Ontario, Canada M6S 2C8

ISBN: 978-1-80419-324-2
eISBN: 978-1-80419-326-6

A CIP catalogue record for this book is available from the British Library.

Typeset in Garamond Premier Pro 12/14.5pt by Six Red Marbles UK, Thetford, Norfolk.

Printed and bound in India by Manipal Technologies Limited, Manipal

SRD

Publisher: Jo Morrell
Commissioning editor: Katie Forsythe
Senior developmental editor: Pauline Bache
Creative director: Mel Four
Editorial assistant: Sarah Ramnath-Budhram
Copyeditor: Michaela Twite
Deputy head of publicity: Karen Baker
Marketing director: Matt Grindon
Typesetter: Six Red Marbles
Production controller: Sarah Parry

This FSC® label means that materials used for the product have been responsibly sourced.

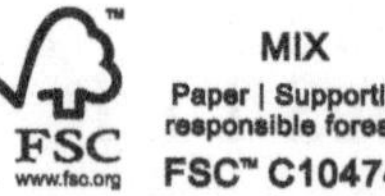

For George.
Whose love and support
made this book possible

'Be the chess player, not the chess piece'
Ralph Charell

CONTENTS

Bold: chapter applies to *all* readers, whatever their little addictions.

PREFACE

We all have a little addiction, or several, nowadays.

And it's no wonder. These days, we have some of the brightest minds trying to make things that are already sticky, even *more* sticky, whether it's a cake or an app.

This means modern life is addictive. Outrageously so. All of the things that were already inherently addictive – sugar, sex, booze, news and buying shoes – also just so happen to generate titanic profits, and thus we have gangs of geniuses who have graduated from Oxford or Harvard (and who will mention so at least once an hour) working on making them *even more addictive.*

It's a fix.

These unfairly gifted humans taste-engineer, finely market, bait clicks, engagement-farm, loop rewards, reduce friction, hide the exits and write irresistible cliffhangers. This reduces those of us who were already pretty helpless in the face of temptation into the bewildered – who wind up a bit too drunk on a Wednesday, with two broken vapes in our bag, wearing an outfit we can't afford, wondering why our screen time reached four hours today, and why the paperback we *really* wanted to read sits ignored in our bag while we obsess over Instagram on the commute.

We've lost control, ever so slightly. Thing uses person, rather than person using thing.

Once we like something – Vinted, roulette, the emotionally unavailable – we want to do it again and again. We are pleasure-seekers, eternal optimists who believe that buying this goose-down duvet could actually change our life, that this meme-making app could catapult us into influencer stardom, or that this CBD oil will stop our anxiety from predicting five-car pile-ups the next time we're driving on a motorway.

I can't think of one friend or family member who isn't addicted to *something*, whether it's getting into credit card debt to obtain the latest tech, gossiping about others (judgement is addictive), *Words with Friends* or get-rich-quick YouTube clickbait (my partner George. Spoiler: we're still not rich).

Truly, most of us struggle with a few things/many things. We are the people who accept Amazon packages we don't quite recall buying ('every day is Christmas for Cath', my ex-flatmate said), who will purchase wine over vegetables on the day before payday, who would take giant Toblerones rather than kindling to a desert island.

Against the backdrop of geniuses hacking into our primal urges, we also have the modern wellness explosion. In many ways, we're watching what we put in our bodies and minds more than ever.

This means that we haul ourselves into the dock after the act. Why can't you just eat one M&M? Why do you keep texting that toxic fuc . . . funhuman? Why are you still on socials at 11pm . . . wait, do you have iPhone claw?

When it all goes sideways, the modern product-makers' caveat is 'but we told you to drink/eat/bet/shop/scroll/use our app responsibly! Please see it in this teeny tiny font on the underside/in the Ts and Cs of our product, whereby we shunt all of the responsibility of its highly addictive design back on to your human weakness. Oh and we donate money to organisations that help cretins like you, so. OK, thanksbye.'

Our little addictions may not be *all* our fault, but they are – inconveniently – all our responsibility. Modern life is not about to get less addictive any time soon; the geniuses at work in laboratories are not going to down tools. If anything, it will grow more sticky. We are the only hope we've got, and we need to get back on our own sides, as the mug slogans might say.

Little addictions don't require long-term abstinence. You're not going to buy a dedicated book on how to quit [insert thing] because, frankly, you don't need to quit it, nor do you want to. Instead though, you might want to shrink or temper your use of this thing before it grows into something bigger.

That's where this book comes in.

We're going to talk about how to define a little addiction (versus a big addiction) and I'll give you some tips for how to dial these down so that they cost you a little less in terms of your time, mental health, energy and money. We're also going to look at some universal themes that span all of our little addictions. More on this later.

Whether your little addictions are scroll holes, wine binges, £50 takeaways, nicotine, people-pleasing, bread, social-stalking your ex, the next episode, biscuit binges or casual hook ups you later regret . . . I'm here to help.

After all, I've been known to do all of those things *in one night.*

Dubious honour, huh. Why listen to me, then? Well, I've already helped thousands of people quit drinking, stop being relentlessly negative and/or refrain from dating like it's a job – I have the beautiful thank-you emails to prove it – and now I am here to help you, no matter what your thing(s) might be. And, crucially, what the thing(s) after that might be. Because they are coming for you, just like a *Game of Thrones* winter.

Little addictions are a moving target, a shapeshifting thing. I used to have a serious little addiction to TV. I once watched eight straight hours of *Selling Sunset* (for those too cerebral to know, this is a reality show about bougie house-selling in LA, with realtors that dress more like Lady Gaga than estate agents).

From 6pm until 2am, I clicked 'next episode' like a lab rat pushing a lever to get a treat. This didn't have any real-life consequences whatsoever, other than causing my eyeballs to sting, helping me work out that my flat was the square footage of a four-car garage and making me feel like shit that I didn't have an infinity pool. (I also wore some bizarre outfits to work over the ensuing days.)

Now that I'm a parent to a toddler, I physically couldn't watch TV from 6pm until 2am. The bedtime routine doesn't finish until 9pm most nights, and even if I tried to binge-watch TV, my body would intervene and make me fall asleep on the sofa. Because, I am very tired a lot of the time. And so, my little addiction to TV has shrunk somewhat, while another little addiction has upsized: S U G A R.

Up until recently, I've been fairly restrained around ice cream, being able to make a tub of Häagen-Dazs last four sittings, but nowadays: gimme that tub, hold my tea and watch while I melt it down in the microwave and chug it in one.

But just because I don't have the time for hours of TV any more, it doesn't mean my 'next episode' lever-pulling is gone for life. It's still there, resurfacing on the rare occasion I have time to indulge it. And even after I wrangle the ice cream thing down, there'll probably be another thing, and another thing, and *another*. Once I've caught one strand of my human fallibility, another breaks loose.

That is why this book covers a total of 15 little addictions. Our current mix of tiny compulsions could look slightly – or even very – different in a year or two.

That's how and why this book is good value. If dominating all of our little addictions is like trying to catch a jellyfish in a bucket, while its tentacles flail and creep over the side, this book is a field guide on how to – humanely, gently, beautifully – catch the entire jellyfish.

INTRODUCTION

I'm not cured of all my addictions. My jellyfish is not sitting obediently in a bucket, its tentacles tucked neatly underneath it.

Here's a list of my former big addictions:

Alcohol
Cigarettes
Love

I'm 12 years sober from booze, 11 years out from cigarettes and 10 from thinking I had to get married in order to be a complete human.

It's well known that if we dominate one addiction, we often find another lesser addiction inside it. In recovery circles, these are called your primary and secondary addictions.

My primary addiction was alcohol, my secondary was cigarettes, my thirdary* was love. But, once I cracked those, I *still* found a set of ever-descending but unignorable Russian nesting dolls within.

Next up were the following:

Overdraft shopping
Validation-seeking sex
Doomscrolling news

I haven't lived in my overdraft for eight years, I'm six years out from having sex to please others and six years from doomscrolling the news (lockdown 1.0 was my rock bottom).

Here are my remaining little addictions:

Nicotine (lozenges, rather than vapes)
Social media (Instagram is my drug of choice)

---

* Not a word, but let's suspend disbelief

Screen time via the phone-checking cycle (WhatsApp – Gmail – Instagram – repeat)
Biscuits (get in my face)
Binge-shopping
Tea (non-caffeinated, mint)
Chewing gum
Television (less pronounced now, but still kicking)
Caffeine
Ice cream (a near nightly habit)

I still have work to do on all of these. We're in this together.

Big addictions

Addictions come in varying sizes and with different proportions of consequence. Usually, with big addictions, the way to deal with them is to quit altogether. None is easier than one. Moderation is a fantasy.

These are the no-brainer addictions with big consequences; the ones that have the power to get us fired, dumped or arrested. They're the ones people beg us to forsake; the Godzillas of the addiction world, that stomp over everything we hold dear and can even threaten our lives.

With some big addictions, the ubiquitous nature of *the thing* can mean that quitting altogether is unlikely (as with love, screen time or certain foods), in which case a long break can be enough to loosen its grip. Like my year-long dating sabbatical, which I wrote about in *The Unexpected Joy of Being Single*.

As Gabor Maté, author and addiction specialist, says, addictions feed the here-and-now hunger, not the psychological appetite. The appetite often remains, even after we've fixed the hunger for a certain thing. Oftentimes, what happens after a big addiction is vanquished looks like a dissolution, a dispersion of sorts.

We're ultimately OK, nobody is worried about us now, but we're also not totally OK. We're not dissimilar from human Velcro strips who walk around the world and find that things stick to us – where did this family pack of Haribo come from? Who downloaded Tinder on to my phone? Whose shopping bag is this?

Even if we've cracked our big addictions, the miniscule dolls hiding within – the fourtharies, fiftharies, sixtharies – the little addictions that in no way threaten our lives or livelihood or relationships, can still cause problems. As the saying goes, it doesn't have to be a problem for it to be a problem.

For others, they've never grappled with a big addiction at all. This might be you. But little addictions are universally experienced. Everyone has – or has had – a little addiction, if not several. I'm willing to die on that hill of a statement.

It's a human in denial, or just an outright liar, who claims they've never been hooked on anything whatsoever. And, of course, that's not you, because of the very act of buying this book.

Little addictions

The influence of little addictions is more of an insidious drip-drip rather than a dramatic whoosh, so it's easy to dismiss them as no biggie. Littles are the rainfall showerhead, rather than a gushing tap. But you still get wet.

It's not going to kill me when I spend two hours a day on social media, nor will I lose my house; I may actually receive a reward loop for it (c/o likes and increased work contacts), but I do also know that I feel a damn sight better when my use is a tenth of that.

My fiancé (such a creepy word) will not cancel our wedding because of my propensity to stuff three mini snowballs into my mouth before walking around with a coconut moustache. However, it's not great for my self-pride, nor my borderline high cholesterol.

My current obsession with *Yellowjackets*, whereby I think about it at least once an hour, having devoured 16 hours of it in the past fortnight and signed up to an entire new streaming service to access season three . . . that's not going to threaten my job as an author.

But I do have a book to write, which it is interfering with. My choice to press go on season three, and to consume 24 hours of telly in total *will* mean that when I'm staring down the barrel of the final deadline, which is alarmingly soon, I will have to pull late nights.

Hate consequences. And just like death or taxes, they're inevitable. Even little addictions have consequences, which incrementally snowball.

Why me?

Good question. Well, I help people grapple with addictions without the teeth-gritting deprivation. At least, that's what I'm told. Readers say that my books get them to the other side with lesser amounts of craving and white-knuckling, and maximum bounties of freedom and happiness.

Here are some common threads my reader letters and reviews mention:

a) I'm one of you, not a guru.

b) I will not try to deny the unignorable pleasures of all of the above. To say that nachos or box-set binges are unenjoyable would be disingenuous. Insulting, even.

c) I dangle everything you have to gain from the change, rather than chasing you with a big stick of guilt.

d) I have been a journalist for 20 years, so I am trained to hunt out the latest research, dig up the lesser-known data and quiz the luminaries in this realm. I do the job of all the reading and research, so that you don't have to.

My skill base is taking the complex things geniuses are saying, simplifying them and making sure they're actionable before arranging them to give you an overarching view.

My not being an expert has a positive flipside: I have no singular theory to peddle. No specialist angle to prove.

You'll get a multitude of expert takes for the price of one book; I spoke with two dozen experts in total. Which means you can choose what you like, keep what works for you and chuck the rest (in recovery speak, this is 'take what you like, leave the rest').

That's me dealt with.

Why you?

As for you, you're probably here because the negatives you're experiencing from your thing, whatever that might be, are starting to outweigh the positives.

You didn't buy this book because you're loving your monthly credit card bills or texting suitors you don't like very much or needing to vape to feel calm. You bought this book because, even though buying a £150 Reformation dress or being mid-cookie-jar feels good in the moment – and isn't threatening to kill you or even hurt you slightly – overall your current thing is making you feel *bad*.

So, you want to do less of it.

Most addictions look like this:

Stage 1: FUN
Stage 2: FUN + PROBLEMS
Stage 3: PROBLEMS + FUN
Stage 4: PROBLEMS

Once an addiction becomes big, it's probably in stage three or four. It's a pursuit of ever-diminishing returns.

Little addictions live in the liminal space between stage one and two. A slippy-slidey, in-between realm where the problems have only just made themselves known, and the fun still dominates the picture, but they're creeping in all the same.

None of these little addictions are dire, so we mutter 'must do better' but still mostly ignore them. We set an hour's limit on WhatsApp and then tap 'ignore limit' in order to bust through it.

Nonetheless, these little addictions can grow into medium, then big addictions. On some level, you already know that.

Congratulations for tackling it so early on. That takes some serious self-awareness.

Getting to know our little

This book is going to dig into the 'what' and the 'why' of the most common little addictions. Knowledge is power, and once we know everything about our adversary – the 'what' – we become like an athlete who has studied tapes of their upcoming opponent's matches, who now knows everything about their killer moves or weak spots. Forewarned is forearmed.

The 'why' takes a look beneath the hood, at the engine driving our use of this thing. Often the 'why' comes from a place much more primal, and much less modern, than you might expect. The thing we're using may be modern, but the urge for it is ancient.

We'll unpack the evolutionary psychology that has led us here. Oftentimes, knowing about the 'why' that powers our reach enables us to instead grab alternatives that satisfy the same primal desire.

Behavioural scientists have been banging on about the *thing beneath the thing* for decades, with good reason. We don't want social media, per se; we want acceptance by a tribe. We pursue and hoard items because of our impulse to hunt and gather. We don't want junk food as such; we want to feel energised.

The hardwired desire to nest in our home has us buying cushions we don't need. The subconscious drive for opportunities to procreate (even if we don't want kids, consciously) can trample our ability to make shrewd decisions about love and sex. This is why sometimes our loins can stir even when our higher brain says to defer.

Universal truths

Given all addictions at their core have the same modus operandi – person reaches for external substance/thing/activity/other person in order to change an internal state –much of this book is not specific. It's universal.

Once you dismantle all addictions, although the outer casing may differ, you'll often find the same nuts and bolts. The same deep neuropsychology is at work, whether it's a compulsion for chocolate or Candy Crush.

I recommend you read all of the 'Universal Truths' chapters. They're about tactics and wisdom that overarch *all* addictions. So, each one of you might want to take a look. They're flagged in bold on the contents page.

You'll more than likely then flick directly to the 'little addictions' (in regular typeface on the contents page) that resonate with you. That's cool. But if you're curious, it might help to also skim the other 'little addictions' too.

Even if a section of the book doesn't apply directly to you, it could help you understand someone you love and their urges. Your partner's porn use, for instance, or your sister's fixation on gaming.

Your little addiction might be niche and not specifically named here (I know someone hooked on watching chess tournaments, and another person obsessed with saunas), but you will still find many tools dotted throughout that *will* work, even if they're buried in the ultra-processed food or nicotine chapters. Many of the 'micro tactics' at the close of each chapter are potentially transferable.

Modern life is addictive

We'll also tackle our unique conundrum, in that life has never been as addictive, as moreish, as accessibly hooky, as it is right now. Thanks, life!

Back in the 19th century, they didn't have to deal with this shite. Nobody was dangling the 'next Oscar Wilde play in 5, 4, 3 . . .' in front of a farm worker who needed to be up in six hours.

Access to their own calorific downfall was inhibited by both budget and access, rather than there being a whole primary-coloured aisle in the supermarket of affordable treats with which to clog their veins.

Dealers literally sold horses rather than baggies of horse, and even the gentry didn't have devices in their pockets with which they could borrow and gamble away £5,000 within the time it took for their carriage's steed to have a toilet break.

Consumer life is now always on, ever more, instantly there, same-hour delivery, watch it now. If we want more we can get it, and we can usually get it right now via a virtually frictionless app. Which is why we've got some serious work to do. Resisting this will be an inside job.

We'll be pulling back the curtain to reveal the wizard, by hearing from whistleblowers from the worlds of retail manipulating, game testers, vape marketing and much more. You won't *believe* what some of them have to say.

Although it's easy to blame the Silicon Valley app developers or the food designers or alcohol industry for making life just so damn addictive, they're just doing their jobs, albeit very well. At times they can be ruthless, but conscientiousness is not part of their job description; profit margins are.

Our real nemesis is our own brain. And no matter how highly schooled or

IQ-ed our brain is, it will crave more of what makes it feel good. Even if that good feeling is temporary, and the consequences are permanent. Our hunter-gatherer brains, unless cajoled to do otherwise, will always prize the short-term buzz above the long-term gain.

In the 'Field Notes' sections (also flagged in bold on the contents page), I'm going to go out into this fiendish modern world and find out everything I can about this brand new conundrum. This is my most investigative book yet. I've spent weeks on the road, have had my brain scanned, visited two labs styled up like bars, handled human tissue samples, worn a white coat, tried on an EEG cap and have said 'explain it to me like I'm 12' to experts whose IQs are at least 20 points higher than mine.

We can borrow a lot from the world of big addictions here, downsizing those tools for our little addictions. I've shadowed the team from a five-star rehab, spending 48 hours there and emerging feeling zhuzhed.

I have analysed hundreds of academic studies which, I must say, do not usually make for scintillating reading. To give you a taster, one was called: 'Caffeine-containing, adaptogenic-rich drink modulates the effects of caffeine on mental performance and cognitive parameters: a double-blinded, placebo-controlled, randomized trial'.

This is also my least personal book. Some readers will exhale at the ceasing of the overshare. But wait. I will still be oversharing a little. Along the way, I'll be disclosing data, such as how many vibrators I own, that time my boss called me a c*nt, why I'm useless at smoking weed and what my partner and I have had 37 arguments about.

Does she have no shame, I hear Middle England mutter. No, not really. Shame leads to noplace good. You can keep your shame.

Along the way, I've found out things that I genuinely believe are transformative. That have transformed my life too.

What's going on inside our brains

It helps enormously to understand what exactly is going on in our brains and *why* our brains are behaving that way.

Key to this will be understanding what's really going on, neuroscientifically speaking, when we experience that 'want it but also don't want it' battle.

Medieval dramas, particularly morality plays, often described this tug of will as having an angel on one shoulder and a devil on the other.

The reality is, this push-pull is often due to a clash between two particular parts of our brain: the limbic system and the prefrontal cortex. We'll get into this in detail later, but I like to think of it as having a split-personality brain, with my limbic system as a delinquent that requires calming the fuck down. Neuroscientists concur.

The prefrontal cortex is best described as the adult, rational part of the brain, which plans for the long-term. It wants to do your taxes tonight given that the deadline is tomorrow. Your limbic system, meanwhile, wants to set fire to all the receipts, use that fire to light a spliff, and watch back-to-back *Walking Dead* while throwing bon bons into its mouth.

We'll talk about established science, which shows that the prefrontal cortex is the key to gaining mastery over addictions. Most importantly, we'll cover how to unlock that.

We'll also be getting into dopamine's starring role in all of this. A couple of decades ago, we thought that dopamine was all about 'liking', but now we know it's about 'wanting'. Liking and wanting are not the same thing.

A couple of decades on from the liking/wanting revelation, the tectonic plate of dopamine understanding shifted again, when the multi-million-selling *Dopamine Nation* broke new ground.

'What goes up, must go down,' author Dr Anna Lembke told us – showing that, when we indulge in substances or activities that artificially spike our dopamine levels, our brain fights to return to balance, and thus drags our dopamine *below* baseline after the spike.

What followed was a proliferation of TikToks and influencers misunderstanding what Dr Lembke had put so eloquently; talking about 'cheap dopamine' and selling 'dopamine-fasting' as if it's a juice plan.

We'll be talking about why 'cheap dopamine' is a misnomer, and why 'fast dopamine' is a much more accurate way to describe it. We'll then unpack why 'dopamine-fasting' via a binge-purge cycle is a truly terrible idea.

When understood adequately, 'dopamine-fasting' is great, but here in this book we'll discuss 'dopamine-shifting' as the wiser choice. Because we need dopamine. Mostly though, we need to point ourselves towards the slower kind: 'slow dopamine'.

Dopamine isn't a villain. We need dopamine to keep ourselves upright and motivated. We'll hear from experts saying that our reward systems, which run mostly on dopamine, evolved to keep us alive, fed and striving. Rats whose dopamine is inhibited will literally lie around a cage, not bothering to go and eat the food on the other side. They have to be hand-fed.

'Dopamine-shifting' – while less catchy – is the secret.

The sticky eight

As you know, I've pinned down 15 'little addictions', working these out meticulously with expert help. But within those 15, we've also identified the 'sticky eight'. The 'sticky eight' are those we need to handle with caution.

I've treated these eight with the awe and fear they deserve by frontloading them.

The remainder are also sticky, of course, just not *as* sticky. It's also worth mentioning that almost everything is addictive (although I'd argue that kale, burpees or tax returns aren't). To honour this, we'll talk later about how *even* addiction experts become addicted to the likes of vampire romance or buying classical music. I spoke with one neuroscientist who doesn't keep a TV in his house, given his propensity to sit in front of it, slack-jawed. Meanwhile, a dentist told me that he has clients who get addicted to teeth-whitening.

There are three outliers you might notice, among the notoriously sticky substances (like alcohol, nicotine, cannabis), and the classic process addictions (such as gambling, gaming, shopping, porn).

This trio is more behavioural, namely procrastinating, people-pleasing, and judgement and gossip. These are conditioned in by fascinating cultural and evolutionary forces we'll get into.

We'll be going on a forensic investigation into what we think these things are giving us, and why the brain wants that. And finding other ways to give ourselves the same thing, but usually in a slower way ('slow dopamine'), and with other, better feelgood neurotransmitters in the mix.

This will mean we cajole ourselves into doing less of the 'wrong' thing (which is of our own definition) and more of the 'right' thing (ditto) . . . but we will still feel just as good. Better, even. A win-win, if ever I saw one.

External things *can* help, and we'll be using them along the way, but the beginning of it all starts with us.

Tooling you up

I feel strongly that books should tool you up. Shining a light on something is great – thanks geniuses – but then, what do us mere mortals do with it? Where do we go from here? How do we use this knowledge to make our lives easier, better, faster, slower, more, *less*; whatever it is we're hankering after. This is why there are specific tools for each little addiction, which are called 'micro tactics'.

You'll spot common through lines, such as self-binding, cue-hiding, structure-building, identity change and accountability, although each time they'll be positioned slightly differently. We know these things work with big addictions, so we can whittle them down and use them here too.

This book is here to help you moderate your little addictions down to less of a propulsion and more of a pleasure. Because let's face it, you don't want to – or need to – totally quit shopping, dating apps, PlayStation, Facebook; whatever your *thing* might be. I have no intention whatsoever of quitting my little addictions either (spoiler: the book had other plans).

At the same time, I do also know that my day (and big-picture life) would be better if I could stop thinking this particular knitwear-shop binge will 'complete my wardrobe', restrict myself to three biscuits at a time, resist clicking 'next episode' when it's time for bed and keep my screen time under two hours per day.

We just need to regain mastery. Are you excited? I am. Let's do this.

THE EXPERTS

Dr Alex Korb is a neuroscientist and the author of *The Upward Spiral: Using neuroscience to reverse the course of depression, one small change at a time.*

Dr Judith Grisel is a neuroscientist from Bucknell University, and is the author of *Never Enough: The neuroscience and experience of addiction.*

Dr Andrew Thomas is an evolutionary psychologist at Swansea University.

Dr Emily Finch is an addiction psychiatrist for the NHS.

Professor Philip Murphy is a psychobiologist from Edge Hill University.

Professor Natasha Dow Schüll is a cultural anthropologist from New York University and the author of *Addiction by Design: Machine gambling in Las Vegas.*

Dr Axel Bouchon is a molecular neuroscientist and the co-creator of the Matter Neuroscience app.

Hilda Burke is a psychotherapist and author of *The Phone Addiction Workbook: How to identify smartphone dependency, stop compulsive behaviour and develop a healthy relationship with your devices.*

Josh Fletcher is a psychotherapist who specialises in anxiety (his handle on Instagram is @anxietyjosh) and is the author of *And How Does That Make You Feel? Everything you (n)ever wanted to know about therapy.*

Anna Mathur is a psychotherapist (Instagram: @annamathur) and the author of *The Uncomfortable Truth: Change your life by taming 10 of your mind's greatest fears.*

Chris Lomas is an addiction psychotherapist at Delamere, a residential private rehab.

Paige Keegan is an addiction therapist at Delamere rehab.

Jerome Fagan is a recovery mentor at Delamere rehab.

Gail Sargerson is a recovery mentor at Delamere rehab.

Sally Hopkins is a recovery mentor at Delamere rehab.

Dr Clayton Hickey teaches psychology at the University of Birmingham, and heads up the 'Motivated Cognition Lab' at the CHBH (Centre for Human Brain Health).

Nir Eyal is a behavioural designer and the author of *Indistractable: How to control your attention and choose your life*.

Shahroo Izadi is a behavioural change specialist with a background in addiction services, and is the author of *How Diets Make Us Fat: The weight loss book that finally helps you keep it off for good*.

Professor Alex Miller teaches psychiatry at the Indiana University School of Medicine.

Dr Debbie Crossland is the brains behind bar lab, Wendy's, at the University of Winchester, as well as a lecturer in psychology there. She co-leads the Centre for Forensic and Investigative Psychology.

Patrick Fagan is a behavioural scientist and the co-author of *Free Your Mind: The new world of manipulation and how to resist it*.

Dr Sarah Bayless is a senior lecturer in psychology at the University of Winchester. She specialises in the influence of alcohol intoxication upon recall.

Dr Anna Lembke is a psychiatrist and the author of *Dopamine Nation: Finding balance in the age of indulgence*.

Dr Julia Lewis is an addiction psychiatrist with the NHS in Wales and clinical lead for addiction services in the Aneurin Bevan University Health Board.

LITTLE ADDICTIONS vs BIG ADDICTIONS

Here, I invite you to test the size of your addiction.

It's imperative that you only use this book for little addictions. It's not intended for medium or big addictions.

We're going to be covering 15 different types of little addiction. These are:

THE STICKY EIGHT

Alcohol
Gaming
Nicotine
Gambling
Our phones
Cannabis
Ultra-processed food
Porn

THE REMAINING SUBSTANCE/ PROCESS ADDICTIONS

Dating, flirting and sex
Shopping
Television
Caffeine

BEHAVIOURAL COMPULSIONS

Judgement and gossip
People-pleasing
Procrastination

Ring or tick which ones you feel apply to you (these may change over time).

Then, you need to test out <u>each</u> addiction on the grid, individually, by ticking or ringing the statements that apply.

So, if you list five little addictions, you need to do this five separate times.

Don't just glance down the grid, guesstimating that all of your addictions are little. You might be surprised to find that some of them aren't sizing up at the proportion you expect.

The three little behavioural compulsions that we cover (people-pleasing, procrastinating, judgement and gossip) won't fit as neatly into this blueprint, but most will.

LITTLE ADDICTION	BIG ADDICTION
You wouldn't dream of spending the last money in your bank account on it.	You wouldn't hesitate to buy it with your last wages – and then need to borrow money to survive the rest of the month.
When you're not using/doing it, you barely think about it, other than a fleeting thought.	When you're not using/doing it, you're regularly thinking about how to get closer to it.
You joke about your use of it.	You hide your use of it.
After doing it you feel naughty, but not guilty.	After doing it, self-loathing sets in.
You know you could live without it . . . you just don't want to.	You can't imagine life without it, even though you tell others you can 'take it or leave it'.
You've never Googled '[insert thing] addiction'.	You regularly Google '[insert thing] addiction' (usually on private mode, late at night) and look for proof you're *not* addicted, or for stories from people who are *more* hooked.

LITTLE ADDICTION	BIG ADDICTION
If your family, friends or partner asked you to stop, you would be mildly amused, then decline without needing to justify why.	If your family, friends or partner asked you to stop, you would burn with shame, then refuse, giving a defensive speech as to why you don't need to.
When you hear about people giving up this thing, you are curious and ask them questions as to what it's like on the other side.	When you hear about people giving up this thing, you feel anxious, as if your use of it has been attacked. You wish they'd restart.
When you do the thing, you sometimes do it more than you'd like to.	When you do the thing, you almost always do it more than you'd like to.
In public (if you use it in public), you use it the same way as you would in private.	In public (if you use it in public) you pretend to be more casual about it, and less intense, than you are in private.
You have been known to delete apps or throw away physical items linked to this thing. However, this is very infrequent.	You regularly delete apps or throw away physical items in relation to this thing, only to download or buy more the next day.
If a doctor told you that you *had* to stop this for a medical reason, you would immediately stop. You'd miss it, but your health comes first.	If a doctor told you that you *had* to stop this for a medical reason, you would seek a second opinion and look for resources online that undermine the first doctor's opinion.

LITTLE ADDICTION	BIG ADDICTION
Most days, you manage your engagement with this like a champ. Some days, you don't.	Most days, you cannot manage your engagement with this. You intend to use X at the outset, and you then use Y or even Z.
You've received the odd birthday card, or social jibe, alluding to your liking of this thing.	Many of your birthday cards, or the social jokes at your expense, allude to your liking of this thing.
You wouldn't go out at weird times, go out of your way or buy expensive extra WiFi or data to do or get this thing.	You have been known to go out at weird times, or go out of your way to get this thing. Or you have bought expensive WiFi or data to gain access to it.
Your use over the past couple of years has remained fairly constant, with intermittent ups and downs.	Your use over the past couple of years has become steadily greater.
Score...	Score...

Your score

If you've only ticked or circled statements in the left-hand column, your addiction is a little one.

Some little addictions, due to their more forbidden nature, might warrant a tick or two in the right-hand 'big' column. For instance, you may 'hide your use' of cannabis or porn, even though it's not a medium or big addiction, due to general social disapproval, or your partner not liking it.

As long as you've only ticked one – maximum two – from the 'big addiction' column, and the rest of your true statements live in the left-hand-side, you're still in the little leagues.

You have a medium addiction if you ring three or more statements from the 'big' column.

If your ticks live mostly on the right-hand side, I am sorry to say that you have a big addiction, my friend. I've been there and it's scary to confront.

If that's the case, this book isn't the right resource. Drop it and roll away to a resource that is more proportionately appropriate. I've put a stack of these on page 313.

****

- **The 'sticky eight'** were reviewed and approved by Dr Judith Grisel, a neuroscientist from Bucknell University, who specialises in addiction.
- **The 'test your size' grid** was approved by Dr Emily Finch, an addiction psychiatrist for the NHS. Her notes are below.

Dr Finch says:
'I agree with everything you have included here. The symptoms mentioned with regards to "big addictions" closely mirror the diagnostic criteria I'm familiar with from the DSM (*The Diagnostic and Statistical Manual of Mental Disorders*).'
'I personally wouldn't use the language "little addiction" for the behaviours described in column one myself. I'd be more inclined towards "tiny habits", but even that phrase doesn't quite cover it.'
'It's an essentially human impulse. There are some chocolate biscuits on the table over there and I know I'll visit them two, maybe three times, today.'
'However, that's just the alternative language I would choose myself, and I can certainly see the benefit in tackling what you have named as "little addictions" before they become larger.'

NO GENERATIONAL PRECEDENT

No generation before us has been in this sizeable a clusterfuck when it comes to little addictions trying to grab our time, money and energy.

While learning how to navigate the world, we tend to mimic our parents or guardians; to copy their structures for dealing. This can go either way. Maybe you adopted your mother's habit to never keep 'naughty stuff' in the house, or maybe your parents had a 'treats drawer'.

Historically, every generation encounters a few new sticky temptations that their parents didn't have to contend with. My father, for instance, came of age in the 1970s, and was offered drugs his father had never encountered, such as cannabis.

A generation on, my brother and I would have had to deal with temptations our father never needed to grapple with while growing up, such as gaming consoles and cleverly-marketed sweets that weren't served by the quarter-pound in paper bags.

It's manageable when the new generations only have a *few* new things to learn to resist. It's when there are dozens pushing their way in that we run into problems.

And that's where we find ourselves right now.

How we got here

Our society has advanced rapidly over the past 100 years. Picture 1926 pre-WWII Britain, with cheese wrapped in wax and stored in larders, oil lamps, books and the wireless radio being the in-house entertainment, and only the wealthy owning cars.

But the past couple of decades have gone shockingly fast when it comes to things becoming more addictive, near limitless and almost always accessible.

Let's go back to 1996, whenabouts many of Gen X (me included) were coming of age and learning how to deal with the adult world of little addictions.

If you wanted to gamble you physically went to the bookies. Takeaways were things we literally took away from restaurants, unless you wanted an awkward conversation on the landline with the one Indian restaurant in your town that delivered. We had fish and chips on Fridays (one of the few foods that weren't rationed during WWII, in order to boost morale). Ultra-processed ready meals were largely reserved to barely edible chicken kievs or gross 'crispy pancakes'.

The only internet access in our home was via a dial-up modem in the living room. It took a good few minutes to get online via dial-up, and there was little chance of being furtive about it, given internet use tied up the landline and made a sound that went a little something like this:

bing-sssh-scree-bing-bop-bing-bop-eee

Subtle.

If you were horny, unless you wanted to risk this (usually shared) modem being proliferated by telltale pop-ups or even a charming virus, you paid for achingly expensive subscription-only TV channels, or bought top-shelf magazines such as *Playboy* or *Playgirl*. We didn't have smartphones, so we couldn't look for kicks inside our bedrooms, browsing histories concealed within private fingerprint-protected windows.

What's more, there were certainly no faux social landscapes where you could find out someone fancied you, or experience the heart-stopping fate of being cancelled by a peer group. MySpace wouldn't even exist for another seven years.

If we wanted to socialise, we either went 'down the rec/park', to shopping centres where we'd loiter around Miss Selfridge or HMV (this was a big Saturday out), to house parties or, for the boldly underage/overage, we went to the pub, which all closed at 11pm, or earlier on Sundays.

Aside from the advents of cable TV and dial-up internet, life truly wasn't all that different from this in 1986, or even 1976.

Millennials come of age

Now, let's move into 2006, when many Millennials were in their late teens or early adulthood, and starting to require the art of self-regulation.

We were still watching broadcast telly – at most cable or Sky – rather than streaming, early adopters had only just got on Facebook, and only eight in ten of us had mobile phones, which were either Nokia bricks, the fancier flip-phones by the likes of Samsung or, for the businessy, Blackberries.

The iPhone hadn't been invented yet, and nine in ten of us still had landlines. Nobody had heard of 'screen time', let alone were they wrestling with how to limit it. The idea of somebody spending four hours a day on their flip-phone would have been laughable. We were all playing *Tetris* on said bricks or flips – while dedicated gamers were playing the latest *Super Mario Bros* on PlayStation 2.

There was no such thing as grocery-delivery services within the hour; if you wanted treats you walked to the shop. Nicotine was mostly ingested via cigarette, or vaguely medicalised nicotine gum only available from the chemist's or on prescription. Vapes had only just landed in the UK and were extremely rare.

Dating apps didn't exist yet; Tinder wouldn't be rolled out for another six years, Bumble for another eight. All that existed were dating websites such as Match.com and Mysinglefriend.com. Needing a laptop or PC to access flirtatious chat and potential suitors inhibited the amount you could do.

The 24-hour licensing laws had just been rolled out, which meant that, unless you lived someplace remote, the party was rarely curtailed by a lack of booze. Most towns had a dodgy off-licence selling through the night, usually called something like 'Wine Not', or a petrol station where you could order it through a partition (something I engaged fully with).

Cocaine became much more socially common, caffeinating these all-nighters. Before cocaine, many just passed out. The use of cocaine as a 'sharpener' to sober you up so that you could drink more took hold.

The 'digital natives' of Gen Z

The only generation of age today who even had a notion of what was coming for us – *has* come for us – has been Gen Z, currently aged between 13 and 28 as I write, the eldest of which would have become adults in 2015.

And they – unsurprisingly – tend to be the most shrewd among us, when it comes to knowing about the need to gain mastery over this stuff, given they're 'digital natives', and grew up around the internet.

They talk about things like 'attention harvesting' and 'data mining' and are the target audience for brand-new feature-free 'boring phones' (the 'dumbphone' has had a re-brand, given having one is actually smart).

Gen Z love vinyl, Polaroid cameras, flea market finds, Game Boys, nineties music and shows that are cosily retro, such as *Gilmore Girls* and *Friends*. It's evident that they yearn for simpler times.

They're hopelessly addicted to their phones, true, spending an average of six hours a day on them, but are also the group most intent on moderating this down. Research says that Gen Z are the only generation whose time on social media has fallen since 2021 (the social media time-spend of Baby Boomers is going *up*).

Moreover, a 2025 government-commissioned report found that two-thirds of Gen Z think socials do more harm than good. Based on their own experiences of growing up on socials, 78 per cent of them vow to 'delay their child using social media for as long as possible'.

They're nicknamed Generation Zero for a reason, choosing to largely eschew drinking and partying, spawning headlines like 'What's wrong with young people today? They don't get drunk any more' (*The Guardian*). A recent survey found that 43 per cent of drinking-age Gen Z don't drink.

The foremost little addictions of Gen Z are non-coincidentally things that have only recently come to the fore: vaping and TikTok. The first vape shop in Britain only opened 10 years ago in 2015, while TikTok launched in 2018.

No 'how to cope' playbook

Here's what happens when the speed of technological advancements outstrips generational hand-me-down wisdom. When there are scores – not just a few – of unprecedented items in the bagging area.

We have no playbook of structure, of coping strategies, to draw upon. Which brings us to how we now live, each holding a clutch of little addictions.

'Thirty years ago, we would have inherited structure and habits from our parents,' says neuroscientist Dr Alex Korb, author of *The Upward Spiral*. 'But rapidly advancing technology and modern society broke a lot of the inherent structures.'

'It's just like fruit used to have this inherent structure to it,' Dr Korb said. 'Where strawberries were only available in summer months, but now we can buy them all year round.'

There are only two ways out of this structureless predicament, he says. 'Either societal expectations need to home in on "this is the right way to use this thing" or – what's more likely – we need to do it ourselves.'

Because even when societal expectations *do* bed in (I'm thinking of the 'don't be a dickhead at dinner' trend where everyone places their phones in the centre of the table, and the first one to pick it up pays for dinner), here's what happens.

The technology then upends it, because you now need to scan a QR code to read most menus, and order, and then also pay. And voila, 'don't be a dickhead at dinner' just got jettisoned.

Us 0, Silicon Valley 30.

And so, that leaves ourselves. 'It's on us to create our own inherent, individual structures,' says Dr Korb. 'That's the only way to avoid over-consumption. We need to figure out the right amount of marijuana, or gaming, or streaming, or smartphone use *for us.*'

Addiction experts call this willingly imposed structure 'self-binding'. With big addiction, it looks like the heroin addict who checks themselves into rehab, removing access to dealers, or the porn-fixated who live without WiFi in their house. A pharmacological example of self-binding is the naltrexone implant, which blocks opioid receptors in the brain, blunting the desire for oxycodone or fentanyl.

Of course, with little addictions these solutions are too extreme. Little addicts don't need rehab, abstinence or pharmaceutical intervention. Which is why we'll take the big addiction model of self-binding and downgrade it by several levels, presenting a baby version.

Once we have structures that work, there's an onus on us to teach our kids, nephews and nieces, godchildren, pupils – whoever is young and around us. If we stand no hope against the ruthless attention-grab, what hope do they have?

Yes, the technology and our society will change in ways we cannot even imagine; I'm thinking now of AI. In the 2000s we thought artificial intelligence's push forward would look like *I, Robot,* where bots created for service roles revolted and became evil. Usually, their eyes turned red.

We could never have predicted the world we currently live in, where AI can write books and songs, is used to deepfake celebrity porn, or can be harnessed to defraud us by mimicking the voices of our loved ones. Turns out the red-eyed robots were the least of our worries.

We don't know what's yet to come. What new ways capitalism will hack our fast dopamine, hooking us on substances and activities we cannot yet imagine.

But we do know this: given we're not able to learn how to deal from the generation/s above, we need to learn how to 'self-bind' ourselves within our own lifetimes.

'We need to build the structures ourselves that we didn't see modelled by our parents,' says Dr Korb, 'given many of the temptations at large *now* didn't exist when we were learning from them.'

Now's the time, people. Before this clusterfuck gets any bigger.

OUR BRAINS EXPLAIN EVERYTHING

The first thing we need to understand about the neuroscience of little addictions is this: everything that *seems* irrational probably has a rational explanation.

'Every time the brain appears to not make sense, once you consider the environment in which it evolved, then it usually makes perfect sense,' says neuroscientist, Dr Korb.

It may seem as if our brain is being contradictory, irrational even, when it both wants something and doesn't want it. It wants a cake, yet doesn't want a cake. 'Gimme a beer!' it demands, like Homer Simpson, while another part intervenes, saying 'No, you have a big day tomorrow.'

'Our brains are multi-layered,' says Dr Korb, 'and the reason we experience multiple desires simultaneously, often in opposing directions, is because different parts of your brain want different things.'

That experience of push-pull is a physical neurobiological fact. 'Part of your brain wants to watch another episode, and part of your brain doesn't, literally,' he says.

We think it's our lack of character, or a sign we need to grow more willpower. We feel like weak, fallible, defective humans who need to dig out more grit, like that athlete influencer who gets up at 4am to chug protein shakes and hit the gym.

'Our thinking and feeling and actions are all controlled by different parts of the brain,' explains Dr Korb. 'Which are often pulling you in different directions.'

It's why we end up being 'cognitively dissonant' where we can hold two opposing beliefs in our brain at the same time. 'I want to gamble, yet I don't want to gamble.'

There's something enormously comforting in finding out that everyone's brain does this. That it's just scientifically normal to think one thing, want something else and then do a third thing entirely.

We don't need to stop wanting

'Don't get mad at yourself for wanting to do things that are enjoyable,' says Dr Korb. It's just the reward centre doing its job, and the reward centre runs mostly on dopamine.

Dr Korb calls dopamine the 'molecule of wanting'. 'Many people think that wanting things that are "bad" for them means there's something wrong with them,' he says. 'There's not.'

It's not about amputating the wanting. It's about understanding the wanting, and the reasons for it, and tapping into the other parts of your brain that want differently, and creating ideal conditions for that re-route to happen.

'We don't have to stop the wanting,' says Dr Korb. 'We just need to start enabling the brain to choose differently.'

As we're going to cover extensively in this book, our brains have evolved to seek out pleasure and avoid pain, our reward system is geared to repeat, repeat, repeat whatever gives it a hit of fast dopamine, and we have to work harder to engage the sensible part of our brain (the Croc-wearing prefrontal cortex) above the spontaneous region (the 'Who needs shoes?! Let's dance barefoot!' limbic system).

What's more, self-flagellation for being drawn to pleasure only serves to make us crave it more. 'Many of us believe – particularly in America, with its puritanical roots – that *pleasure is bad*,' says Dr Korb. 'The irony is that when we pile guilt or shame on top of the pleasurable thing, it then reduces how satisfying the thing is, and therefore you want it more.'

This phenomenon, which I'm calling 'the guilt paradox' will be something we come back to again and again. Self-berating does not work.

The evolutionary mismatch

The wiring of our brain is ancient, and incompatible with the way we live now. It evolved in hunter-gatherer times and hasn't changed since, therefore it can't handle the jacked-up rushes our post-modern world offers.

'We call it the "evolutionary mismatch",' says Dr Andrew Thomas, an evolutionary psychologist at Swansea University. 'Our environment has changed at a rapid pace. The first agricultural revolution was only 10,000 or so years ago, which threw us from tight communities of 150 people maximum, into cities filled with people we don't know; cities filled with choice.'

Ten thousand years sounds like *forever*, but in the bigger evolutionary picture, it's an eyeblink. 'Considering humans like us have been around for about 300,000 years, the formation of cities is very recent,' he says. 'Our environment went pretty much unchanged for 290,000 years before that.'

The sprawl of megacities (London, New York, Tokyo) only happened in the last few hundred years. 'Due to the speed of all of this, our evolved psychology has simply not caught up,' says Dr Thomas.

You hear it a lot, because it's true. 'This mismatch has led to Stone Age brains in modern bodies,' he says. And in modern societies. 'This causes a lot of fundamental problems.' Dr Thomas flags dating, diet and tech as the biggest mismatch issues he sees.

The wiring gets overwhelmed

This mismatch means we evolved for environments of scarcity and our brains are *still* built for that, yet we now live in worlds of over-abundance.

Picture this as a metaphor: you buy a historic listed, chocolate-box cottage whose electrical wiring has not been updated since the 1930s. Then you start trying to use that system to run dozens of modern devices. The wiring would be overwhelmed, right? Fuses would trip, safety standards would not be met, you might even have a fire on your hands.

Many of the things we're going to talk about in this book – from tech like social media, to drugs like alcohol and nicotine – artificially overload our brain's reward circuitry.

'Evolution has not prepared our brains for these drugs, so they become overwhelmed and screwed up,' Dr Wolfram Schultz, a neuroscientist at Cambridge University, told *The Guardian*.

'Think about hunter-gatherers still operating today,' says Dr Korb. 'Take the Nenets of Siberia, who wear the hides of the reindeer they herd, relying on their meat to get them through harsh winters; or the Hadza, a tribe in Tanzania who tunnel into subterranean chambers to hunt out porcupines, dig wild sweet pea tubers from the ground and literally carry a "honey axe".'

'We have the same brains as them evolutionarily speaking,' says Dr Korb, 'but they're still living in an environment that places a limit on how much they can eat. When they find a beehive, they'll crack it open and eat as much honey as they can, but none of them are overweight because these foods are hard to get.'

Whereas over in our worlds of Middlesex or Montecito, we have unlimited access to high-fat, high-sugar food, which has been supercharged to make it as blissful as possible.

'Our brains have evolved to tell us "eat as much high-calorie food as you can" through dopamine and other mechanisms,' Dr Korb says. But our access to it is now near limitless.

Our brain's innate design has no hope. It still has a honey axe in its hand.

Add in capitalism

Then, you add in capitalism. 'This is where it gets sinister,' says Dr Korb, in that the systems we live in are rigged against us, because: money.

Profit-turning companies don't want us to find moderation, they want us to throw more money at bingeing. Capitalism doesn't care about our mental health, family life or waist circumference; it only cares about converting us to their brand.

'Food companies could design ultra-processed foods that are both delicious *and* satisfying . . . but they don't,' says Korb. 'They design it so that we want another – and another – because it's not quite satiating enough.'

This creates a fire hose of dopamine. 'We then have an unnatural flood of stimuli that are dopamine-delivering,' says neuroscientist Dr Judith Grisel. 'What happens next in the brain is that it gets insensitive. And so, we then want more. Which is why we can't wait for 90 seconds in the doctor's office now without getting on social media.'

This problematic dovetail between the ancient blueprints of our brains vs the design of modern-day consumables will play out in almost every little addiction we discuss.

A dog and a teenager plan a party

Then, within our brains themselves, there is another push-pull at play, which we touched on earlier, with the Croc-wearing adult (the prefrontal cortex) needing to wrangle down the barefoot delinquent (the limbic system).

'The limbic system is like a teenager, and it can get really upset when it doesn't get its own way,' says Dr Korb, 'while the prefrontal cortex is the adult in the room, who will pipe up and say "Er, maybe that's not the right decision".'

What the hell, let's add in a dog, just to dial up this chaos some more. Oh, and it's the seat of addiction. Great.

'The striatum is like the "dog" section of the brain. It's pleasure-oriented and habitual – doing what it's been trained to do,' says Korb. 'The striatum is the seat of addiction, because it's what compels you to act.'

The striatum (dog) means well, and doesn't consciously conspire for your downfall, but given that it is spontaneous, fearful, habit-based and pleasure-driven, it's probably not the member of the household who should be making all the big decisions.

Like a dog left unchecked, the striatum would eat a whole roast pig, and then need to vomit to be OK. It thinks a squirrel in the garden is a mortal threat. It does not own a long-term goal planner.

'The striatum is triggered by the emotions in the limbic system,' says Dr Korb. Yes, you heard that right: the teenager is telling the dog what to do. Which probably means telling it to dive into a TikTok clickpool or pour Nerds directly into its mouth.

There's hope, though, in the shape of the 'adult in the room'. 'Luckily, you *can* use your prefrontal cortex to teach your limbic system – and striatum – to make better choices,' says Dr Korb. 'Our cravings are like the barks of a dog. The dog can bark as much as it wants. Whether you give it a treat or not? That's your choice.'

We'll be learning how to engage the prefrontal cortex later. If you don't, then it's like you're giving permission for a teenager and a dog to plan a party. And they will.

'The striatum and limbic system are like your brain's autopilot, and they're perfectly happy to live your life without your conscious input,' says Dr Korb.

I'm trying to imagine this party now. A ball pool full of bones and a goody bag of space cake.

Early pick-up predicts addiction

The younger you are when your striatum learns that you like 'a thing', whether it's a Game Boy or shopping beyond your means, the more likely you are to get addicted to it.

'Younger people are better at learning anything, and that includes addiction,' Dr Grisel told me. 'Yes, the brain "learns" addiction, even though we associate learning with positivity,' Dr Grisel says. 'The earlier we start anything, the more we take to it, whether it's learning a language, playing an instrument or playing a sport. The earlier the child picks up the substance, the more plastic and malleable their brains are,' she said, 'and the more likely they are to learn to use it in an addictive manner. Our brains have more neuroplasticity at 15 than 18.'

But, luckily, this very neuroplasticity is on our side too, given it *does* mean that we can change our brains. The brain we have aged 45 is very different to the brain we had aged 25.

We can – and do – consciously alter our own brains in our own lifetimes. We pave new neural pathways, expanding our capabilities, every time we learn a new skill such as driving, or become a parent, or start a saving habit, or self-bind against watching TV before 8pm.

Work from us is inevitable in this process. But it *is* possible. And that's why we're here. To learn how.

WHY WE LOVE UNCERTAIN REWARDS

Now, we come to another fundamental truth underpinning many addictions – 'reward uncertainty'.

A few of my experts told me that substances offer pretty certain rewards. It's physiological. Caffeine and nicotine stimulate, alcohol gets you drunk and cannabis gets you high.

Not everyone finds the 'reward' rewarding, of course, which is why we don't all enjoy the nicotine or coffee buzz, or the feeling of being drunk or stoned. The meaning of the physiological output is individualised. But the automatic 'input substance + physiological output' chain reaction is largely universal and robust.

'Reward uncertainty', however, mostly comes into play with our 'process addictions': our phones, gaming, gambling, shopping, porn, flirting, dating and sex. Uncertain rewards were already baked into all of those activities. For example, when shopping it feels like the outfit will change your life upon acquisition (but the result varies), gaming even with old school backgammon and chess has uncertain results, gambling has been serving uncertain rewards from the spit and sawdust days at the tracks, and even the very first flip-phones were charged with the innate unpredictability of people.

But nowadays, those organically uncertain rewards have been artificially supersized and manipulated, with clever marketing strategies (pop-ups, countdowns to trigger FOMO), algorithms loaded with a seemingly random schedule of treats (throw them an incentive to keep 'em playing!), the infinite scroll (maybe there's an even better person/item/video?) or apps which synthetically leverage that which we're already fascinated and unsettled by – what people will do or say (make comments visible to all!).

Reward uncertainty's power over us has been known about for almost a century. Academically, it's more often referred to as a 'variable schedule of rewards' and its sway over our behaviour was discovered in the 1930s, when a Harvard graduate called B F Skinner devised the Skinner Box. He didn't call it that (he called it the 'operant conditioning chamber'), but he went on to become a bit of a rock star in the academic world, so other people did.

It was a simple box, fitted with a lever/pecking button, which dispensed a treat. Skinner put rats, mice and pigeons in there, to see how rewards shaped their behaviour. He thought rewards would reinforce learning – and they sure did. But then he had a brainwave. How about mixing it up, and not giving a treat every time?

Well, the pigeons, mice and rats became obsessed. When the treat was certain, not so much. But when the treat was uncertain, they pressed that lever, or pecked that button, compulsively. They even ignored water, food or socialising with other pigeons or rodents.

If there was a pattern to the reward, the birds or rodents would soon learn that pattern and lose interest, says Professor Natasha Dow Schüll, a cultural anthropologist from New York University. They would peck or press ten times when they're hungry, and then go back to their lives, she says. 'But if you run it randomly, they will abandon their life and just stay there pecking.'

'We have evolved to figure out puzzles, and puzzles drive our behaviour,' Schüll says, 'because we're inspired to pursue them, figure them out.' Reward uncertainty throws the brain a puzzle it can't possibly work out. 'It becomes a raw encounter with chance,' she adds, 'and so, we get stuck in the puzzle.'

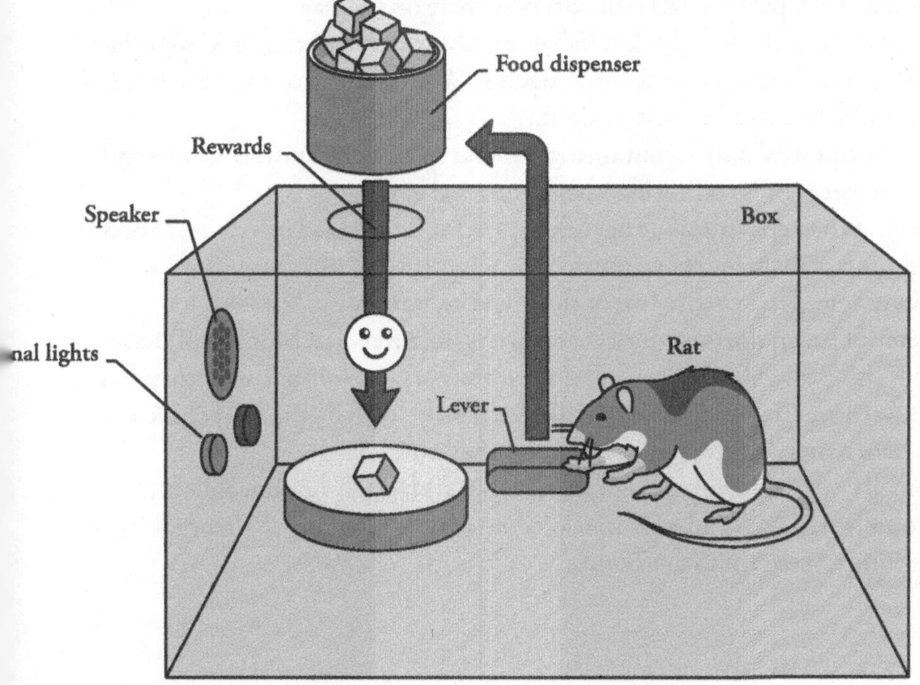

ALCOHOL

Sticky eight

This is my second lab that is styled up like a bar within two months.

I have to say, I prefer this one to the last. The last bar lab was like the place you might have a functional pint while waiting for a plane; where there's only two lagers on draught, no artwork on the walls, no frills, no messin' – do you want a pint or not?

Whereas this bar lab, situated at the University of Winchester, is more like *Cocktail* (the '80s Tom Cruise film) muddled up with the interiors section of Oliver Bonas. It's all neon-pink signs and deep blues, velvety cushions and golden birdcages, soft lighting and a Tears for Fears soundtrack. It's the brainchild of Dr Debbie Crossland, who teaches psychology here at the university.

This is somewhere you might sit and have an ironic cocktail – or mocktail, in my case – with your friends, like a Cosmopolitan or a Virgin on the Beach. We've left the departure gate, friends; now we're on holiday.

Record scratch Wendy's bar/lab doesn't serve retro cocktails. Only ethanol, literally, which is the purest form of alcohol. With a mixer, of course, because you wouldn't want to drink it straight.

The optics at Wendy's, containing popular spirits like Smirnoff, are only for show – to get people feeling like they're in a real bar.

Back at the departure gate bar lab, located at Edge Hill University, Professor Philip Murphy told me that the dozen or so optics, ranging from rum to whiskey, were also a ruse. 'Most of those just contain water,' he said.

Some of the important work that experts (like Rebecca Monk et al) have done at this bar lab has been around the power of cues – visual, olfactory, aural – and how those cues nudge us to drink. See drink, smell drink, hear clink, glug or pop; *want* drink. The brain is elementary that way.

'Smell is actually more salient than you would guess,' he said. Salient, I have now learned, is academic-speak for 'attention-grabbing'. Salience denotes something important to our brain.

'Think about where the nose is situated – right under the frontal lobe – so it has a direct route into the brain,' he says. Murphy tells me that they'll wipe alcohol around the glass, even though the drink itself contains no alcohol, to test the potency of the cue. The upshot? Very potent.

Back at Wendy's in Winchester, they're showing me their secret weapon. Edge Hill has cameras in the bar lab to study drinking behaviour, but Wendy's has something much more fun. We step into the next room and they unfasten a panel to flip it down. One-way glass, just like in a detective drama. So that they can watch the ethanol drinkers without them feeling watched. (When we're watched, or feel watched, we tend to behave better; this is called the 'Hawthorne effect'.)

The two experts showing me around Wendy's –Dr Crossland and her colleague Dr Sarah Bayless – specialise in the nexus between alcohol imbibing and eyewitness testimony, work which is groundbreaking for crime investigation. 'Alcohol myopia' is, in particular, of great interest, which they use the bar lab to study.

Alcohol myopia is a narrowing of cognitive function. It means we're more likely to engage in extreme behaviour. Our focal point is the immediate short-term, rather than the long-term, and we can become more emotional or have an inflated view of our self or abilities (my ability to perform karaoke springs to mind. Since getting sober I have spared the public this horror show). This is what I've read about it, and I ask Dr Bayless if it's correct.

'Yes, all of the things you've said would fall within alcohol myopia,' she says. 'Our attention could be described as a spotlight,' she continues. 'When you're intoxicated, that can narrow. We tend to take fewer elements of our surroundings in, and can perhaps miss relevant peripheral details.' Which is why these studies are so important to the police.

What happens when we drink is a contradiction of sorts, she says. 'We may be hypervigilant and focused on immediate concerns, like getting home after a night out, but lowered inhibitions can lead us to make choices we wouldn't normally consider sober – such as accepting a lift from someone we've just met.' This hypervigilant + unsafe mash-up sound like my entire twenties. 'Where's my phone, where's my bag?!' *Drinks into blackout and loses both.*

Professor Murphy told me that the alcohol itself is also something of a paradox. It's a depressant that we experience as a stimulant.

'Alcohol depresses the central nervous system,' he said. 'But given it also depresses the part of the brain that inhibits, we experience it as a stimulant.' He adds that the disinhibiting effect is what we find pleasurable.

I can relate to this, hugely. Back when I drank, that disinhibition was what got me hooked. It felt like it unclenched me, untightened my ever-present social anxiety. Not only that, but it dimmed the lights and turned down the volume on a world I experienced as overwhelming.

The problems arrive when too many of our inhibitions are removed. Like when I disinhibited to the level where I thought it was reasonable to take my top off at a wedding (it's *too hot!)* and demand a cheese sandwich.

But that's me, and you're you, and given that you've already tested out the size of your alcohol addiction and proportioned it as 'little', it's unlikely that we have the same experiences.

You have probably *never* put your personal safety at risk in order to access more booze, by going to a house party in Brixton with randoms, and then discovering that they keep pet snakes, but staying anyway because they also have cider. I woke up on their sofa (a leather one – not ideal) with a yellow python eyeballing me from across the living room.

Creative accounting

I'm going to guess that, since you're reading this chapter, you want to drink a little less.

The first thing you need to ascertain is what moderate drinking looks like, whether you fall under that category and, if not, how far away from it you are.

Moderate drinking is defined by the NHS as a maximum of one to two drinks a session, with three or four days a week off boozing. One in four Brits are *not* moderating, given they regularly drink over the lower-risk threshold of 14 units per week (which now applies to both men and women; the male threshold used to be 21).

This statistic is based on self-reportage; the true figure is likely much higher. We have a nationwide tendency to downplay how much we drink, says Alcohol Change UK. 'If we compare the amount people say they drink in surveys with how much the Government data tells us is actually sold,' the charity writes, 'then it turns out we drink about 50 per cent more than we say.'

So, you can probably take that one in four and double it, quite safely.

Sometimes we just don't know that we're busting through our weekly units. Personally, I know many highly intelligent people who don't know what constitutes a unit. Many still think it's one drink = one unit. I've had two conversations with friends in the past week that have gone like this:

Friend: 'I drink one beer a night – two at weekends. So that's well under the threshold.'

I nodded and smiled. It's not up to me to burst his bubble. But the reality is that a standard 330ml bottle of 5 per cent beer – or cider – is usually 1.7 units. So, even though he looks like a moderate drinker upon first glance – and compared to what I was drinking, he is the very image of self-restraint – he's not one, given that he's actually putting away around 17 units a week, and not taking the recommended days off.

Another friend of mine said she was 'only drinking a couple of bottles of wine' per week. She does take a few nights off, so go her, but that's 20 units, and well into risky territory.

Wine pours are notoriously miscounted; most home pours are probably 250ml, mine certainly were, which is three units. But they might be creatively accounted for as 1.5 units.

The only glass of wine that is 1.5 units is 125ml, a mere thimble. Most pubs don't even serve this measure unless it's for prosecco or champagne – a 'small' glass of wine is usually 175ml. When the NHS says 'one or two drinks per session', they're talking about the teeny tiny 125ml, or one shot of vodka with a mixer.

Well, this is boring. I know it is. But it's the first hurdle we need to clear, given many people who would class themselves as moderate drinkers are unfortunately not. You need to know where you're starting in order to get where you're going.

I was also shocked to learn what the NHS defines as a 'binge': just six units of alcohol, which is three pints of regular draught or three double G&Ts. I'll be frank, back in my drinking days, six units was a mere appetiser; my biggest nights out could involve twenty.

So, you won't find any judgement here. I considered 30 units a week as a success, and most of my weeks looked more like 50. I kept a 'unit diary' in a little golden notebook and wrote 'why are you so bad at this?!' and 'this needs to stop!' in spiky prose alongside my week's units.

Nowadays, you can just keep track of your units via an app, but not all apps are created equal, and some unit-counting apps will actually nudge you to drink *more*. More on that later.

Even moderate drinking is not good for us

There is still a lot of misinformation flying around on this matter, the reasons for which we'll get to, but, for now, it'd be remiss of me not to dispel this myth.

You have every right to choose to drink, but you also have a right to the facts. Just as we'll discuss with sugary treats, and cannabis, and nicotine, this thing is definitely not good for you . . . there are no health benefits pre-loaded into small amounts of alcohol, and any claims of this are deliberately misleading smoke and mirrors, or just outdated information from before we knew any better.

If you drink anything at all, even one alcoholic drink a week, you're taking a risk, say the NHS and WHO.

But *wait*, I can feel you thinking. And you'd be right to question this. Because we've been told differently our entire lives, particularly when it comes to the hero-worshipped glass of red wine. We've all seen the 'a glass of red wine keeps the doctor away' headlines.

The alcohol industry bankrolls clinical studies

Here's what's gone on, and it's why we're all so confused.

It's previously been fed into the cultural tap water that a small amount of alcohol is safe, desirable, even protective health-wise, given a 'J-shaped curve' on studies comparing the life expectancy of moderate drinkers vs teetotallers. The tail of the 'J' showed that those who drink a little lived longer than those who drank nothing.

'Moderate drinkers live longer than teetotallers!' the headlines cried joyously.

However, and crucially, these studies didn't compare moderate drinkers with *lifelong* teetotallers.

They compared the moderate drinkers with people who'd quit drinking due to ill health (like a brush with cancer), or to people like me (who was once Balham's version of Henry VIII, mainlining fried chicken, draining several bottles of wine a week at my worst and smoking my face off. I didn't behead any spouses though, so: yay me).

Of course a moderate drinker is going to be healthier than me, even though I quit drinking altogether aged 33.

The J-shaped curve theory has since been jettisoned by the medical world. A Canadian meta-analysis of 107 such studies involving nearly 5 million people upturned this 'moderate drinkers are healthier' theory.

Once they separated out the studies that were responsibly done, ie, those that only looked at true lifelong teetotallers vs moderate drinkers, the tail of the J disappeared. With it, so did the apparent health benefits of a small amount of alcohol.

The lead author on the Canadian study, Dr Tim Stockwell, said: 'It's been a propaganda coup for the alcohol industry to propose that moderate use of their product lengthens people's lives.'

Hang on, what's the alcohol industry got to do with medical research? *Everything*. Brace yourselves.

Historically, the alcohol industry has been intimately involved with clinical studies that have espoused the supposed health benefits of boozing; funding them and even authoring them. This means that the alcohol industry has largely controlled the narrative around booze. And it still does.

In 2020, the University of York found that, in the past century, 82 per cent of clinical studies into alcohol were 'authored or funded by' the alcohol industry.

It's good, of course, that they're paying for research. But not when it influences which studies get the money and, therefore, shapes the output.

This same study found that studies bankrolled by Big Alcohol are – what a shocker – more likely to find positive outcomes. Some even lay claim to alcohol causing 'biologically implausible' health benefits, said the researchers.

A solution needs to be found, and quickly, because this in-funding is gathering pace, rather than slowing. 'You're not going to take money from the NHS or, say, primary school funding, to put into alcohol research,' says Dr Clayton Hickey, who teaches psychology at the University of Birmingham. 'It makes sense that the industry pays for it. However, it does create a "moral hazard", whereby the two sit too closely together.'

Where the government is failing to act, the medical industry is stepping in, but at the expense of advancement – and themselves. Dr Hickey was recently involved in a bid for a study into gambling addiction. The whole thing fell apart because it was funded by the gambling industry, and two thirds of his peers felt the moral hazard was too great.

C'mon policymakers. We need to find a way to take the money from the industries that profit from addictive things and *also* ensure the studies funded remain impartial. Surely that's not impossible?

The brain neighbourhood you want

Let's move on to some better news. A little addiction to alcohol lives in a different part of the brain to a big addiction, which means you can potentially prevent this move.

'One of my favourite studies about alcohol showed this,' says Dr Alex Korb, author of *The Upward Spiral*. 'They took social drinkers and showed them pictures of their favourite alcoholic drinks while scanning their brains. In these non-addicted drinkers, the nucleus accumbens activated, which is involved in wanting and pleasure.'

Then they performed the same experiment on those with a clinical (big) addiction to alcohol. 'There was no activity in the nucleus accumbens,' he says. 'Instead, the activity was in the dorsal striatum, which is the habit circuit of the brain.'

Habitual motor skills, such as typing, driving or playing an instrument, are also stored in the dorsal striatum. Automaticity is its thing.

When it comes to drinking urges, the dorsal striatum is more about feeling compelled, says Dr Korb. 'That compulsion arises because their brains now associate unpleasant feelings with *not* drinking.'

Those with big addictions experience this literal neurobiological shift, whereby drinking no longer feels like a choice and starts to be a compulsion. Why? Our brains are designed to spare us discomfort, whether it's in our best interests or not.

I relate *hard*. I thought I needed alcohol to socialise in my teens, then I thought I needed it to relax in my twenties, then I thought I just needed it to *exist*, in my early thirties.

This is why it's important, if you want to shrink your little addiction, to choose carefully *when* you drink. If you're already drinking habitually, that horse has already left the stable. But it hasn't entirely bolted yet.

What you do on discomfort is key. Routinely drinking on negativity – say, to medicate anxiety about a relationship you need to end or to segue from stressed to unwound after the working day – will start to encode the drinking within the brain as a habit you *need* to feel OK. Your drinking will then move to the less desirable neighbourhood: one of habitual requirement to relieve discomfort.

'Drinking: feel OK. Sober: feel bad' the dorsal striatum will start to learn. 'Once the habit circuit gets involved, we're set on a treadmill where we derive less and less enjoyment from drinking,' says Dr Korb, 'yet feel we have to keep doing it.'

It's a self-perpetuating prophecy, says Dr Korb. 'The more you do it, the more appealing it becomes,' he says. 'Then, when we don't drink, our brain becomes stressed and prompts us to drink. It's a brain loop.'

The incremental stress effect is real. Stanford neuroscientist Andrew Huberman went viral when he released a YouTube video called 'How alcohol actually increases stress levels, rather than relaxing you'. In it, Dr Huberman revealed that even moderate drinking changes the brain circuitry, making drinkers feel more stressed all the time.

'People who drink regularly,' said Huberman, 'maybe just on the weekend, two to four drinks, well those people experience changes in their hypothalamic-pituitary-adrenal axis, that result in more cortisol, more of the so-called "stress hormone", being released at baseline, when they are *not drinking*.'

As we'll discuss later, cortisol isn't the anti-hero everyone makes out, and is more accurately described as the 'stress *and* arousal' hormone. But in an ideal world it goes up and down naturally, over the course of the day, rather than remaining elevated.

Nonetheless, it follows that if you want to continue to drink, then occasional, non-habitual drinking is the ideal target. Maybe just at certain events, such as parties or weddings.

But not *all* social events. Because another dead giveaway that your drinking is in the process of moving neural neighbourhoods is this; you start to think you need drinking to do something; say, dancing and dating.

That list – a manageable one – then grows, to include work networking and house parties.

And, oh look, it just expanded again to become *any evening out with other humans.*

This is where my drinking took me.

Structure in a drink-pushing world

There's hope. The only catch is, our brains will rail against it. 'Whenever we want something, our brain is really good at coming up with logical reasons we should have it,' says Dr Korb.

'Your brain will collude if you want another drink,' he says, 'throwing in an enabler like "well, today was a really hard day, so yes, you *should* have another drink". But the action you take can be different from the thought in your head.'

You need to build a set of parameters, says Dr Korb, and make them non-negotiables. 'Some people can drink without it ruining their lives,' says Dr Korb, 'precisely because they have strict parameters. That they're only going to drink with other people, or they'll never drink before 5pm.'

Sticking to them is the tough bit. Our drink-pushing culture – although it has vastly improved in the past five years – collaborates with our brain in throwing us reasons and opportunity to drink almost constantly.

The hotel offers mimosas from 7am, or the dining table has a wine glass on it even though it's lunchtime, or there's half a bottle left in the fridge, and everyone on telly seems to be drinking too.

Our modern world encourages drinking more, faster, and why not now, because it fattens profit margins and, frankly, the businesses only care about their take-home net, rather than your take-home hangover. The eatery can charge you a lot more for a fabled red than a fizzy water.

Peer pressure adds another layer. Drinkers hate to lose drinking company, and will attempt to pull you back in, just as crabs will stop other crabs from escaping a bucket. It's called 'crab mentality' and means that, even though you're trying to change your life positively, and your drinking-less doesn't impede their drinking-hard, it will still cause affront. People will take your desires for your drinking and replace it with *their* desires for your drinking. 'Go on, I can't drink alone!' or 'It's my birthday/engagement party/leaving do, so you have to.'

I don't have any ire for these drink-pushers – I used to be one myself – but for you, remember that it's absolutely a case of 'your body, your choice' even if it *is* their birthday.

In my experience, the more you stand your ground, the more they'll back off. Repetition is the secret.

The impact upon the brain

We're going to do a deep dive into engaging the prefrontal cortex later, on pages 247 to 262, and *for you*, reading that chapter will be utterly crucial.

We've known for some time that the prefrontal cortex is inhibited when we drink, and that it even loses density in long-term big addiction. This makes us more impulsive and up for risk-taking when we've had a drink.

'Ordinarily, the limbic system's emotional decision-making would be downregulated by the prefrontal cortex,' Dr Bayless says. She calls the prefrontal cortex the 'controller', who keeps an eye on things, making sure all the systems are running correctly.

Without it, decision chaos tends to reign supreme. 'You might throw a punch instead of walking away,' she says.

'Or lower your threshold as to who's safe to get a lift with home,' Dr Crossland adds in. Overall, this means our ability to make solid choices is impaired when intoxicated.

Memory is also affected. Big drinkers, like me back in the day, will experience what's called 'blackouts' where chunks of the evenings are lost altogether. The lesser version of this is called a 'brownout', which I ask Dr Crossland about.

'You have gaps in your evening,' she says. 'You might remember turning up, chatting to your friends, but then once you start drinking, it's like, "OK, I remember this bit of the evening. I remember that bit of the evening, but what happened in between, I can't remember." ' A 'brownout' is a piecemeal version of events, generally caused by a couple of drinks tipping over into what the NHS would define as a 'binge'.

Thanks to a recent stunning finding, we now know what many suspected to be true; that the 500-strong 'neuronal ensemble', which has the power to inhibit binge-drinking, sits neatly within the prefrontal cortex. Given the brain has around 86 billion neurons, and the prefrontal cortex itself is a third of that, homing in on just 500 is profoundly important.

It's like this: before this discovery, we knew that there was some buried treasure someplace in the United States. Now, we know the exact square mile.

Ozempic and binge-drinking

There has also been the illuminating finding from takers of GLP-1 agonists (Ozempic, Mounjaro and Wegovy, to us laypeople) who are reporting that not only do GLP-1 agonists soften the urge to over-eat, they also dampen the urge to over-drink.

As a result, there are now a bunch of clinical trials testing out whether a spin-off of GLP-1 – a weekly injection of 'semaglutide' designed specifically for those who over-drink – can work to treat alcohol addiction.

Human trials are currently small, but animal studies have shown great promise, and much bigger trials are pending. The latest human study found that the injections resulted in a 41 per cent reduction in alcohol consumption. So, we could be on the verge of a to-market intervention which dramatically reduces harmful drinking.

I have mixed feelings on this. I would never take it personally: why would I? I now have zero cravings for alcohol. I do think others who are less happy and settled in their long-term recovery might partake though, in order to resume drinking.

'Is it worth having an injection every week,' asks Dr Grisel, in long-term recovery herself, 'for the sake of having one or two glasses of wine, instead of your usual seven or eight?'

But, on the other hand, it's great as a tool to arrest the onslaught of someone drinking themselves into an early grave – as long as the eventual goal is abstinence, because you can't be on weekly injections for the rest of your life.

It's likely that if semaglutide is ever approved for prescription, it'll only be available on the NHS to those with clinical alcohol addiction. For non-chronic drinkers, it would be a private affair. Private access to Ozempic or Wegovy is around £250 a month for the injections alone, so it's likely to be similarly priced. Like any drug, these will also come with side effects.

Besides, your drinking is not at the level where you would need or want this, if your addiction tested as 'little'. You still have the ability to choose when and how you drink; the neurobiological compulsion has not yet kicked in.

My solution was teetotalling – for me, none is easier than one. Your solution will look different; maybe *very* different. And I'll be over here, rooting for you to find it.

Dear ex-big addict,

(Sorry little addicts, I'm cheating you out of a letter here, but this is too important to go unsaid. I've given you a bumper edition of 'micro tactics' in recompense.)

There's an important nuance we need to discuss; the nuance of not currently being addicted, yet still being vulnerable to re-addiction.

Oftentimes, the pat phrase 'Once an addict, always an addict' is wheeled out, but that doesn't cover the complexity of this.

As we already know, the brain learns addiction.

'Unlearning it is very difficult,' says Dr Clayton Hickey. We don't unlearn addiction when we quit drinking, we learn sobriety instead. A whole different pathway.

'You establish control over that former addiction by not placing yourself in a situation where you can activate that learned response to alcohol again.'

So, I ask him if I'd understood correctly: that learned response to alcohol is still in my brain, even though I'm 12 years sober?

'Yes,' he says. 'And it'll always be there, but you will not put yourself in the same circumstance. Learning to be sober was very difficult for you, but it got reinforced *in* in the same way as the addiction was. The longer you're sober, the more likely you are to continue to be sober.'

If only we could think of a snappy way to say all that, I joke. 'Once an addict not always an addict, but always the great potential to re-addict.' Hmmm, that needs some work.

'Yes, if only we could make that into a phrase,' he laughs. 'I don't like "Once an addict, always an addict" either, but there is a kernel of truth in there, which is this: What you learned as an addict is still there once you're not an addict, but that doesn't mean you are still that addict. You are now that person plus all this other stuff, because your life has progressed and you're doing it differently.'

The two can co-exist – not an addict + the addiction still living on in your brain.

This is why people can be thriving, then think they can pick up again, believing it will be different this time, since they're different. But their use of alcohol eventually, perniciously, ends up being the same.

There's also something called 'persistent sensitisation'. In *Dopamine Nation*, Dr Lembke cites a haunting study with rats who were given daily cocaine. When they were on the daily cocaine, the rats exhibited a particular running pattern, darting across the cage in a frenzied manner, unlike the other rats, who ran around the periphery.

What happened next was surprising.

'One year later – a veritable lifetime for a rat – the scientists reinjected the rats with cocaine one time,' Dr Lembke wrote, 'and the rats were immediately running as they had on the final day of the original experiment.'

She calls this the 'abstinence violation effect', and tells me over email that she's experienced it herself. 'It happened to me when I went back to reading romance novels,' she wrote, referring to the vampire, fairy and witch romance and erotica she once grew overly attached to.

We're not rats, and alcohol is not cocaine. But these substances can alter the brain forever, nonetheless.

I'm not trying to scare you. You are not teetering on the brink of anything, you are not unsafe, you are not about to fall into a vat of cider and you *have* got this. You are firmly on a sober path, and all that learning, as Dr Hickey emphasised, is just as strong as your addicted path was.

But with this nuance – the addicted path is *still there*. It's not magically erased itself, leaving an empty plot for you to build a brand-new moderation highway.

All you need to do is stay here. Don't go back over there. It's not worth the risk.

Love,
Cath x

ALCOHOL MICRO TACTICS

Start a unit diary

The absolute easiest way to do this is via an app, which has all the units of each drink already encoded. I recommend *Try Dry* by Alcohol Change UK or the NHS's *Drink Free Days*.

Swerve 'dark apps'

Be aware of what the Institute of Alcohol Studies calls 'dark apps'. These are seemingly trying to help you with your drinking but are a wolf in sheep's clothing, given they're created by 'industry actors' such as Drinkaware, who are predominately funded by the alcohol industry.

'Ninety-three per cent of the industry-funded apps contained misinformation strategies,' said the IAS experts. They nudged users to drink more, by only including smaller servings of wine as options on the unit calculator, or via 'social norming' messages (*Everyone's doing it*). Examples of 'dark apps' cited were *MyDrinkaware*, *Cheers!* or Australia's *DrinkWise*. Always check who made your app, noting that the names of these are liable to change.

Replace 'I can't' with 'I don't'

'I don't drink during the week' will be much more attractive to your brain than 'I can't drink during the week', which is why saying 'don't' rather than 'can't' is a pillar of behavioural science.

'When our brain actively chooses something, we release more dopamine than when something is thrust upon us,' says Dr Korb. Remember, dopamine is the 'wanting' molecule, which means its involvement can make us more likely to succeed, providing we point it at healthy pursuits.

Consider an alcohol-free home

Given your status as a little addict only, you can probably resist the motley selection of spirits gathering dust-fur in the cabinet, or your housemate's/partner's (frankly wrong) tequila-spiked beer. But, if you're trying not to drink at home, maybe try removing the cue of your *favourite* alcohol. If it's just sitting there, chilling in the fridge, you will probably drink it.

Make moderation a part of your identity

One of the reasons that the book *Atomic Habits* has sold millions of copies is because of this simple yet potent truth: identity change leads to behavioural change. My partner demolished his little addiction to alcohol, going sober overnight, by starting to describe himself as a 'non-drinker'. Saying it like it's already happened – 'I don't drink more than two beers' – could make it more likely to happen. 'Fake it till you make it' as the A A bumper sticker slogan goes.

CBD gummies could help

This research is in its infancy, with more trials underway, but one fascinating study has found that CBD can reduce alcohol cravings. The most recent cited a dose of 800mg (gummies go up to 1,500mg) and found it 'significantly' reduced cravings, even after a deliberate 'combined stress- and alcohol-cue exposure session'.

Play the tape forward

People in recovery from big addictions swear by this tactic. It's all about fast-forwarding to what our life might look like if the little – or large – addiction continues or even gathers pace. Draw it, write it down or visualise it like a film.

Feel the sober fear and do it anyway

We talked earlier about how to avoid your drinking moving into the dorsal striatum, the region linked with compulsion. A way to ensure this doesn't happen is by making a list, right now, of things you think you *need* alcohol to do, from your birthday to attending a wedding, and then deliberately doing these things without alcohol.

An excellent way of ensuring this happens is by signing up to a longer-term alcohol sabbatical, like the three month 'Sober Spring' I founded and set up with Alcohol Change UK. It runs from 20th March to 20th June.

Buy treats with the extra money

When I quit drinking, I suddenly had a lot more money. A night out previously would have cost around £25 minimum (I'm told that's now double), but now I could go to a pub quiz and spend £2 on a pint of lime and soda, plus £1 for a game of pool afterwards.

Instead of saving all of this money, I consciously spent some on fun, unusual alcohol-free experiences. Immersive theatre, gigs in secret locations, 'dark yoga' in the crypt of a church. Therefore, my circuitous nightlife routine of 'drink, dance, eat, hangover, repeat' became replaced by something much more interesting.

Don't leave a wine- or beer-shaped hole. Fill it by baiting the moderation with a reward.

Create a core-value pin board

This is borrowed from Delamere rehab (the rehab centre that I'll tell you more about later). It does an exercise with guests where five core values are chosen. Whittling it down to five is surprisingly difficult. I think this tool can be shrunk and used for a little addiction as well as for a bigger one.

I've written this version myself, but essentially these are the intentions you most fiercely want to angle your life towards, the values you want to pin down as constants – the things you would love to have mentioned in your obituary.

My five were honesty, curiosity, creativity, loyalty and determination. If my funeral features a eulogy where I'm described as all of these things, I'll probably arise from my coffin to do a spectral jig.

The exercise of picking my values created a key-turn in my brain. I realised after having done it that my big addiction to drinking pulled me out of alignment from all five of my core values, which was why I was so miserable as a drinker.

When I was a drinker I lied frequently, stopped reading and learning, cheated on partners, betrayed friends, left tasks incomplete, kicked back at work with Facebook, then urgently had to scrabble to catch up – which is why I felt so wretched. I was pulled out of alignment with my core values.

If you relate to this misalignment, even if it's subtle, your desired new drinking structure will be built upon these newly sharpened values. 'The reason you don't want to drink another beer is often because doing so undermines something important to you,' says Dr Korb.

Maybe one of your core values is 'professional'. And when you drink at work events, you find yourself behaving a little unprofessionally. Thus, your desired drinking structure might involve no longer drinking at such events. Or maybe you choose 'patience', with your kids firmly in mind. If you're snappier with them on a hangover, mild or otherwise, that consideration might be relevant.

Choose just five core values from the words below. Then reflect upon whether your alcohol use helps you stay in alignment with them or pulls you away.

Accountability
Achievement
Adventure
Ambition
Authenticity
Balance
Beauty
Belonging
Bravery
Cleanliness
Community
Confidence
Connection
Contentment
Creativity
Curiosity
Determination
Dignity
Diversity
Empathy
Environment
Fairness
Fidelity
Forgiveness
Friendliness
Fun
Future generations
Generosity
Harmony
Health
Home
Honesty
Hope
Humour
Improvement
Independence
Inspiration
Integrity
Intelligence
Kindness
Knowledge
Love
Loyalty
Modesty
Openness
Order
Parenting
Patience
Pleasure
Popularity
Professionalism
Reputation
Responsibility
Safety
Self-respect
Sharing
Skill
Spirituality
Spontaneity
Stability
Success
Talent
Teamwork
Temperance
Travel
Trustworthiness
Wealth
Wellbeing
Wisdom

GAMING

Sticky eight

I crawl into bed for a kiss and cuddle with my partner. He pushes me away, choosing to place his *Star Wars* game in his face instead.

'I can't right now babe, I need to buy R2D2; he's only 1,200 crystals.'

I mean, the signs were there. When we met, he told me that a farming game had 'saved him' during lockdown. It felt like misplacement of the 'saviour' variety, only this saviour model featured corn on the cob with googly eyes.

And then, when we had our daughter, my brother (a fellow gamer) bought him a T-shirt with a console controller on it saying 'I levelled up to Daddy'. They both laughed a little too hard.

My sister-in-law and I exchanged looks. I was perplexed; she was more knowing. She was already a gaming widow, and this served as a foreshadow that I too was about to become one, as my partner started to medicate the stress of early parenthood by popping balloons on a screen.

Balloon-popping served as a gateway drug to *God of War*.

'Is this going to be a problem?' I remember asking, seeing him tip into a second glazed hour, as I breastfed our newborn. 'No, no . . . gaming used to be an issue for me, but now I have it under control,' he said.

It turns out that 'an issue' was a bit of an understatement. He used to steal money from his parents' wallets in order to hit the arcades. For eight hours. This later became full days spent in internet cafes in basements, mired in a fog of cigarette smoke.

'Wow,' I said, when he told me. 'Gaming was for you what drinking was for me.'

We're now three years on and approximately 37 arguments about gaming later. And that self-awareness of a former gaming addiction has been tucked in by denial and shushed to sleep.

When I told him I was writing this chapter, he said, 'Be sure to tell them gaming can cure depression.'

'Says who?' I enquired.

'Says me,' he said.

The amazing side of VR

Let's kick it off with some positives. Virtual reality gaming can relieve pain, as found by a study out of the University of Washington. Taking dozens of burns patients – many soldiers – experiencing chronic pain, they plunged some of those patients into an immersive virtual reality game called *SnowWorld*.

'*SnowWorld* is the opposite of fire,' lead researcher Hunter Hoffman said. Those who enter it glide through the icy world past a frozen waterfall, meeting woolly mammoths and chucking snowballs at snowm . . . people.

The results were remarkable. The burns patients who accessed *SnowWorld* via the VR headset while undergoing painful procedures, such as wound-dressing, reported much less pain. This wasn't just experiential, it was factual; their MRI scans showed drops in pain-related brain activity of between 50 to 97 per cent.

Hoffman and colleagues also performed a follow-up experiment, using a game called *SpiderWorld* (er, I'll go to *SnowWorld* instead, thanks) to distract adolescents undergoing burns procedures. They compared it to a control group who played *Mario Kart*. The immersive VR game still worked in reducing pain, despite the less soothing, furry-legged content; whereas sadly, traditional handheld console games like *Mario Kart* did not. Bah.

The most addictive games

Of the most downloaded games, there are two stand-out genres:

1. **The handheld elemental**
   Bite-size, normally 2D and usually played via a phone, for free, with in-game ads mostly leveraging revenue. An obvious example of this is *Candy Crush*, a sweet-matching game that has been crushing resistance since its inception in 2012, in which time it has barely changed. Why change that which is played by 200 million people (as of 2024) and worth $20 billion?
   From my research, other examples of the dovetail between the handheld elemental + very sticky include *Block Blast!* (Tetris with some twists), *Township* (there goes the farming game again), *Subway Surfers* (endlessly running little dudes) and finally *Offline Games – No WiFi*

Games (sounds like malware, but is legit old-school content; think word searches, snake and hangman).

The popularity of the latter download has exploded in the past year, with more than 10 million players acquiring it. It's either a *kinda* good thing, indicating a growing appetite for WiFi-free gaming, or a very bad thing, indicating an unwillingness to be without gaming, ever. Or, it could be both.

2. **RPGs (role-playing games) – including open worlds**
   Generally paid or subscribed to – after a free intro – and played on larger devices with player-designed characters who are moved either via a pre-ordained pathway through a set world, or freely about an open world.

   There are even player-created worlds within worlds; we're talking user-generated theatrics that can be spicy or disturbing (*Roblox* – keep your kids off it), or building a bespoke *Minecraft* city (much more wholesome).

   Some ultra-popular games in this (very large) sub-category include diving down to sunken shipwrecks for treasure (*Sea of Thieves*), or the monster-slaying one my brother was addicted to questing on (*World of Warcraft*).

Of course, this splice into two is a blunt tool, to say the least. You could carve gaming up into dozens of genres, from 'sandbox shooter' and 'stealth' to 'tower defence' and street, rally or off-road racing. But for our purposes here, these two overarching categories will suffice, given each hit distinct buttons.

Special mentions for the kookiest games I came across while researching this:

- *Unpacking*, which is literally what it sounds like. Why you would want to relive unpacking after a move, I truly do not know.
- *Plague Inc.* You help spread a plague of your choice with a running tally of infected and dead. Has been played a (worrying) 700 million times.
- *Bacon.* You throw bacon at everything, from a fish, to a martini, to a hairdryer, to trigonometry. Admittedly hilarious. It has 192k reviews.

The lure of the repetitive

Repetitive and consistently small reward-seeking, as per the 'elemental' games, is a behaviour that's been genetically coded in, says evolutionary psychologist Dr Andrew Thomas.

How? Why? The need to forage. It seems like a reach, but it's not. Addiction experts like Dr Anna Lembke say the exact same thing (see page 118).

'The urge for small, repetitive, reward-bringing movements has been reinforced in genetically,' says Dr Thomas. 'Think about how traditional societies would have sourced their calories. You don't want to be the kind of organism who is only motivated to pick one berry.'

Candy Crush is not real food, obviously, and we're apparently 'crushing it' rather than picking it, but when you think of the actual process – clicking on the sweets to get them to vanish – it's uncannily similar to picking berries from a bush.

Role-playing from your sofa

The RPGs and/or open-world universes are addictive for different reasons. The rewards are more intermittent, but much bigger. We need to be patient, persistent . . . but luckily we're wired for that quest. This may remind our 'Stone Age brains' of hunting.

'Both sexes hunted, actually. It's a myth it was just males,' says Dr Thomas. 'But women tended to hunt smaller game, such as rabbits or birds, while big game-hunting was traditionally performed by groups of males.' They went off in a group (sound familiar?) and might come back empty-handed four days in a row, but when the reward did come, it was huge. Maybe they'd come back carrying a deer, producing more meat than their village could eat.

'These two suites of evolutionary behaviour, these dual processes, were essential,' he says. You needed some people digging up the tubers, like a cow consistently crops grass, and others motivated to wait for a long time for something unpredictable, but also amazing.

RPGs tap into much more besides. You tend to customise a character (or vehicle, or both) right from the get-go, and even though many of these characters or items are off-rack rather than couture, this still taps into 'loss aversion' (which we go into more on page 243). In short, once we feel like we 'own' something, we'll fight like hell to keep it.

In many RPGs you collect more exclusive items too, such as keys or a set of wings or roll cages, either via in-game currency (which you win via battles or races), or – once they've got you – with real hard cash. This collection of belongings, paint jobs and magical clothing then activates our hardwired-in hoarding urge (covered in the Shopping chapter, from page 228), which is both ancient and undeniable.

Then there's the social prestige of advancing yourself within MMORPGs (massive multiplayer online role-playing games), whether that comes from being known for your witty repartee on the chats, from having slain a dragon others could not, or being within the top 10 in the world.

Imagine how intoxicating receiving a 'We need you for this quest! Log in already!' WhatsApp is for an awkward 15-year-old boy who's unpopular at school, or an increasingly housebound fiftysomething woman. It's another world, literally, where they feel heroic, seen, important.

Immersing yourself in the universe is how game play becomes most satisfying, with the knock-on that this is when it seems reasonable to start spending real money. This goes all the way from the £5 fashion bundles being dangled to teenage girls on *Roblox*, up to serious £££s for tools, weapons, enchanted outfits, or virtual real estate. Die-hard users of MMORPGs report on Reddit threads that they have spent thousands.

Players buy and sell from each other too. A rarefied 'blue party hat', which added no magic powers whatsoever, still sold within *Runescape* for $4,500, while a very convincing incarnation of Amsterdam built brick-by-brick within *Second Life* fetched $50,000.

Some elite players even have agents – or make millions – being sponsored to play via streaming platforms, such as Twitch. But most just sink money into the game, activating the 'sunk cost fallacy' all humans are vulnerable to, whereby we don't want to lose what we've invested time, money and energy in, whether it be social currency on chat boards, a fetching blue hat or a dispiriting slide down a leader board.

Can you really 'swipe the stress away'?

Candy Crush's slogan is 'swipe the stress away', but what actually happens in your brain while you game?

The biggest meta-analysis of gaming studies that I found looked at 116 separate studies. And the outlook was, mostly, surprisingly good (I checked; the gaming industry had no part in funding this study). It found that dedicated gamers experience structural brain changes, citing regions associated with focused attention, while action-oriented video games (such as racing or shooters) also boosted powers of 'selective attention' (role-playing games didn't have the same effect). Some regions of the brain associated with visuospatial skills also showed 'volumetric increases', the study said.

Indeed, many of the experts I interviewed were gamers.

Professor Natasha Dow Schüll, a cultural anthropologist at NYU, likes a game with social bonding and a hero's arc. 'I have a soft spot for some of the quest games, where you go on raids and you've got a team and it comes to a natural end. You feel like, "Wow, I went on this adventure with people". I don't think we need to demonise *all* digital entertainment.'

The games that are problematic, she thinks, are ones that create 'repetitious ludic loops' ('ludic' means play). Pop balloons – more balloons appear – repeat. 'The better ones provide a narrative arc, which means they're the opposite to the ludic loop. They have the saving grace where there's transformation and change.'

Meanwhile, Nir Eyal, behavioural designer and author of *Indistractable*, calls games 'works of master craftmanship', which are no less valid than quality books or films.

'Gaming can be really good, or really bad,' says psychotherapist Josh Fletcher, author of *And How Does That Make You Feel?* He has skin in the game – literally – as a gamer. 'I sit down and tune into the most beautiful artwork games – *Clair Obscur*, *The Legend of Zelda*, *The Witcher 3*.

Again, the phone doesn't feature in Fletcher's use. 'I don't play anything on my phone, I think that's an entirely different thing. It can become a compulsion, rather than the intentional, high-quality ceremonial feel you can get at a console.'

Fletcher credits gaming with helping his mental health. 'I can immerse myself, escape my inner critic, work on my hand-eye and activate my parasympathetic rest and digest.'

The lead author of the meta-analysis, cognitive neuroscientist Dr Marc Palaus, was careful to note that it wasn't all good news. Other research in the 116 studies linked gaming to 'negative effects on social information processing' or a 'lower verbal IQ'. He also pointed out on the visuospatial skills gained that 'these effects do not always translate to real-life changes'. Someone on the leader board of *Forza Motorsport* could be a truly terrible driver on the actual roads.

However, this jars with a small but remarkable study, which analysed 33 surgeons. It found that the surgeons who had been gamers in the past, playing for at least three hours a week, were 42 per cent better at their jobs than those who had never gamed.

Gaming produces more addictions than cocaine

There have been a number of lawsuits against major game developers in the US and Canada over MMORPGs, with parents claiming their kids refused to eat or sleep, such was the height of their child's addiction. One of the games targeted is *Fortnite,* the controversial shooter game. These lawsuits are still ongoing, with the parents' lawyers citing the legal precedent of 'duty to inform' which was historically used against tobacco companies to leverage pay-outs. The legal actions argue that these game developers should have told users how addictive the game is. The gaming companies are defending themselves against the claims, saying they are meritless and that there are parental controls in place.

It won't be the last game in the dock. Data-crunchers found that *Minecraft*, *League of Legends* and *Candy Crush* actually generate more online searches for addiction support than *Fortnite*. In the UK, 15 per cent *more* people Googled 'video gaming addiction' than 'cocaine addiction' in 2022.

It's thought that one of the most addictive aspects of *Fortnite* – with some experts saying it's as addictive as heroin – is that it's entirely free to download. Once you advance, you can purchase in-game items, but that's optional.

Free-to-download models are increasingly popular, with most games dangling a free introductory offer, getting gamers on the hook and then attempting to tie them into subscriptions or 'packs' for play.

My brother, Chris Gray, who freely admits to a former 'deep addiction' with gaming, tells me that within gamer world, players are called minnows, dolphins, whales or kraken. Minnows play for free, or less than a tenner a month.

Dolphins are spending £10–£100 a month, while whales spend thousands. Kraken, the rarest of all, can blow tens of thousands.

'They'll bait minnows in with a free introductory offer or download, and then try to get you to dolphin up,' says Chris. 'You connected your credit card to the game back when you accessed the free offer or download, so those details are already there, and it's then easy to lose track of how much you're spending.'

'In-game currency is cleverly disconnected from real money,' he says, 'given they use golden coins, or bundles, or summons that keep tiering up the longer you play – starting with £5 for 10 summons, rising to £20 for 30, then £79 for 100.'

'Reward uncertainty', the gasoline for fast dopamine that we talk about on page 32, is very deliberately built into the game, says a professional games tester, talking to me under the pseudonym Harry Mills. 'The crystal bundle you just bought will rotate and change colour before settling,' says Harry, much like a roulette ball circling a wheel.

He says gacha games are huge right now because they tap into that, and were modelled on 'mystery gacha vending machines' in Japan (supersized adult versions of the ball machines kids put 50p into, winning a random ball with a toy in it). Gacha is extra-sticky because gaming and gambling are fused. In gacha, there's a mechanism whereby you pay to pull for heroes, much as you might pay to pull a fruit machine. 'The problem with gacha is, the more you spend, the better you'll be,' says Harry. Free players just can't compete.

Chris agrees, saying gacha is what everyone's hooked on right now, and it entices people to spend thousands. 'Whales walk through battlegrounds utterly untouchable, while krakens can collapse an entire game, making everybody else leave.'

Harry may know exactly how games hook users, but he still got addicted to games himself. 'There's a reason they call *Everquest* Evercrack,' he says darkly.

The picture emerging is that gaming is a mixed bag. It depends how you do it, when you do it, where you do it. Gaming can mitigate loneliness in the short-term, since it is interactive, especially with games featuring chat boards or games where you banter with co-players over headsets. But over the long-term, as a little addiction grows to become a medium or big addiction, it's been shown to create *more* loneliness. Whether the loneliness is cause or effect is hard to prise apart, but what we do know is this: gaming certainly doesn't cure it.

'Video games have both positive aspects (on attention, visual and motor skills) and negative (risk of addiction), and it is essential we embrace this complexity,' Dr Palaus said. It can be an addiction like any other, he went on to tell *Wired*. 'Roughly speaking, there are no big differences between video game addiction and other addictions.'

There *are* ways to leverage the positives and minimise the negatives, though. Especially the risks of addiction upsize. We'll talk about these in the 'micro tactics', which will hopefully help us to advance to the next level.

'Knowledge is the key to survival.
The real beauty of that is it doesn't weigh anything.'

Survivalist Ray Mears

Dear little gaming addict,

I've only ever gotten fixated with one game, but I swear it helped during a terrible time.

I'll be revealing my mid-forties status now, but it wasn't the years I spent playing *Gran Turismo* and *The NewZealand Story* on my brother's Amiga (I was a girl, and girls weren't supposed to be gamers). It was a much more boring game, and my form of stimming: a beta black-and-white rocket game (*Descent*), where you landed this rocket in increasingly craggy and challenging surroundings.

I played it aged 11–12, when my brother and I lived with a stepfather who hated us (openly calling us 'the lodgers'), arguments raged downstairs and the living room was out of bounds to us past 7pm. During which, my brother and I found solace in games. And drinking, on my part. But before that – games.

Bracing for the door-slams that would vibrate through the house, I would soothe my mind with the repetitive act of landing this grayscale rocket over and over. If you didn't land it just right, it would explode. I could handle the stress of that within the game, at a time when I couldn't handle the stress of my real world.

Maybe you relate. And I get it. Maybe you too have escaped within a game, at a time when it felt urgently necessary to do so. Escaped to a world where your only problem was how to slingshot more pigs or save Princess Peach.

As with any little addiction, a lose-yourself escape can begin to mutate into a life-limiting time suck, as your use increases, and we start to think it's reasonable to pay real money for more time, power-ups or enchanted shields.

That's when we start to get into bother. When losing ourselves in the game results in losing our real life. When enchanted shields become more important than the enchanted pony our niece wants us to draw. Or when real friends become sidelined for fellow gamers with tags like Dragon Slinger and Bad Bunny.

Because, while we're spending all that time developing a character, having adventures, planting flowers or striking up friendships in-game, we're not doing it out-of-game.

We often get several lives in a game. But out here in the real world, we only get one.

Love,
Cath x

GAMING MICRO TACTICS

Find games you can pause
Games tester Harry downsized his self-apportioned 'medium addiction' to games by moving to games you can pause. 'Games that you can't pause engender obsessiveness,' he says, 'not to mention driving big spikes of bad feeling into relationships. If your partner asks you to come down to dinner, or your housemate wants a chat about a bad day, you don't want to choose the game over them.'

Games without events
Both Chris and Harry agree that games that host battles, events or tournaments where you have a certain log-in time and people are depending on you, are the most life-devouring. Chris cites *Raid: Shadow Legends* as a particular time-eater. 'Those can eat up three or four hours a night . . . even an entire weekend,' he says.

Psychotherapist Josh Fletcher agrees. 'I only play single-player games for this reason.'

Leader boards are also egotistically addictive, says Chris, who *also* wants me to tell you that he has been in the top 10 in the world on some of them (Chris's addiction to leader boards: intact).

Fill vacuums in advance
Little addictions, especially bitesize ones such as gaming, thrive in a vacuum. They're going to twerk around joyously in that unscheduled downtime, trying to get you to come dance with them. While travelling or relaxing, you can easily tell yourself 'just five minutes' on a handheld elementary, or 'just a half hour' on an open world, and find yourself blinking out of a rabbit hole hours later. Consciously decide beforehand – even writing it down on your day's to-do – how you're going to spend a lunch hour, train journey or evening.

Add a layer of accountability
Accountability is a pillar of recovery from big addictions because it works. You could share your desired usage with your partner, housemate or a gaming buddy

who's also trying to reduce. Even committing to sharing snapshots of your total screentime usage that week with them (all major consoles – as well as smartphones and tablets – track hours played).

Play on trad consoles

An easy way to self-bind your little gaming addiction is to go fully old-school and delete your games from tablets or phones, promising yourself you'll only play on a console from now on, even if it is a handheld.

It's obvious that this shift provides an obstacle between us and the game, given it's no longer in our pockets, and our gaming experts agree. This is why Eyal has deleted all games from his phone, while Fletcher will only play on a Steam Deck. 'Playing on a phone is a bad idea,' Fletcher says.

Consoles have inbuilt limits – use them

Inbuilt parental controls handily allow you to set a daily or weekly limit for yourself on the following consoles: PlayStation, Xbox and Nintendo Switch, mostly through on-console settings, but Switch's is controlled via the downloadable 'Parental Control' app, for which you'll need to sign up as a fictional parent to yourself.

NICOTINE

Sticky eight

He brings an imaginary vape to his lips, taking a deep inhale. 'It's the perfect storm,' says Professor Clayton Hickey. He blows out luxuriously, swirling his hands to denote smoke. 'Vapes don't have to create this cloud, but they do.'

And there's a very good reason for that, which we'll come back to.

I'm at the University of Birmingham, talking with one of the country's foremost experts in dopamine. Dopamine, as we'll also come back to, used to be thought to be the 'liking' neurotransmitter. We now know better, in that it's the 'wanting' neurotransmitter.

Dopamine is the molecule that carries the 'want' – whether you want a trad cigarette, a blast on a forest fruits vape pod or a nicotine pouch. When you zoom out further to look at the big picture, dopamine is the fuel that drives all addictions, little and large, not just nicotine. We'll talk about that on pages 171 to 189.

But we're talking about nicotine right now. And the new ways we're getting it into our bloodstream.

Over one in 10 Brits now vape, the highest amount in recorded history. In 2012, there were 0.8 million vapers; now we're looking at 5.6 million, a sevenfold rise. We don't know how many people use other nicotine products.

Vaping isn't as harmful as smoking cigarettes, of course, but here's the rub; almost half of the vapers are *not* ex-smokers.

This brand-new market, who perhaps never would have smoked, is because of the rollout of the vape, otherwise known as the e-cigarette. Dr Anna Lembke, author of *Dopamine Nation*, calls them, 'chic, discreet, odourless, rechargeable nicotine delivery systems – leading to higher levels of blood nicotine over shorter periods of consumption than traditional cigarettes.'

Nicotine marketeers are after kids

There's a reason why every vape shop looks like it could potentially be a phone shop (normally spelt 'fone') selling kawaii phone charms or unofficial Star Wars-themed phone cases. Some not far from me me are called things like Wicked Vape, Electric Wildfire and Naughty Smoke.*

I went on a field trip to these shops, to see what the deal is. Plumes of fire, cheeky devils and anime comic wallpaper are their marketing vibes. Black walls make the glossy neon products pop. Lines range from Vampire Vape with a cartoon vampire, through to Bad Juice, which has skateboard-brand vibes, and the cutesy cereal-esque Breakfast Club. The flavours could be for jelly beans or fruit rolls, from Unicorn Shake to Rainbow Candy and Cinnamon Crunch. Some also sell actual sweets.

I am not their target customer. You do know who is, don't you? Don't make me say it. It's forehead-smackingly obvious.

You could, of course, argue that my confirmation bias led me away from the rose gold £24.99 vape units, or made me skim over the Prosecco Blush pods (I made that up, but I'm sure it probably exists) and trained my eyes upon the products aimed at my niece and nephew, respectively 12 and 16. And I'm sure there *were* other products in the store; it just so happens that I noticed the most alarmingly infantile ones.

A worker at one of the stores I visited caught me taking pictures of the Breakfast Club boxes, styled up to look like kids' cereal boxes.

'Shocking isn't it,' he said, rather than scolding me.

I sensed an ally, so asked him some questions. He asked to be pseudonym-ed as Xena Warrior Princess (yes, he was taking the piss and, yes, I have to honour it).

'The bulk of the nicotine market does now feel aimed at teens,' Xena said. 'I just work here, and I vape too,' he continued, 'but I also disagree with how bloody blatant it's becoming. I ID everyone who looks to be under 25 and won't serve if I see schoolkids gathered outside the shop, waiting. Sometimes I wonder how far they'll go, with the cartoons and the candy-this, candy-that.'

This deliberate marketing is working, too. A quarter of schoolkids aged 11–15 have tried vaping, and nearly one in 10 do it regularly, says the NHS.

* Real names of shops have been changed for legal reasons.

These companies aim to get them hooked young, and keep them hooked. I spoke with a whistleblower who works for a top 'nicotine delivery system' company, who wishes to (thankfully) be known as 'Steph'.

'We talk about "lifetime use" in our company,' she says. 'And while older consumers are definitely our market too, and they have more money to spend on sexy sleek units, the "lifetime use" of a teen is of much greater value.'

When the legislation throws nicotine companies an obstacle, they just pivot. 'Disposable vapes have just been banned for sale,' Steph told me (in June 2025). 'When we heard about the change in legislation coming, we had many urgent meetings about how to keep the low-income, disposable user,' she says. 'These are mainly teenagers.'

Disposable vapes were banned because they were often unregulated, and throwaway vapes confiscated in playgrounds have been found to contain lead, chromium and nickel; all heavy metals that can be devastating for health. There's now a 'Disposable Alternatives' tab up front and centre on many nicotine sites, with some comforting text about how these will taste just like their favourite disposable, and flogging non-disposable pod kits from just £4.99. It reminds me of the razor handles they'll sell for rock-bottom prices, just to get you on the buying ladder of that brand.

Most of these sites use automatic age verification services, and obviously if you buy in-shop you need to show ID (particularly to Xena Warrior Princess), but it's obvious that kids can just ask older teenagers or siblings to buy them, just as they used to in the '90s with cigarettes.

This is where it gets sinister. It's now very, very easy for a 12-year-old to hide a growing nicotine addiction. Cigarettes *stank*, and so it was unignorable when a kid started smoking, even if they chomped three Juicy Fruits and sprayed a liberal amount of Lynx.

Even vapes throw up telltales; the units themselves, the smoke billowing up from the garden, and they're *not* odourless, with most carrying a certain sickly-sweet aroma. But now – pivot! – there are pouches and pearls, which can easily be hidden from parents in pockets (school blazers inexplicably have about eight pockets in which to conceal contraband) or tucked in the side of the mouth while waiting for a Sunday roast at Harvester.

'These products were deliberately designed to make nicotine consumption frictionless,' Steph says. 'For all, not just teens. It doesn't matter if you're on the tube or at a gig or watching TV with your family, you can still get your nicotine going.'

Nicotine taken through the mouth is more addictive, because of the speed of its access to the brain, says Professor Philip Murphy. 'You get quicker access than you would do through a patch on the skin.'

And the amounts of nicotine involved are now becoming scary.

****

Full disclosure: I am addicted to nicotine and I *like* nicotine. Which may undermine everything I've just said. And yet two seemingly contradictory things can exist at once. I am both a user of nicotine and alarmed by what's going on with the marketing and the spiralling nicotine content. I'm a parent but, even if I weren't, I would feel the same way.

My nicotine story: I quit smoking in 2014 but have since remained addicted to nicotine replacement therapy (NRT), in the shape of lozenges, ever since. (I am the only weirdo I know addicted to NRT. Everyone else vapes.) I quit my nicotine lozenges for three-ish years, when I was pregnant with, and then breastfeeding, my now-toddler. Like a total dunderhead, I then re-addicted myself deliberately – I'm not even kidding – having got myself free.

I blame the fuzz-brain of perimenopause, slash the work–parent juggle, slash undiagnosed neurodivergence, or see all of the above, who knows. I told friends and family that my restart was because I find that the nicotine (or more accurately, I *tell myself* that the nicotine) 'helps me focus'.

I'm on a routine 1–3mg a day, depending on how much I need to 'focus', which is the equivalent of one to three cigarettes. So, I too partake of these 'nicotine delivery systems'. Mine just happens to come in the shape of a 1mg mint, which I buy from Boots, rather than a 'bubble crush' pod that claims it'll 'dance on your tongue'.

However, in a handy enabling twist for my own use, it turns out that my 3mg daily intake is *nothing* compared to what vapers, pouchers or pearl-users could be putting away.

I discovered this by accident, and now that I've researched it some more, I'm horrified.

****

I was driving home from Norfolk, where I'd been to see one of my best friends. It's a four-hour drive at the best of times, and I was starting to flag, and I still needed to go through the Dartford Crossing, with its HGVs that glide silently alongside you, eerily close, like whales that could kill you with a flick of their tail.

Nervous driver, me? Yes, yes I am. And I'd run out of nicotine, so how was I supposed to 'focus'? I need it to work, and I need it to drive, OK?

So, while I was at the services for a ~~pee~~ pit stop, I looked for my nicotine lozenges. No luck. But they were selling nicotine pouches behind the counter in WH Smith.

'What milligram are those, can I have 1 or 2mg?' I asked the server.

'Er, I don't know what milligram they are, but these say "low"?' she said, holding up a Nordic Spirit packet.

I nodded, and the deal was done.

Back in the car, I still couldn't figure out what strength they were as the packet didn't seem to specify, so I popped this little pouch, which looked like the silica pouch at the bottom of new handbags, into my mouth.

It also tasted like the bottom of a handbag might.

The nicotine, once it hit, was so intense and so jarring, that it made me feel sick. I spat the pouch into a tissue before I even left the service station car park, continuing the drive without it.

Once home, I analysed the packet. I still couldn't see the mg strength. Usually, this information is emblazoned in font size 20 on my packets of nicotine lozenges.

I ask Steph about all this. 'The legislation says that the nicotine content should be clearly displayed,' she says, 'but "clearly displayed" is open to interpretation. We make it as small as possible.'

Finally, I found it, buried in the small print, in a font size that is the same size as 'harmful to aquatic life'. It said: Nicotine content: 6mg.

Six milligrams? And that was considered 'low'? That's usually two days' intake for me. No wonder it hit me like an HGV.

The average cigarette contains between 8 and 20mg of nicotine FYI, but we only absorb 1–2mg of that nicotine. Basically, 1mg is like smoking a light cigarette, like Marlboro Lights, whereas 2mg is like having a Marlboro Red.

The highest-strength gum or lozenge you can buy in chemists in the UK is 2mg of nicotine (of which you absorb about half. Vape pods are the same rate of absorption).

So, 6mg is *a lot*.

Curious, I plugged in 'How many nicotine pouches are recommended a day' into Google, and the AI overview told me this:

'Most users consume between four and 10 pouches.'

(The source of this average usage figure? Northerner.com, which sells nicotine pouches. Nice one, AI, on finding an impartial source.)

I then found out the 'high' nicotine pouch can be up to 20mg.

Sellers of pouches claim that absorption rates are 25–30 per cent of the total mg, but an independent medical study observed that the 'bioavailability' was more like 44 per cent.

A 44 per cent absorption rate of a 20mg pouch would be like chain-smoking *nine* Marlboro Lights. The same study found that one nicotine pouch can increase the heart rate by over 22bpm, which is probably why it made me feel instantly sick.

Were we to follow Northerner.com's lead and put away 10 of these pouches a day, that's like a 90-a-day habit. What the actual *fuck*.

It's highly unlikely that you are using this amount, I realise, as a little nicotine addict. I'm sure you're probably only using the equivalent of 20 cigarettes a week, or 40mg in pods weekly, as a light user.

But the reason I'm telling you all this is twofold. First, to show that the 'nicotine delivery' industry is ruthless, it is after our youngest cohorts and it *is* getting them. If that doesn't scare you, you are ice-cold, my friend.

And second, merely knowing about all this can act as a handy insula activator, a brain region that, as we'll discuss on page 232, is crucial in generating disgust, and can even turn the urge to partake off. Disgust is a vehicle which can carry us away from overuse of our little addictions.

The perfect storm of cue-reward

When e-cigarettes were first invented, they resembled actual cigarettes; they had the golden filter tip and the ashy end, and even glowed when you pulled on it. Yahhh – out came the 'smoke' (technically: vapour).

Nowadays, vape units have distanced themselves from actual cigarettes as much as possible, because: cancer (my own father died of lung cancer, c/o smoking, aged 65). Modern-day vapes don't look anything like cigarettes. Now, they tend to be neat little boxes, fitted with buttons and lights, which deliver rewards. What does this remind you of? (See page 32.) Then there's the 'smoke', which is entirely optional. Along my journey of vaping research, I saw a lot of products claiming 'big smoke' as a selling point.

This brings us back to Professor Clayton Hickey's comment that vapes create the 'perfect storm'. By which he meant a perfect storm of cues; cues that provoke us to use. The cues built into vapes include the light, the buttons, the specific, repetitive noises made when you pull on them and, of course, the representation of smoke. 'Vape units don't necessarily have to produce huge clouds of vapour,' says Professor Hickey. 'So why is it there?'

It behaves as a visual cue, triggering craving in both ourselves and others, which then bigs up sales. 'That visual cue probably makes the product more commercially productive,' he says. 'It's like how, when you walk into a restaurant, the cues of alcohol in context can create the "now I want a drink" urge. With drugs like nicotine, which are commercially sold, you'll see these "neuroeconomic nudges" built into the product.'

The artificially added smoke becomes a 'neuroeconomic nudge', selling more vape units. It's a marketing gimmick, increasing our chances of future addiction. 'They're not deliberately being evil; it's just capitalism,' Professor Hickey says. 'It's up to us to be aware of these built-in nudges.'

Is nicotine bad for us?

Culturally, nicotine is largely regarded as next door to coffee. No big deal. I certainly didn't think – until now – that nicotine harmed my health, other than making my heart beat a little faster, just as a flat white might.

Brace yourselves for the imminent denial-lifting. I wasn't prepared to learn any of this either. And once you know it, you can't un-know it.

It's necessary here that we only take studies that look at the nicotine itself, given I don't know how you're getting it. Maybe you're partaking via gum, pouches, pearls . . . who knows. Not all pods or liquids are created equal either in terms of chemical compounds.

So, purely nicotine.

The only other use of nicotine has been as an insecticide. Its handiness in keeping insects away from crops faded out after WWII because farmers found cheaper pesticides that were *less* harmful to the animals who accidentally ingested it while buzzing about or hopping around crops. The United States then banned it as a pesticide in 2014. Too many dead bees and bunnies.

I know.

It gets worse. One medical meta-analysis that took in 90 studies on nicotine alone (excluding tobacco use) found that nicotine can adversely affect your heart, lungs, stomach and reproductive health, and it also has carcinogenic potential. It's even been shown to progress tumours.

Holy shit.

My belief that it helps me focus seems to bear up, though. 'Brain imaging studies demonstrate that nicotine acutely increases activity in the prefrontal cortex and visual systems,' the same study said.

As we've mentioned, the prefrontal cortex is the advanced adult of the brain. However, the study's authors then rained on my parade, by calling this sharpened cognition merely 'apparent'.

This dirge from the 'bad nicotine news bears' (proposed garage band name) concludes by saying that nicotine ought to be used for smoking cessation only, and that widespread sale of nicotine-for-fun needs a crackdown of regulation.

Bloody hell.

Thankfully, I then found a cache of good news, in another 2018 study, which showed that the cognitive enhancements aren't just 'apparent'; they're real. The authors concluded, having taken in a wealth of evidence, that 'Nicotine has cognitive-enhancing effects, including improvement of fine motor functions, attention, working memory and episodic memory.'

I don't know what episodic memory is, but I assume it's something to do with TV episodes.

All that memory-enhancing doesn't quite explain why, even with a lozenge in my mouth, I consistently go upstairs only to murmur 'why am I upstairs?' And then go downstairs and promptly remember why I went upstairs.

Our bodies aren't meant to ingest nicotine

More bad news, in this dizzying club sandwich of news.

Our bodies are not designed to smoke or ingest nicotine, Professor Murphy told me. 'All you're then doing is continuing to smoke, or take nicotine, to avoid the withdrawal from not doing so.'

The use of it carves out the craving for more. The drug *creates* the withdrawal. We would never want it if we didn't start. 'It's an artificially acquired addiction because none of us are born wanting nicotine,' he adds. So nicotine addiction is unlike many of the other little addictions we'll cover in this book, like food, sex or pleased people.

This is one of the reasons, I think, that it's so disturbing to see nicotine industries targeting kids and teens. They're ice-cream-scooping out a need within them that wouldn't exist, had those kids or teens never tried nicotine. Creating a lifetime consumer, who will always now feel they need nicotine to feel OK, when they would have felt perfectly fine without it. As a society, we should rail against that.

But on a personal level, you and I are adults. Adults who need to decide for ourselves whether we're willing to risk all the health harms unveiled here, for the feelgood buzz and mind-sharpening.

It's a loss/gain equation that only we ourselves can crunch.

Dear little nicotine addict,

While writing this very book, I realised that my little nicotine addiction is now medium.

The hallmark of that shift? You may have spotted it earlier. I've started feeling like I *need* it to do certain things. Like driving.

Funny how I managed the remainder of that drive (2.5 hours, many of them M25-hairy) without nicotine, so clearly I don't *need* it to drive, but I still tell myself that I do.

This 'need' story that we script means that our habitual use of [insert thing] moves into the dorsal striatum, like we discussed with alcohol on page 40. Which is when trouble begins.

My relationship with what I 'need' nicotine for has changed this time around. I used to think I needed it to socialise, much as I once thought I needed a drink and cigarette in hand to socialise.

Interestingly, sometimes the meaning we ascribe to a drug is the opposite of what it actually does. When I smoked, I'd categorised cigarettes as a 'relaxant', when they do the physiological opposite.

This 20-year-strong 'relaxant' belief was the reason I steered all my socialising to pubs with beer gardens, or to bars with pretty pavement terraces, and then badgered my non-smoking friends to sit under the climate-change-accelerating outdoor heaters, in order to have my two socialising props handy.

But, I naturally reframed nicotine when I restarted, after pregnancy and breastfeeding. This was because, during the restart, I could feel that nicotine had a similar effect to me as caffeine. Of course it does, it's a stimulant.

Which meant I began only using it at times I would use caffeine, and for similar reasons; the coffee for the long drive, the tea for the afternoon push through. I didn't take nicotine after 3pm and prided myself on taking a couple of days off in between packets to 'prove' I wasn't addicted.

(Question: is the juncture when we need to 'prove' we're not addicted the exact moment when we also begin to become addicted? Discuss.)

That couple of days off between packets died off a few months ago. I demolished this rule with a casual wrecking ball of 'no need for that'. But it was one of the necessary structures I'd built to inhibit my use. Such demolition is always a sure sign of a medium addiction starting to dig in.

But, given I had already changed the meaning I ascribed to this drug, from 'relaxant' to 'stimulant', that means I can do so again.

'A drug can acquire a new meaning to the same person,' says Professor Murphy. 'This isn't uncommon. This changed meaning can result in a changed response to the drug.'

That gives me hope. Hopefully it feels empowering for you, too, no matter what you do next.

Love,
Cath x

NICOTINE MICRO TACTICS

Place it next door to coffee

There are many parallels in the physiological effects of nicotine and coffee, so why not place it in the next-door cupholder? I don't know about you but I don't tend to cane coffee when I'm socialising; in fact, I don't drink it at all, since it only serves to caffeinate my social anxiety.

Stimulants are not relaxing, end of, so let's all re-categorise nicotine accordingly.

Try a body scan

'I teach guests how to "body scan",' says addiction therapist Paige Keegan. 'We all have hotspots where we store stress and anxiety, but we're often not aware of where,' she says. By lying down, closing our eyes, taking deep breaths and clenching and unclenching muscles, Keegan says we'll often alight on unexpected areas of tension. 'One client found it in their knees.' She says stress is commonly kept in our chests, which could help explain why vaping is so damn popular.

Water for your vagus nerve

I quit nicotine lozenges cold – without much craving – when I found out I was pregnant, via the 'drink a glass of water every time you want a cigarette' old wives' tale. As with so many ancestral hacks, it seems to now be evidence-backed, since I was recently advised by a doctor to 'drink loads of water' after a big procedure (unrelated to this book), because 'drinking water stimulates the vagus nerve'. I was intrigued enough to look into it.

Oft-described as the 'information superhighway' of the body, the vagus nerve is best visualised as a tree, stretching from the gut to the brain, then branching out. ('Vagus' is Latin for 'roving' and this nerve does indeed rove.)

The vagus nerve is having a starlet moment, attracting much quackery: TikTok and the like are awash with ways to reset your vagus nerve, from humming and ear-massaging and eye movements, to the Goop-recommended 'vagus nerve oil' (just $48!) through to cold-water immersion and – bizarrely – blowing on your thumb.

There are even now electromagnetic bracelets and headsets that claim to be able to 'bio-hack' the vagus nerve. Experts are sceptical.

Unless they're Josh Fletcher, and then they're downright withering. 'Don't listen to any of this "quick fix" bullshit you'll see on TikTok about stimulating your vagus nerve with an ear massage,' he says. 'There's zero evidence that you can reset your vagus nerve on demand. I'm disappointed when I see therapists who should know better putting this out.'

You may not be able to reset it, but there are empirically sound ways to 'stimulate' it, and one of these is by drinking water, according to a 2002 study into 'cardiac vagal control'. Another more recent study of 53 people found that if you add ice to the water, the 'vagal enhancement' effect is boosted.

Use patches to get yourself off vapes

I snorted with disbelief the first time I saw the Nicorette ad that suggests you use *their* nicotine to get off the vapes. 'Don't vape. Quit for good' the tagline goes.

Talk about jumping from the fire back into the frying pan. But, actually, there's solid evidence that this could work, as Professor Murphy said, given patches are much less addictive. 'Patches can be very useful in withdrawing from other nicotine sources,' he said. 'Have you tried them?' Not yet, I say, but I will.

We have no data on how many people get addicted to patches, but put it this way: do you know anyone? No, nor me. So that anecdotal dearth speaks for itself.

Do the vape ritual without the vape

Reams of studies show that rituals help relax us. Some people even use zero-nicotine vape liquid (heads up: these often contain trace amounts still), yet remain addicted to the ritual of the vape. Bizarre!

Not bizarre. This is because the ritual of ducking out of a social situation or workplace, stepping outside, taking a juicy deep breath and then exhaling luxuriously, is genuinely relaxing. Says every expert ever.

We're giving the vape way too much credit. The vape is just relief adjacent to something that would already be relaxing.

Commit with a deposit

Solid banks of evidence (one study I've seen included 250k participants) show that financial incentive is a powerful motivator for behavioural change, particularly when it comes to smoking, vaping or nicotine cessation.

So, whatever your goal might be, a strategy might be to promise to give a friend £[insert a months' disposable income for you] – or even punchier, *actually hand it over* to them as a holding deposit – and if you don't achieve your goal within three or six months, you will never see it again. Of course, this depends upon you being rigorously honest, but: I believe in you.

Inspired by this (and terrified by the laundry list of harmful effects of nicotine) I just texted one of my best friends saying: 'If I haven't quit nicotine within three months, I will give you £300.'

Fidget toys for vape-quitting

'With vapes, some psychologists have said that the act becomes reinforced in because it's something to do with your hands,' says Professor Murphy. We all know that socially awkward feeling of not knowing where to put our hands. Now that fidget toys are widely socially accepted, a squishy, bendable pencil or fidget spinner could help.

WHAT WE CAN LEARN FROM THIS FIVE-STAR REHAB

I've never felt the urge to check out a rehab before, which is pretty peculiar given my obsession with all things addiction.

Actually, that statement is not entirely true, but here's the nuance: I wanted to check *into* a rehab, and desperately so, when I was slip-sliding all over the place trying to get sober back in 2013, aged 33.

Why? Because I just didn't see how I was going to resist the many alcohol-based temptations and pressures in the civilian world. I wanted to be locked up and released with 28 days sober in my tank.

And so I went to my GP after a bank holiday bender, shakes and nausea at large. I had sat in a bath with a knife the night before, drafting a potential suicide note in my mind. I then got out of the bath, placed the knife on the counter and dripped my way to the kitchen to get more wine, defeated by what I regarded as my own cowardice.

The next day, I made the emergency GP appointment and told him all of this, hoping he would send me away. Because, frankly, I thought that would be the easier route. I didn't know how to continue living with alcohol, but I didn't know how to live without it either.

I was in that liminal space of wanting to stop drinking, but also wanting to continue drinking. It's called cognitive dissonance, whereby you can hold two conflicting desires in your mind at one time. And given I was being offered alcohol everywhere from the supermarket ('try this new seasonal liqueur!') to baby showers ('it'd be rude not to toast the mother-to-be'), which never happens when you try to quit any other sort of drug, I wanted to check out of the outside world and check into a temptation-free one. Unfortunately, I couldn't afford the price tag of rehab and nobody else was offering to pick up the bill.

Only a handful of people in my life fully supported my tentative quest for sobriety, including my parents, another family member and my best friend. As for the rest? 'You're not that bad' and 'just take six months off instead' were the starring phrases.

Not that I'm blaming them; my desire to *maybe* not drink had only just sparked, so had all the staying power of a budget birthday candle. Any little puff in its direction – 'one drink won't hurt, Cath' – and it was extinguished. I fantasised that rehab would be an airtight space where my birthday candle could become a blaze.

This is why I've often maintained that, along with *ourselves*, there are two main obstacles people face should they want to go alcohol-free:

1) Our booze-championing culture
2) Other people

And so, that day, I *begged* that GP to send me to residential rehab. However, because I hadn't actually made an attempt on my own life (I'd only thought about it, in that bath and on bridges) the GP said the NHS couldn't help. He prescribed me a super-strength vitamin B complex (heavy drinking leeches our body of it, particularly B1), suggested AA meetings and sent me back out into the world advising me to 'taper'.

Tapering is reducing drinking slowly, in order to avoid needing a medicalised withdrawal. While he meant well, tapering was probably the most dunderheaded thing to suggest to a person who has roundly failed at reducing her drinking for 21 years. 'I've been trying to taper for decades, Doc,' I wanted to say.

Since then, tales of other friends who have been to rehab have upturned my salt lamp rosy imaginings. My mind was conjuring a fusion of a deluxe spa and the rehab in *28 Days* (the Sandra Bullock film), replete with a boating lake, yoga studio, trees to climb, gingham picnic blankets and cuddly staff members. (Sandra would probably be there too, actually. Maybe after graduating from rehab she returned as a staff member. It happens.)

'Rehab is not a floaty yoga retreat, Cath,' I was told by a friend who had actually been; and not only that, to three different ones. 'There's no chia pudding or singing bowls. It's intense, brutal even, and you're often treated like a child.'

Recovery *is* a second childhood of sorts. But she – and others – have told me of dictatorial rules, a lack of any news from the outside world, plus the confiscation of your phone, laptop and any sex aids (which bizarrely, can include electric toothbrushes).

Then there were tales of unappealing Dickensian food, being woken at 6.30am by air-raid-style horns, not being allowed to watch films over a 15 rating, bunk beds in shared rooms and forced participation in *everything*. The reality of rehab sounds more like being in the army – or prison – than my 'but which kaftan should I pack?' fantasies.

All that, together with the dismal reputation of success rates, made me sceptical of rehab centres and their efficacy. I'd heard data quoted about one in five people achieving a year's abstinence after a residential stay.

A friend of mine actually had this stat quoted at her in rehab, as a desultory clang of doom. The 25-strong group were told: 'Only around five of you will make it . . . the rest will relapse again and again.' And the counsellor delivering this speech was not, you'll be surprised to hear, Sandra Bullock in a kaftan.

Since then, I've dug around in the research myself and found that this 'one in five' stat is just one tiny piece of cloud in a jigsaw puzzle. In fact, I couldn't even find the original source of it; I could only find it cited elsewhere.

The larger picture is much more hopeful, much more blue-sky. I found a 2022 meta-analysis of residential rehab studies, taking in a total of 17 studies from the UK and beyond. It reported that success rates (here defined as total abstinence) reported at a year post-treatment do vary wildly, yes, but none are as dispiriting as one in five.

Abstinence rates a year later pendulum between roughly one in three (a US youth rehab) and an impressive 88 per cent (a study in the Czech Republic), depending on which finding you look at. One study – specifically following veterans, so not randomized – actually had a 100 per cent success rate.

The spooky alignment

Before all this digging, as I said, I had a total lack of interest in exploring a rehab facility, let alone reverse-engineering one.

That was until I heard about Delamere, a £7m residential rehab set on the outskirts of a cute village in Chester, and mostly grabbing headlines because of the price of a stay (the lowest-rung room is £18k for a 28-day stay), even though this price tag is pretty standard – cheap, even – for a luxury rehab.

The first thing that attracted me to Delamere was this: the activities it includes are spookily aligned to the activities that helped me when I was getting sober. The centre also champions a personalised approach to recovery, rather than trying to create a conveyor belt of people shaped like cookies, something I feel strongly about. My own recovery followed no pre-existing pattern. Oftentimes, even if a person's recovery looks 'by the book', we all do this in a slightly different way.

It resembles a supersized Grand Design among 90ft trees – one that Kevin McCloud might say 'blends seamlessly with the hillside'. Think warm wood and vast expanses of glass with a meadow of wildflowers beside.

Finally, there are, indeed, singing bowls and chia pudding (I didn't see any salt lamps but I'm willing to bet my entire essential oils collection that there are some).

The plan was for me to spend 48 hours hanging out there, in order to extract the tools they use to dismantle big addictions. Then miniaturising them, so that you and I can use them for our little addictions. Here's what happened . . .

I become the crazy horse lady

Before I even arrive at Delamere, I'm fairly sure I get a reputation as the crazy horse lady. I bang on about experiencing the equine therapy so much, and when will this be, and I can't see it on the agenda, and if the equine therapy person is busy, maybe I could just go into the field and introduce myself to the horses? . . . that I receive an email from the loveliest, kindest member of staff who says:

'I do apologise for not being able to add equine therapy on to your schedule. This takes place each Monday at an offsite location and so isn't something that we could easily offer. There are horses close to site but, unfortunately, they do not belong to us, and we are asked not to feed or stroke them.'

My friend Hannah and I find the parting line of the email so amusing that we riff off it for a long while, planning scenarios where I turn up to Delamere wearing a riding hat and jodhpurs, armed with a ready-peeled carrot.

Our final plan is that I canter in astride a hobby horse.

My interest in the equine therapy was for good reason: I wrote about this at length in *The Unexpected Joy of Being Sober*, but I had a moving, nay *magical* experience with some horses on a day I was experiencing suicidal ideation. This was back in the dark days of 2013, six months before I quit drinking.

I had spent the sunny day wandering around a heathland, telling myself I was getting some 'fresh air' while drinking white wine out of a sports bottle, crying and having arguments with people in my head. And then *this* happened (abridged from the book):

There were three grown horses and a yearling in the field on the heath. I didn't have any food, and yet they all came to me. And stayed with me. Bowed and let me hold their beautiful strong heads. Breathed me in, licked my open hand.

The mother even let me stroke her yearling. I spent an hour in that field, with those horses. They pulled me out of the mire of my own mind, and into that field with them, when I needed it most.

It's no secret that animals are empathic, but even thinking of this now, 12 years on, I still can't believe it happened. Animals don't usually let you near their babies, even their year-old ones, let alone hang out with you for an hour.

Lesson one: trees and animals

The first thing I notice about Delamere is how many trees there are. So, so many. There isn't a window in the building that isn't filled with greenery, at least in part. And this maximum nature exposure isn't by accident, it's by design, as are the fields of horses (don't touch those, Cath) and cattle flanking the site.

'Being among greenery has been shown to lower the heart rate and blood pressure,' says Chris Lomas, Delamere's foremost addiction psychotherapist, who is very smiley, tall and clever.

Forest bathing, or as the older among us might say, 'a walk in the woods', has been proven time and time again to lower cortisol, the stress hormone, and activate the parasympathetic nervous system, like Lomas just mentioned. Forget column inches; column *miles* have been written about this, so I won't labour the point.

'OK, so what's with the horses then?' I ask Lomas.

'You co-regulate with the horse to some degree,' he says, 'whereby your heart rate meets the horse's.' This makes sense, given my calming hour in the field.

Evidence has found that this co-regulation sorcery extends to dogs. The mere body weight of an animal sitting on us can activate 'rest and digest', hence why autistic societies worldwide recommend 'therapy animals'.

This is probably partially why we're so attached to our pets, and why fake 'emotional support animal' ID tags sell out online, with dog owners trying to game the system that regularly parts us from them.

Lesson two: we need more than talking

As I walk around the clean, airy centre, I notice how much is geared towards physical health. There's a sleek gym and a yoga studio, while they also teach breathwork, and host regular walks in nature.

Talking therapies – and groups – aren't enough when tackling addictions, in both my view and Delamere's. The centre provides one-to-one therapy, of course, as well as group sessions, but there's a deliberate schedule of bodywork alongside it.

This is because, as Bessel van der Kolk famously broached in *The Body Keeps the Score*, trauma is stored in the body, not just the mind. And if you've ever been at the mercy of a big addiction, trauma probably features in your emotional luggage, whether it pre-dated it or was a consequence.

Mostly, trauma pre-dates the addiction. 'Rough estimates are that 80 per cent of addictions are related to traumatic events,' Lomas reveals. 'This trauma leads to hyper-stimulation of the amygdala, which is like the fire alarm of the brain. The amydala then triggers an auto-response of physiological armouring, or emotional dysregulation.'

Talking therapy provides what they call 'a top-down approach' to trauma, but to achieve emotional regulation, we now know that we also need a 'bottom-up' one in tandem, which is achieved via the body.

Of course, genuinely traumatic events (rather than what TikTokkers often define as 'trauma', which is often just life's rich tapestry of headfuckery) such as domestic unrest, a car crash or medical strife, can all create little addictions as well as big ones.

We often talk about these life events to psychologically unpack, but forget about the body's storage of them. Breathwork, exercise, meditation, massage; *anything* physically relaxing is the way we 'bottom-up' our way to emotional regulation.

'When you concentrate only on talking about previous trauma or addiction, you're reactivating the amygdala repeatedly,' explains Lomas. 'Re-stimulating those unpleasant memories doesn't help to actually process them, or change the schemas linked to them.' (A schema is a mental framework upon which we hang our beliefs and behaviours.)

'In fact, there's an argument that top-down alone can actually make things worse,' he says. 'But once you learn to regulate the body as well through bottom-up, and you're getting into that resting and relaxed state, you can get underneath that physiological armouring and beneath that fire alarm of the amygdala.'

Mind and body in tandem is the key, he says. 'We start to change and contextualise those traumatic memories, processing them in the hippocampus and shifting the schemas into a positive direction.'

Lesson three: schemas are like coat hangers

I'm still not totally sure what schemas are, or why they matter, so I ask him to explain. 'Schemas are beliefs about the world, which then lead to automatic behaviours,' he explains. This 'automatic behaviour' could be a little addiction.

Often our schemas are wonky because they were built in childhood, he says. 'As kids we don't have brilliantly developed brains, and we have to make assumptions really quickly, and so we build schemas. But those schemas may be misled, or may not work any more when you're thirty-eight rather than eight.'

I'm now thinking back to eight-year-old me, who watched adults pour themselves big glasses of rum and Coke after rough days, exhaling deeply. 'A-ha, so that's how you relax, gotcha' became one of my schemas, like a coat hanger upon which I hung my own beliefs about drinking, and my later behaviour.

Your schemas will be entirely personal to you; maybe sugar was used to bait good behaviour when you were little, so the schema laid down was: 'I deserve sugar when I've been good.' And so now, you crave chocolate when you're working late.

Or if gaming was the only way your family of origin relaxed together, the schema created could be: 'Gaming time is family time,' and so now you want every Sunday to be a PlayStation day, and you still feel cheated if it's not.

Our schemas aren't necessarily right or wrong, they just *are*. But once we're aware of them, we can begin to challenge and change them, consciously rewriting the meaning we award to alcohol, sugar, gaming ... whatever it might be.

Lesson four: interoception's side doors

I push out into the courtyard of Delamere, where cherry blossom trees wait to bloom. Hanging from a tree are cardboard hearts with handwriting on them (things the guests want more of), twizzling in the breeze.

Looking back at the handsome U-shaped building, with its many doors, I realise it's a handy metaphor for top-down and bottom-up processing. If we think of ourselves as a building, then using top-down processing only would be like only having one door in and out. One door is insufficient, risky even.

Bodywork is one way to create more doors, interoception is another. Often referred to as the 'sixth sense' because it's the through line between body and mind, interoception is – at its most basic level – knowing when you're hungry, thirsty, itchy or hot. At its most advanced level, it's knowing that little addictions at work in the brain *also* manifest in the body.

'Interoception is what Bessel van der Kolk would call a side door,' Lomas says.

Ordinarily, receptors inside the tissues and organs help us sense what is going on, but our interoceptive sixth sense can become muffled or blunted, often by trauma, sometimes by modern life, sometimes by other factors. Neurodivergent 'meltdowns' are often attributed to a lack of interoception skills, say experts.

Interoception 101 is tapping into the senses when your mind is in freefall. So, when you sense yourself being sucked into a whirlpool of panic, or catch yourself re-playing a negative thought over and over, wanting to reach for a little addiction, you can engage your sixth sense of interoception by – ironically – coming back to the other five senses:

'What can I smell, what can I see, what can I hear, what can I taste, what can I feel?'

Often just using three is enough to move yourself out of your head and back into your body. Right now, I'm feeling anxious about a talk I'm giving to the guests of Delamere later in my stay. So, I tune back in to my senses.

I can smell the cinders of a 'fire ceremony' where guests burn things they want to let go of, I can feel the breeze on my skin, and I can see snowdrops bowing their lovely heads. The anxiety softens.

Lesson five: the power of sound

I meet some of the other guests at a sound bath. (I like that Delamere calls its recoverees 'guests' rather than 'patients' or 'clients'.)

For the sound bath, we lie down in a crescent shape, coddled in blankets, heads closest to the singing bowls to get maximum vibration for our buck. Jerome Fagan, a recovery mentor and former guest of Delamere, is leading the sound bath. Jerome is sharply dressed and has a dry line in Northern banter.

At first, I was surprised that he used to be a priest, but that now makes perfect sense. As he plays the Tibetan singing bowls, the soundwaves play the reward centres of my brain like a harp. When the rain stick starts, it's like an orchestra of pleasure.

Singing bowls, gongs, didgeridoos and rain sticks are often classified as hippy claptrap, or derided as the items posh teens bring back from gap years for performative display – 'I did a culture thing, look bruh!' – but this is all unfair. The science behind sound baths is robust.

Sound baths encourage the brain to move out of beta brainwaves (alert, active, problem-solving; us on a work day) into alpha brainwaves (relaxed, yet still alert; us on the sofa) or even better, into theta (a dream-like, creative, meditative state; us lying on a remote beach) by using the science of synchronisation, which is all about vibrational energy transfer. Our brain follows the frequency of the soundwaves, essentially.

A Korean study, which analysed brainwaves via an EEG, found that just five minutes of singing bowls produced a surge of theta brainwaves of, on average, 118 per cent.

Sound baths effectively place you into a meditative state without effort, even if – like me – you're hopeless at meditation and have a brain full of squabbling cats. It's an aural hack into a more monk-like brain, without the daily commitment to a meditation cushion and subscription to Headspace.

Lesson six: the window of tolerance

I'm still blissed out when I learn about this game changer. It came from Sally Hopkins, a recovery mentor at Delamere, whose sunny, capable energy is like Penelope Pitstop meets Nicola Coughlan.

'The "window of tolerance" is how much a person can withstand before they become emotionally dysregulated,' she explains. And it's when we're dysregulated that we're more likely to pick up [insert addictive thing], whether our attachment to it is little or large.

'We all have days where our window of tolerance is tiny,' Hopkins says. 'We spill a drink or lose our car keys and it feels like the worst thing that's ever happened. Whereas we'll have other days when the exact same thing happens and we're like *shrugs*. Every day has natural challenges, but on the days where our window is a sliver, which is anyone in early recovery, these challenges can floor us.'

Our power comes from knowing about it.

I'll now observe throughout the day how large my window feels, and have taken to telling my partner, 'I have a very small window of tolerance today', so that he'll be more understanding if I fly into a tailspin because I broke a jar of gherkins, while acting like I broke an international peace treaty.

Lesson seven: reward system activation

Delamere is designed for guests to find new ways of activating their reward systems. Guests play games, have film nights, set exciting goals. A lot less stick and a lot more carrot. That worked for me too, given one of my strategies was pointing myself towards 'sober treats', and Chris Lomas explains why.

He says that when we have a primary addiction, or what we're calling a 'big addiction', our pleasure in all other pursuits fades. 'The reward centre, or dopamine system, becomes desensitised to other pleasures in life, and is comprised of only one big cog, or the primary addiction. If there's a primary *and* secondary addiction in place – say cocaine and shopping, or alcohol and sex – then there'll be two major cogs in there.'

Once you remove that one big cog – or two major cogs – we enter a danger zone.

'That danger zone is around seven to fourteen days in,' Lomas says. 'Around that time in rehab, people feel generally better, but also start thinking they're bored and want to leave. What's actually happening is that their reward system is recalibrating, but that big cog – or two – has been removed and is yet to be replaced with something new.'

We might then cross-addict. 'The natural proclivity is to replace the lost cog/s with that or those of equal size,' he says. This can look like a romantic relationship, or an over-dependence on the gym, or heavy use of sugar, or nicotine, or phone use, or judgement.

Tiny cogs are what we *want* to input, to replace that previous system. It's tempting to think he's describing little addictions. Those are small cogs, right, that make us feel good? But he's talking even tinier and more meaningful, more wholesome and, annoyingly, usually more effortful.

'Things that give us hope,' he says. It's about having dozens and dozens of cogs, otherwise known as alternative ways of feeling good. 'This means that our reward system still works even if one – or a few – fail. Say, if we injure ourselves at the gym.'

And those cogs need to be as differently shaped as possible, differently coloured and made of different matter. 'We want their type to spread widely, across mind, career, family, body, home, friendships and long-term planning,' Lomas says.

Lesson eight: personifiying your little addiction

I'm talking with Paige Keegan, an addiction therapist at Delamere. If she had an aura, it'd be green; I feel more relaxed after about 10 seconds in her presence.

Within minutes, she's said something that makes me want to punch the air. 'It really helps to separate our addiction out from ourselves and give it a character, colour and name,' she says. 'It taps into configurations of self, which I trained in.'

This one gives me joy as it was so effective for me. Way back in 2013, I used 'Addictive Voice Recognition', a technique developed by Jack Trimpey in the '90s, calling my addicted-to-alcohol voice 'Voldemort', the villain of Harry Potter fame.

It was apt, because my big addiction felt silken but evil, the wannabe architect of my downfall. But maybe your little addiction to biscuits feels like a blundering Cookie Monster, or maybe the urge to vape is a small yellow anxious bird called Deirdre.

Separating the urge to do the thing away from *yourself* adds a layer of objectivity and, thus, choice. You can even give it a form, as well as a voice. One of the creative classes taught here at Delamere is 'giving form to addiction'.

It's led by Gail Sargerson, a recovery mentor who wears double leopard print, which I fully approve of, and if she had a theme tune, it'd almost certainly be a dancey one by Fleetwood Mac.

'What does your addiction look like, how does it speak to you?' she asks.

I tell her about Voldemort. She laughs, then tells me of some of the things former guests have drawn. 'One woman drew around her hands over and over, layering them, because her addiction felt like hands pulling her in.

'But some of the most powerful pieces I've ever seen have been from guests who aren't traditionally "good" at art,' says Sargerson, 'who can't draw a realistic tree. Their pictures have just been of stick people, but there's been a profound truth at the centre of it.'

****

A month on from my stay at Delamere, I still feel the afterglow. Delamere encouraged me to dust off some forgotten tools, as well as inviting me to try some new ones.

Just this morning, I went for a wild swim – and have only humblebragged about it to every single person I've come into contact with since. As I was bobbing around in the battleship-grey English Channel, I decided to supercharge the cold water therapy with some interoception.

I really took in the spinning wind farm on the horizon, the waves slapping on the shore, the bite of salt in my mouth. And by the time I got out, I wasn't just feeling sharp and clear, as is the usual after a wild swim.

I also felt still.

REHAB TAKEAWAYS

Forest bathing on the hop

If you can't spend time in an actual forest, a great hack involves atomising some oils. Dr Qing Li – a world-class immunologist who specialises in 'forest medicine' – told Goop that the phytoncides (certain tree aromas) are the aspect of forest bathing that exact the 'greatest effect'.

They used hinoki cypress oil in the studies, but other phytoncides include pine, cedar and oak.

Borrowing someone's pet

Given that horses aren't easily available to hug, the good news is that just borrowing someone's dog – or housesitting a cat – gives a similar parasympathetic activation, with Harvard Medical School saying that several studies back this.

DIY sound bath

An in-person sound bath is definitely going to bliss you out more, given the physically present soundwaves, but it's hard to align that with the urge for a little addiction. Luckily, on-demand incarnations (available on whatever music streaming service you use) will work to a lesser, but still lovely, degree.

I like *Sound Bath Escape* for a two-minute Tibetan singing bowl bath, available on Spotify to everyone. Over-ear noise-cancelling headphones do amplify the immersion, so use those if you have them.

Go barefoot

If you need to find zen quickly, this is effective. 'Standing barefoot regulates the heart rate in a similar way to equine therapy,' Lomas says. 'In fact, we should spend more time barefoot here at Delamere.'

Just scrunching your toes into some sand or grass will do the trick. Our feet are meant to touch natural surfaces, after all; shoes are a relatively modern quirk.

Find 50 tiny cogs

If you, like me, are too reliant on a few – or several – little addictions, it's time to replace that machinery with dozens and dozens of tiny cogs instead. I'd suggest shooting for a list of 50 wholesome ways you find meaning, pleasure and purpose. My list includes items like 'finding a new song I love', 'amazing-smelling toiletries', 'doing one miniscule house task a day', 'reading each night, if only two pages' or 'giving a stranger a compliment'.

While making the list, I even eye-rolled myself. Your list will feel cutesy – maybe even cottagecore – because they are, and that's part of why they work.

Draw your little addiction and give it a name

We talked about drawing, naming and personifying your little addiction, so I've left a blank page opposite for you to do so.

'Giving your little addiction a character adds a layer of compassion,' says Keegan. This means that you can speak softly to your little addiction. Suddenly you're no longer telling *yourself* you can't vape or eat a third biscuit, which feels restrictive and punitive; you're telling Deirdre the bird, or Cookie Monster, that they can't.

It sounds infantile but, I promise you, it works, given it separates your little addictions – a 'configuration' of you – out from your core self.

Draw and name your little addictions here:

GAMBLING

Sticky eight

My first casino visit was when I was 29, and I couldn't have been more disappointed. I was expecting mafiosos padding around, molls blowing on dice for good luck, heavies escorting card-counters out, martinis gliding around on trays balanced by wait staff wearing sequins, crowds watching an average Joe on a roulette winning streak, whooping with joy when he did it yet again.

It's fair to say I'd glue-sticked together a montage in my head of every Vegas film I'd ever seen.

It was more of a bored, cigarette-scented, bad-carpeted thunderdome, where all human emotion had gone to die. I'd dressed up, expecting evening wear, but everyone else was in leisurewear, and not the good kind. The roulette sat unused and sad.

Visor-wearing seniors chain-smoked while playing the slots. The croupiers had no banter, they just looked like they were about to fall asleep. When my friend and I took a grinning selfie of us sitting at the blackjack table, a security guard pointed at the 'no pictures' sign.

No pictures, no chat, no sequins and, indeed, no whooping.

****

I'd accidentally observed something that is the centrepiece of one of my expert's work. I'm here with Natasha Dow Schüll, who is an associate professor at NYU, a cultural anthropologist and the author of *Addiction by Design*. She spent over a decade intermittently hanging out on- and off-strip in Vegas, living with a family of high-stakes poker players. She's arguably the world expert in this topic and I'm fascinated by every single word she says. 'Cut me off if I go on too long,' she says, but I literally cannot.

We're both working parents of girls. Her daughter is texting her repeatedly, trying to get into the room during our call to retrieve some clothes. I tell her that here in my world, my laptop is perched shakily on my three-year-old's xylophone to bring it to Zoom height. It feels like a perfect metaphor for the precarious balance of working and parenting.

We're talking about the key of C major. It's the key of 'Twinkle Twinkle Little Star'. I know because I've played it on this very xylophone many times. It's also the key of many famous lullabies, such as Brahms' 'Lullaby'. It's *also* the key that slot machine makers tend to use, Schüll's research found. I wonder if app creators use it too. Probably.

It lulls the people in the seats into what she calls a 'mindless' state. That's what the gambling industry wants, says Schüll.

During that decade, Schüll interviewed casino designers and pored over hefty layout manuals to discover other tactics used to create what she describes as 'little sanctuaries to envelop you'. They lower the lights and ceilings (cocooning), making cave-like nooks that use sound cones for noise reduction. It almost sounds more like the design philosophy for a spa than a casino. Schüll came across one instance where they atomised lavender into the slots area, to make it more relaxing.

'They'll even use curves in the carpet to lead you to the destination they desire for you,' she says. 'The carpets – and layout – usually have no right angles, because what do you do when you come to a crossroads in life? You *think*. You've got to decide, "do I go left or right?"'

It's not what the adverts show, nor the movies, this curved, cocooned, lullaby-keyed *don't think* vibe. 'You can still find that high-end tuxedo version in little pockets but, overall, the vision has outlived the reality,' she says. In some casinos, 90 to 95 per cent of the revenue is coming purely from slot machines. 'Nothing about slots feels dangerous. They call to mind youth arcades or elderly blue-haired ladies who go to Atlantic City to play. Yet it's the most pernicious form of gambling.'

One of the most unexpected findings of her research was that habitual slot gamblers dislike winning, because it yanks them out of what they call the 'machine zone'. 'That was their native term,' she says of the many gamblers she interviewed, 'for that self-suspension that they were seeking.'

Similarly to someone looking for oblivion in a K-hole or the second bottle, the 'machine zone' is about escaping from the clock, the wallet, the housework, other people, work, *yourself*. Winning ruins that self-suspension for the addicted player, she found. 'The machine freezes, makes loud sounds and plays music, coins start pouring out, people look at you and come over. Everything you've been trying to escape *comes back*.'

Something that puzzled her during her research was that 'machine zone' sounded a lot like 'flow'. 'Flow is defined as an optimal human state linked to creativity and wellbeing,' she says. The concept and term were coined by psychologist Mihaly Csikszentmihalyi in the 1960s, when he became fascinated by artists who were totally immersed in their work, forgetting to eat or drink, feeling suspended in the sweet spot between skill and difficulty. Just as with the gamblers, those in flow can get very irritated when interrupted.

'Every aspect of "machine zone" maps perfectly on to flow,' Schüll says. 'It may not be that different from performing a surgery or rock climbing, in that perfect balance between challenge and control. Yet instead of it feeling rejuvenating and creative, "machine zone" is devastating and depleting. I came to realise this is because it's like an algorithmically formatted flow.' A *negative* version of flow.

She thinks it's the self-suspension of the zone that people become addicted to, whether they're on a slot machine or an app. They're not looking for life-changing jackpots; at the very most they're just playing to win to play some more. 'Whether you're playing in person in a casino or on your phone on your commute, they're just different on-ramps to the same zone,' Schüll says.

Only, the apps are much more dangerous, given they're frictionless, and there's no need to go to a physical place at all. Historically, if you lived within 50 miles of a casino, your chances of becoming hooked on gambling doubled, she says. Now, the casino is in our pockets, five inches from our hands.

I don't know what odds *that* creates, but it sounds like they're bad for us, and good for the apps.

The algorithmic recliner

The app creators want to soothe you into laid-back mindlessness, just as the casino designers do, and so they use many of the same design principles; dark colours, chirrups in the key of C, curves rather than right angles.

The algorithm is even spa-like too. 'A slot machine engineer that I interviewed drew a graph plotting money spent against time,' she says. He drew a wavy, ever-downward line. The more time you spend, the more you lose, but it happens slowly. 'We want you to recline on our algorithm like you would recline on a comfortable couch,' he said to her.

Reclining is much more inviting than the 'spiky mountain of volatility' provided by the green felt tables or high-stakes sports bets, she says. Which is probably why the algorithmic recliner tends to be where gambling companies make their big bucks.

'A constant flow of repetitious little bets is so much more addictive than traditional sports betting,' Schüll adds, referring to going down the bookies to put money on a certain horse, or match, or game, or fight. 'One study showed that you don't become addicted to sports betting for eight to ten years, but with these other repetitious forms, you get pulled in within two or three.'

Repetition means reinforcement and, as always throughout this book, reinforcement means learning, which is the fastest route to addiction. 'Whether you're pulling the lever, pressing the button or doing the crack, every time you repeat it is a moment of Skinnerian reinforcement,' says Schüll. 'Tedious processes have an incredible hold on us.'

We find them soothing – think of knitting, stroking an animal, cycling, chopping, whatever your stim is. Repetitious actions have become genetically coded in because they're very useful for our survival. As our experts keep saying (see pages 54 and 118) about scrolling, tapping and clicking, these probably remind us of foraging or farming.

'Survival of the repetition-resilient.' Those who could do a small action hundreds of times over and over for small returns would have benefited themselves and their tribe. Picking one piece of fruit and then stopping, or giving up on grinding the wheat? Not so useful.

Then there are those more driven by the big spiky rewards. 'There are still people who like the volatility, but they need to be willing to have long dry spells and then a sudden win,' Schüll says.

This sounds a lot like big game stalking, says evolutionary psychologist Dr Andrew Thomas. 'Being motivated throughout a long wait for a potentially amazing outcome? Sounds just like hunting, the complementary process to foraging.'

We get stuck in the puzzle

Whatever type of gambling you're into, this world is also where Skinner's reward uncertainty (the rat or pigeon in the box, on page 32) really comes into its own. Schüll tells me that she even found archival footage of Skinner himself from the 1960s, saying: to help you understand what a Skinner box is, let's go to Atlantic City.

'Wow,' I say.

'*I know*,' she replies. Skinner is a David Bowie-level icon for academics – and now also, for me. I might pin up a portrait of him on my fridge.

Just as she said on page 33, the reward uncertainty of gambling presents a puzzle to our brain; only it's a puzzle we can't work out, given it's an encounter with chance. We get stuck in the puzzle. 'We're creatures of learning, but we cannot learn chance,' she says.

The gambling industry knows that and leverages it for profit. Then, just as the alcohol industry does, they sidestep responsibility for their addictive product with the omnipresent slogan of 'gamble responsibly' in the UK. I'm preaching to the converted with Schüll.

'It's the same story in the States,' she says. 'There's even this entity called the International Center for Responsible Gaming. Just as the alcohol industry maintains that alcoholics don't come in bottles – they come in people – their message is that problematic gambling doesn't come in machines or technology, it comes in people.'

Our views on this are so aligned it's uncanny. 'They then fund philanthropic efforts into researching these "poor people",' she says, noticeable heat in her voice. 'But what they're doing is trying to cordon off. To assert that there's no continuum, no spectrum, and that the rest of us consumers can just gamble freely.'

It's othering; establishing them versus us. Which has been used in propaganda since *forever*. 'It's very smart,' she says, 'because who can be against personal responsibility?' says Schüll. 'But it's not about responsibility. It's a deliberate public relations campaign.'

Addiction is an interplay between person + thing; both Schüll and I vigorously agree on this duality. If they're asking *us* to be responsible, then the industries themselves need to be responsible – for creating technologies or substances more likely to addict.

The things that have enabled us to survive – love, food, other people – are at the heart of all addictions, says Schüll. 'It's almost like those who get addicted are just *too* good at them. They're not outliers; they're people that we need to understand, in order to understand *ourselves*.'

This is why sectioning off addicts as this separate group makes no sense, she adds. 'A continuum, a spectrum, which we're all on. All of us have the very same drives. Addicts are just doing it in a more intense way.'

A big gambling addiction can be catastrophic, it must be acknowledged. I spoke with one expert, Nir Eyal, who helps companies design 'habit-forming products', but refuses to work with the online gambling industry.

'We have rich people with rich person problems spending too much time on Twitter,' Eyal says, impassioned. 'Meanwhile, people are losing their houses and lives, and they weren't rich people to begin with. We don't talk about that enough, the fact that they now have a casino in their pocket and can gamble all of their money away on sports betting. Gambling destroys lives and families.'

But you only have a little gambling addiction. So, let's get back to that.

Loss-chasing

In Britain, the Gambling Commission says nearly half of us gamble regularly (defined as within the last four weeks). The most popular form is the National Lottery or other 'charity lottery draws' (played by over a third of Brits), followed by scratchcards (12 per cent) and betting (10 per cent) and, finally, online games (7 per cent).

We've already spoken about this on page 31, but the younger we are when we pick up a substance or activity, the stickier it is. Plus,we're riskier when we do it, with data showing that gamblers aged 18–20 are more likely to bet more than they can afford, in a bid to 'chase their losses'.

If reward uncertainty is the engine, the 'loss chasing' adds F1-level horsepower. It's an attempt to recoup our losses, which lives next door to 'sunk cost fallacy'. The more money we put into the hole, the more likely we will keep putting money into the hole. The more we loss-chase, and the more we repeat the pattern, the lower chance of 'extinction', as behavioural scientists call it.

'Extinction' is the opposite to addiction creation – this is when a compulsion is *not* created. Maybe we buy a scratchcard once or twice, then never again. We have undergone 'extinction'. That is what the gambling industry definitely *does not* want.

They want us to continue to exist on their savannah, running after our losses. Think about a lottery syndicate that runs for decades, made up of a group of friends who have created their chosen numbers from their birthdays. This syndicate will run forever, probably, because can you imagine if they suddenly stopped and then their numbers came up? It's unthinkable.

The narrative that circulates around winning the lottery is this: it's a curse. The press loves to point at lottery winners who lost all of their loved ones, ended up with a gram-a-day cocaine habit, had plastic surgery that went very wrong and had to sell all their fancy houses to pay off debt collectors. A lottery win is Pandora's Box, they want us to believe, and inside you will find the worst winged horrors of the universe. But this is a suburban myth, peddled to make us feel better about our two-up, two-down terraces (I'm not being snooty, this is literally my house).

There *is* older research that showed a thrilling rise and then a boomerang return after a lottery win, with happiness levels reverting to the pre-win baseline. I've cited this study myself – it was compelling stuff – as have hundreds of other journalists. But the current reality is this: that small 1978 study has since been debunked by more recent findings, particularly a Swedish study that looked at the largest sample size I've seen (3,362) *and* large winnings ($100k+), ultimately finding that the happiness surge was 'significant' and held true for over a decade.

What's also true is this, and I don't need a study to back it up, because it's just common sense. If you won the lottery today, from this day forward, you would no longer know if people genuinely want to be your friend/date you/marry you even. Everyone is a potential bounty hunter on the make.

Royals obviously experience this from their first breath, while celebrities experience it from their breakthrough performance. But at least they have people around them who know how to navigate it, or they've had a while to work up to it.

A lottery winner is an ordinary human airlifted into this situation overnight. I cannot imagine anything more discombobulating or paranoia-inducing, socially. I already have wobbles where I think most of my friends and family secretly hate me (hiii, low self-esteem).

There must also be a keen sense of 'what now?' We've been striving, reaching, grafting, hustling our entire lives to get to the promised land of this very place – the apex of never needing to worry about money ever again – and now we've got here via what amounts to a cheat code . . . Now what? I moan about the hustle, while also knowing that I love the hustle. That life *is* the hustle.

That's my devil's advocate dance, done. Do you feel a little better? I know I do. Because let's face it, we're incredibly unlikely to win, which is why the press love to report on, and the public love to read of, the 'lottery curse'.

Meanwhile, I have gathered that the secret to downsizing a little gambling addiction is all about avoiding the lure of the 'machine zone', which seeks to make us dumb and numb. In the upcoming 'micro tactics' we'll learn how to keep our wits about us while gambling, while also retaining the fun. Much of this orbits adding friction back in to a world which has now become utterly frictionless.

Dear little gambling addict,

Omaze is my one and only little gambling addiction. Over the past three years, I have spent £275 on the chance to win the likes of a James Bond-esque house suspended over the edge of a north Devon cove, with steps leading directly down into the water.

(That particular home now lies empty, since the winner and local lore say it's doomed to fall into the sea within five to ten years.)

Even while researching this chapter, I threw more money into Omaze's pot, having clicked on the website for research, and then finding myself seduced by the chance to win a gleaming £4m beachfront house in my home county of Sussex. 'I already live in Sussex, it'd be stupid of me not to . . .' went the justification.

Show me a sexy house and my wallet just opens. Interiors are my porn. Besides, I always feel good about it. Because hovering over the button I click to enter is an angelic reminder that 'every entry you make' sends more money to charity. This time, I'm helping those with motor neurone disease. *polishes halo*

While draws by companies like Omaze are often classified as 'charity raffles', even by the likes of the BBC, Omaze are open about them being no such thing. They are definitely for profit, with on average 17 per cent of the revenue going to a named charity partner.

While entering to win the Sussex house, I was moderate at first, choosing the second from lowest rung: 40 entries for £25.

A marketeer friend has told me that price plans often fall into 'gets you fucking nothing', 'just right', 'even better' and 'no fucking way', in order to funnel us exactly where the businesses want us to go: the happy middle. Which is exactly where I go.

As I'm clicking through to pay, I tell myself that I have friends who chuck £50 a month at subscribing for Omaze, so I'm the very model of moderation. It's always so handy when you know people worse than you.

Pop! I'm offered a 'special offer'. A special offer just for little me! I'm told I can have 60 extra entries, so that makes 100 entries in total, for just £10 extra, which is 75 per cent off, people! Incredible. My head is spinning from all these numbers.

Obviously I click yes, so I end up spending £35 instead of my intended £25. I wonder how many other people do the same. Millions, I bet.

I feel tantalised. I'm already imagining myself reclining on those linen sofas, savasana-ing in the yoga studio followed by the private sauna, then firing up the Ooni pizza oven for a beachside dinner. I am salivating like one of Pavlov's dogs.

Just as with the lottery win, Omaze seems like a cheat code for the dream life, but the reality can look different. The *MailOnline* visited all 14 of the raffled Omaze properties in 2023, to see how the owners were doing. They found that 10 had been sold and one was being rented out. Only three were occupied by winners.

Interviewing one family who'd put their £4m house on the market just eight weeks after they'd won it, the *MailOnline* heard from Uttam Parmar that: 'It is a fantastic house in a beautiful Cornish location but . . . it comes with a price to keep it and we can't afford to.'

Omaze has upped the £100,000 cash gift that comes along with the house to £250,000, given the serious costs of upkeep and the rash of critical articles that followed this reveal.

You might own a stunning house outright but your monthly outgoings are likely to become more expensive, not less. There's no mortgage, stamp duty or legal fees to pay, but given the hugely elevated gas, electric, water, home insurance and council tax bills, the £250,000 is needed just to hang on to it.

The irony is, once I research my Omaze habit, I find out that both my halo and I would have been better off going down to the corner shop and buying two dozen lottery tickets to play The National

Lottery, which I could then use to choose or build my own dream house.

Of all 'charity raffles' or lotteries, The National Lottery is the most virtuous. Only around 1 per cent of The National Lottery's net is profit taken. I mean, that's of around £7.8 billion, so they're not *poor*, but it's one of the better donators, giving 28 per cent to good causes.

Plus, the odds of winning are better. An investigation run by *The Telegraph* reverse-engineered one Omaze draw and estimated that the chances of winning one seemed to be 'much lower' than winning The National Lottery. Just to frame that in some numbers far too big to be comprehensible, the chances of you winning the lottery are around one in 45 million.

Put it this way: our odds of being attacked by a shark are one in 11.5 million.

In their 'right of reply', Omaze told *The Telegraph* that they can't possibly calculate the odds, given it changes with the number of entries to each draw. *The Telegraph* acknowledged this in their calculations too.

I don't know, though. The National Lottery is much less appealing to me. That alternative of 'win lottery – find house – buy house – furnish house' sounds like a lot more work. I just want a furnished, gorgeous house that's paid off and ready for me to move in, OK? I want the house thing solved in one frictionless swoop. All I want to do is book the movers. Which is why I find Omaze so irresistible. Experts call this the 'let me dream on' effect, and it infuses most forms of gambling with intense anticipated pleasure.

It's no coincidence, I imagine, that I found buying a house very, very hard. Unlike many of my friends, whose parents gifted them a deposit, it took me until age 40 to save it up. That's not 'poor me', I know many of us never get there at all, and if that's you, I feel for you. But what's also true is that Omaze presses an emotional button within me. And so I, in turn, click and press, hoping an easy house will churn out.

What is it that drives you to gamble? This is the most important question for us to ask ourselves, because it could also enable us to deactivate that button.

For myself? As long as I'm only spending around £100 a year on the entries, and as long as I can still afford that amount, I don't really care if the chances of me winning an Omaze house could be severalfold lower than the odds of me being attacked by a shark. Let me dream on.

Love,
Cath x

GAMBLING MICRO TACTICS

Stick to in-person gambling

App and online gambling is the most problematic, the Gambling Commission reports. Users aren't driven by fun, excitement or even the money, research found. The reasons cited are usually 'coping' or 'escapism'. Both are worrying hallmarks that a little addiction has become medium or large.

The social interruptions of in-person gambling are a good thing, says Schüll, as other people snap what she's coined as the 'ludic loop' (a circle of elements creating the most addictive types of play). 'The first stage of the ludic loop is isolation, where you're alone and don't have stopping cues from other people,' she says. I definitely relate to this starting point, with my drinking. It was when I began drinking alone that it shifted into medium addiction territory.

Even if you're *technically* at the track, races or bingo hall alone, this method should still work, plus you'll also get that rush of a collective experience.

The best lottery to play in the UK

If you want more thrills and less spills financially, here are the odds, according to an article in *The Sun*; Lotto carries the worst odds (the classic National Lottery), with odds of winning the jackpot being one in 45 million (EuroMillions is even worse, at one in 139 million). Thunderball (£1 to play) has much more attractive odds of one in 8 million, while the Health Lottery (also £1) has even better odds of one in 2.1 million.

The same source said that the biggest chance of winning smaller sums (that are still in the thousands) come from playing the People's Postcode Lottery, but it's also the splashiest; its subscription model means that – at the time of writing – it costs a princely £147 a year to engage.

Use a separate bank account

It used to be 'the house always wins', now it's 'the app always wins' given it's very easy to lose track of how much you're spending when the transactions are buried within grocery shops and parking charges. Even if you try to manage it by keeping it in a separate 'pot', those pots are terrifyingly easy to top up. (I know, because I do it all the damn time with my Deliveroo pot.) Now that it's an absolute doddle to set up a new bank account (a Monzo application takes about 10 seconds), that might be an idea. Your denial about your spend will be ripped away, and you're much more likely to be moderate. Denial is like a duvet: removing it from yourself is much easier than having someone else do it for you.

Play to win, rather than *play to win to play*

As we've covered, it's a red flag if you no longer care about the winning, and almost start to feel irritated by it. As it is when you always leave all of the money in the app, or put it back straight into the machine or on the table. These are all sure signs your addiction is upsizing, so try to stay in that space where a win is taken *out*, meaning extra shopping or fun money, rather than left in to become extra *play* money.

Install your own right angles and friction

'Adding friction back in is precisely the way to go,' Schüll says. She cites time limits on apps, which will bring you to the right-angled crossroads of a pop-up saying 'Ignore limit?' This means you're in with a chance of being plucked from the zone by your prefrontal cortex coming back online, which, as we'll cover later, makes 'which is more important?' value judgements.

One Sec, a science-backed app that makes you take a deep breath before entering self-designated apps – meaning your breath behaves as a speed bump – will also engage the same process. That 'pause, reflect, continue?' is what you want to add in.

OUR PHONES

Sticky eight

Our phones have more power over us than any other inanimate object in our life.

That statement may feel like hyperbole and, admittedly, I do enjoy throwing on some drama as if it's a feather boa and a musical soundtrack. But it's true. Our phones have the power to change our financial lives or break our smitten hearts. To intro us to our first nephew in one send of a squashy-faced pic or tell us a friendship is over in a text of surprise resentment.

Love it when people break up with you over text, platonic or otherwise, don't you? It's just the best. It recently happened to me and I counted nine (nine!) pejorative adjectives in just one little text. It was an achievement, really. I received it at 9pm and I was still awake at 2am.

Of course, it's not the phone itself that wields this power. It's what lies within. And blood-chilling experiences like this, which we've all had – friendship *over* – only increase its sway.

'It's the source of so much pleasure and pain,' says psychotherapist Hilda Burke, author of *The Phone Addiction Workbook*. 'You could pick it up to find out that you've gotten your dream job, or that someone's died.' I flash back to finding out via text message that my beloved grandfather had died.

'Before smartphones, someone might have come to your door with bad family news,' she said. 'Or you would find out you'd got the job by receiving a letter.' But now it's all being funnelled through this one portable conduit.

Death, love, rejection, validation, riches, poverty; it's no wonder we can't put down our phones. In fact, it's a wonder that we're not *more* obsessed.

'If ever nuclear war is announced, we'll probably find out via a notification,' says Burke, her voice darkening. 'And that ping will sound the exact same way as if our friend's been proposed to. It's very interesting that it's the exact same sound.'

Our brains are primed for either 'executive attention' or 'alarm attention', Burke continues. 'And having notifications set to vibrate and ping have the same resonance to our brains as a baby crying, or a fire alarm going off. It doesn't matter how deeply you're working, you will jump to alert.'

We grab our phones, only to find out that Anthropologie has a sale on. 'Truly, with most people's phones, even though there's the *potential* for wonder or devastation, the reality is that there's not much interesting stuff coming in,' says Burke. 'Those alerts aren't actually book deals or proposals.' It's not like we're Dua Lipa.

I ask Burke if having our notifications on ping is a bit like COS coming around and ringing your doorbell every time they release the new season's stock? 'Yes,' she laughs. Or like *The Guardian* ringing your landline every time they publish a new article you might like? I'm on a roll now. 'Exactly, that's exactly it.' (*God*, my references are middle class.)

Unlike our parents, who got large spaces of the day free from being terrorised by their phones or emails, and the uncertainty of 'what lies within' (unless they carried around a PC in a wheelbarrow, plugging it in at random cafes), we don't.

Unless we begin creating these bubbles of freedom for ourselves. Because nobody else is going to do it for us.

The Persuasive Technology Lab

Just as Eton churns out prime ministers (20 so far) in our democracy, which is *definitely* not built on nepotism, the Persuasive Technology Lab at Stanford has famously populated Silicon Valley ever since the iPod was a mere glint in Steve Jobs's eye. Its graduates include the minds behind some of the most irresistible apps on our phones. Think Instagram, Facebook, Gmail, Snapchat and LinkedIn.

Alumni of the lab studied under the forefather of persuasive technology, B J Fogg, who is lionised by tech bros worldwide. There are probably posters of him in frat houses in the Bay Area. The lab is now called the Behavior Design Lab, probably because in today's wokelight, 'persuasive technology' sounds like something regrettable that a creepy pick-up artist might use.

I'm actually a fan of B J Fogg myself (although don't try to talk to me about bitcoin, Brogrammers) so my stereotyping of him is playful. And, right now, I'm here with someone who studied underneath him – behavioural designer, Nir Eyal.

Eyal is calling me from Paris, and his cafe backdrop is so Parisian it looks AI-generated. Some might say he is from the dark side. Indeed, Eyal wrote a book on how companies can create habit-forming products (*Hooked*). I must say, he is the very embodiment of persuasion. Smart, charming and articulate, Eyal keeps asking me to be more specific when I ask him questions, which is fair, given my questions tend to be tangled – if fun – balls of wool, lobbed in the person's direction in the hope they'll throw me a scarf back. He is the kind of person who delivers an effortless keynote in between his cheesecake and coffee, while I'm the one watching in wonder, with cheesecake crumbs all over my dress.

Eyal is one of many of Fogg's alumni (in addition to Fogg himself) who have now moved over to the brighter side, in that he's now trying to empower us *not* to be persuaded against our best interests while on our phones – via his bestselling book *Indistractable.*

Eyal still works with Big Tech but, given he plays both sides, you could see him as a double agent (or a diplomat, if you're less dramatic than I *adjusts feather boa*). He has joined the more radical ranks of the original Google HQ whistleblower, Tristan Harris, and creator of the infinite scroll Aza Raskin, who have founded the Center for Humane Technology, which is exactly what it sounds like. Fogg himself has since founded the Peace Innovation Lab at Stanford too, exploring how tech can promote harmony, rather than radicalise politically.

Interestingly, most tech whistleblowers are female, but they get nowhere near as many column inches as the men. Take Dr Timnit Gebru, who claims she was ousted by Google for penning a controversial paper on the risks of AI. She warned that AI's colossal language training banks could scoop up racist and sexist language that should have died 30 years ago, ladling it back into the world. Google have maintained she resigned.

Then we also have Sarah Wynn-Williams, formerly a director at Facebook, whose book *Careless People* was a hand grenade of explosive allegations, such as her claims that Facebook 'emotionally targets' fragile teens, which she testified about to the US Senate. She's given the chilling example of young girls who, having just deleted selfies, are then shown beauty ads. To the US Senate, Wynn-Williams claimed that it was common for her colleagues at Meta – the parent company of Facebook – to 'forbid their own children from using the company's products out of concern for their safety and wellbeing'. In response, Meta say she has levelled 'false accusations', and they are now taking legal action against her.

Eyal is nowhere near this renegade, treading a careful line. When I describe him as 'pro tech' he corrects me, saying he's 'pro mindful use of tech'. When I ask him about Wynn-Williams' allegations, which he hasn't heard about, he says, 'There's a lot of misinformation that flies around. It's like how, for a while, everyone thought our phones were listening to us, and that we then got served ads based on what we'd been talking about. This has since been disproven.'

I don't know. I keep my mouth shut because I want Eyal to like me (people-pleaser), but I had a very strange experience once. Having talked about Japanese knotweed for the first time ever in my life with friends over dinner (and inputted nothing into my phone), by the time I arrived home, YouTube was already offering up videos on how to get rid of Japanese knotweed. I'm not part of the so-called 'Techlash', but it shook me.

Eyal is careful to point out that these are champagne problems. 'Thank God we're living in an age of information abundance,' he says. 'That's so much better than information scarcity.' I think of propaganda too, which, even though it still exists in the shape of fake news, is at least counterbalanced by responsible outlets.

'Our grandparents weren't worrying about all the time they were spending on frivolity because they were too busy dodging bombs during World War II, or trying to stretch rations.' Now we have the problem of an excess of calories available, largely created by advancements in tech and mass production. 'Technology doesn't solve our problems, but it does give us better ones,' he says.

Compulsive phone-checking

Compulsive phone-checking is inherently misunderstood. When we see someone staring at their phone in a social situation, the adjectives that tickertape across our brains tend to be: indifferent, then self-absorbed, then rude.

I've even faded out a decades-long friendship for relentless phone use. I say 'use' because it went way beyond checking.

'Do you really need to send that email now?' I asked once. 'Can it not wait an hour while we eat?'

'Yes, I do', she said, with a 'come at me' glare.

I'd sat there for 20 minutes and this was her fourth email that was urgent. It had been this way in every meet-up for three years. As the waiter came over to refill our water, he raised his eyebrows at me in an 'everything OK?' way. I shrugged at him in a 'what can you do' reply. As I walked away, I knew that – while I loved this friend, and still do – I wouldn't see her again.

But this story is different from what most of us do. It's the quick pick-ups that get us. The 'just to see' that we can't resist. Over half of us (55 per cent) can't get through a dinner without doing it. I leave my phone in my bag over dinner, then sneak it over into my pocket, like a drug-user might a baggie of MDMA, to take it with me to the toilet.

When it comes to the compulsive checking, it's not self-indulgence driving it. It's actually discomfort. Once we start thinking about our phones and what could be in them, sweat pricks our palms and the co-mingle of fear and hope rises.

Many years ago, Dr Korb told me that we check our phones because of the stress of *not* checking our phones. Eyal agrees with this appraisal, as does Burke, as does *everyone* I've ever spoken with who knows anything about psychology.

Given the discomfort's foundation is fear of the unknown, it makes sense to start with feeling psychologically safer offline. Reassuring yourself that even if you don't check your messages for six hours, your sky will not fall in. You won't open your phone to find terrible things have happened that you would have prevented by being online. The only way your body will learn to input that 'you're safe' data, is if you *do it.*

Three quarters of us sleep in the same room as our phones, and a third of us check them in the middle the night. I don't even have to say it, do I? If this is you, you already know. And no judgement. This used to be me too, especially back when I was dating, and my WhatsApp was a portal to either rejection or advancement.

What's more, we really need to protect our kids from this compulsive checking. A quarter of teens check their phones more than ten times a night.

The first canary

Tristan Harris was the OG whistleblower on tech. It was 2013, way before 'screen time' even existed as a function. But Harris foretold what was to come. He could see that our phones were beginning to control us, rather than us using them. He was a 'design ethicist' for Google back then and had the courage to send a presentation around Google HQ entitled:

A Call to Minimize Distraction and Respect Users' Attention.

Bizarrely, even though his job title makes it sound like he was leading the charge with ethical concerns, his real job was actually to monetise. 'I was hired to come in and figure out what the business model was gonna be for the company. I was the director of monetisation.' Talk about a misnomer.

He summed up the contents of the presentation for *The Social Dilemma*, a culture-altering documentary that wouldn't air for another seven years, a good yardstick for how early Harris was to sing.

'[The presentation] basically said . . . never before in history have 50 designers – 20–35-year-old white guys in California – made decisions that would have an impact on two billion people. Two billion people will have thoughts that they didn't intend to have because a designer at Google said, "This is how notifications work on that screen that you wake up to in the morning".'

The ripple effect from his bombshell reached the very top. 'Later, I found out Larry Page had been notified about this presentation in three separate meetings that day.'

His reasons for lobbing this incendiary while still inside the room were intensely personal. He felt 'burnt out' and 'addicted' to the very email system he had helped design: Gmail. 'I found it fascinating there was no one at Gmail working on making it less addictive.'

And so, email addiction feels like a great place to start.

Email is the mother of all habit-formers

Email is rarely placed in the same bucket as 'slot machine apps', such as socials or WhatsApp. Yet Eyal believes it's the stickiest one.

'Email is the mother of all habit-forming products,' he says. 'It taps into the hunt, the tribe and the self.' These are the three types of variable reward expounded upon in his book, *Hooked*.

The hunt is about the search for material or information rewards. The tribe is about social rewards. The self is driven by the need for mastery, competence and control.

He says that gaming mechanics are baked into email design, and that slaying new messages in your inbox stimulates neurons similar to those stimulated by playing *StarCraft*.

It's a fascinating take – that dominating your emails could be like crushing candy, or blasting blocks. I wonder if, by constantly striving for inbox zero, or at least inbox all-attended-to (personally, I have 6,438 emails still in my inbox), we're also looking for threat zero. Level: completed. All ghosts in this *Pac-Man* maze: slain.

With message-checking, I have this cycle that I run through dozens of times a day. Maybe you'll relate. It's so well-trodden a neural pathway that it now resembles a compulsory roundabout on my day's commute, rather than a diversion. I open my phone and obediently fling myself around it: WhatsApp – Gmail – Instagram. Sometimes I even catch myself circling it again, a few seconds later, before clicking it locked.

I've turned the notifications for all of these apps off, because I don't want to be controlled, and yet they still control me, beckoning me in with the pull of the unknown. Will they yield treasure or trolls, I just don't know. The irony is I may well check them less if my notifications are *on*.

These apps cost me nothing, financially. But this is the first warning sign, says Harris. 'The classic saying is: "If you're not paying for the product, then you are the product".' Advertisers are the customer and we're the thing being sold.

Our hidden desires are for sale, too. A friend of mine was working for a Big Tech company around the same time Harris was disrupting Google HQ. When I asked her what she was doing there, she said, 'We're reading people's emails to find out if they want a red coat, and then sending them advertisements for a red coat.'

'Really?!' I said in disbelief.

'Really,' she confirmed.

I shrugged this off as sci-fi melodrama back then, but now, of course, we know that this is exactly what happened. Gmail only stopped doing it in 2017.

The device always wins

We talked about how much our brains love uncertain rewards back on page 32. Do me a favour and take a look at the diagram of the Skinner Box again. What does this remind you of: a little box with lights and a microphone, which dispenses random rewards when we tap, click or press? I'll wait.

We're not pigeons, rats or mice, but we become hypnotised all the same.

Because the repetitive action coupled with the variable reward is *intensely* addictive. Slot machines were human-sized spin-offs of the Skinner Box, with Skinner himself saying so, and now phones have been modelled on slot machines. So much so that Harris calls phones the 'slot machines in your pocket'.

'When we swipe down our finger to scroll the Instagram feed, we're playing a slot machine to see what photo comes next,' writes Harris. 'When we "pull to refresh" our email, we're playing a slot machine to see what email we got. When we swipe faces on dating apps, we're playing a slot machine to see if we got a match.'

Whether it's a lever, a button or a 'pull' arrow, the net result is the same. Say it in a perfume-ad voice: *fixation*. Pressing 'post' on a picture is like rolling a dice, to see if you win favour from your followers.

'Chance has been captured and formatted,' Professor Schüll, author of *Addiction by Design*, told me. 'Other people's minds and desires become part of this large pool of chance. Do they like me back?'

'There's an affinity between a pigeon pecking with her beak at a little red light, waiting to see "When is that pellet going to come out?", and a person pressing buttons or screens on slot machines or phones.'

I tell Schüll that yesterday I sat and literally watched someone 'typing…' for one whole minute, before shaking myself out of the trance and placing my phone down. We spoke about the 'machine zone' back on page 95, which gamblers become sucked into, and the phone zone is remarkably similar. 'It's hard not to have a glimpse of the "machine zone" if you have a phone,' Schüll says.

'Those three little dots are like watching the reel spin,' she says. 'It's the uncertainty of what they'll say which makes it so compelling. People become puzzles.'

Her research on the 'machine zone' revealed that hooked gamblers dislike winning a jackpot because it pulls them out of the lullaby-like rhythm. Now, think about how rude a jolt it feels when you're scrolling and somebody rings you. Your phone, by ringing, is doing what it's designed to do, yet it feels like an invasion on a private moment.

Our phones are no longer phones; they're doorways to another zone.

The snarls of social obligation

I was naive enough to think that most of us turn notifications off nowadays, but not so, with 67.5 per cent of people keeping them on. You crazy cats.

Those keeping notifications on are probably doing so in an attempt to wrangle the coyote of chance. On Facebook and Instagram, we don't have the ability to 'screen all comments', and this is by design – comments are either all on or all off, other than from individuals we have restricted. This means that leaving a recent post unattended is akin to inviting people to graffiti the outside of your house by leaving a load of pens in a bucket and a sign saying 'Comment here'. *Of course* we feel an urge to repeatedly check what is being written, for all to see. It'd be weird if we didn't.

Then deliberate features such as 'seen', 'online', 'delivered' and 'read' corner us into replying before we're ready. *Shit, they've seen me.* We'll talk a lot later (in the People-Pleasing chapter on page 216) on how urgent we feel it is for us to stay within the tribe. These functions that make us visible are hitting that ancient button.

If we don't send a quick reply, we feel rude . . . then *very* rude. For me, it's like an imaginary countdown starts in my head the moment I receive a message, even unsolicited ones, and I have to beat the clock before I'm regarded as a subhuman ghoster, or uppity ingrate.

We treat every message as if it's time-sensitive, and yet it's mostly all in our heads, says Eyal. 'I've had clients describe the "guilt" they feel about not responding quickly as British guilt, Jewish guilt, Catholic guilt, but the fact is it's human nature.' *Person* guilt. 'It's important to remember that feelings aren't facts,' he adds. Just because we feel rude, doesn't mean we are.

We set unachievable standards for ourselves that we don't impose on others. I have never in my life sent someone an email and then stared at the screen, brow furrowed, until they reply. (If you have, we can't be friends.)

Similarly, we apparently 'invite' people to do things all the time, when all we've done is allow the app access to our contacts for ease. *It* invites people to connect on LinkedIn, converse on WhatsApp, run together on Strava . . . not us. Yet, when we receive the invite, we imagine the person deliberately choosing us. These apps are smart. They know how to turn social obligation into a tug rope. Thankfully we're smarter.

The IQ-lowering effect of interruption

Not when our phones are around, though. They lower our IQs by merely being present.

So said the now infamous 'brain drain' experiments done by the University of Texas (UT), which found that, even if a phone was turned on to silent and in a bag, it impacted a student's exam results. This negative impact supersized when the phone was within the exam-taker's field of vision.

Exiling the device to another room was the answer. 'The researchers found that participants with their phones in another room significantly outperformed those with their phones on the desk,' the UT press release said.

But that was way back in 2017, so maybe we've gotten better since then at focusing around our phones? 'Fraid not. A more recent meta-analysis of 22 studies confirmed the brain drain when phones are in the immediate vicinity, 'even if they are not actively used'.

Studies on kids taking tests found that they score 15 per cent lower on exams when phones are in the room, even if it's not theirs. This is the equivalent of nearly a year of lost learning (a year is 20 percentage points).

One of the reasons for this is how long it takes us to recover from an interruption. The University of California found that after an interruption (a phone call, or a message), we take 23 minutes to recover our focus. Surprisingly, a spin-off study found that the interrupted group still completed an everyday cognitive task (writing emails) within a similar time frame, and with comparable accuracy, but the mental load was markedly different. The interrupted group 'reported significantly higher stress, frustration, workload, effort and pressure'.

It follows that, if we want to be less stressed, particularly when we're doing deep work, our phone should be in another room, while we should also consider resisting email-checking whenever we can.

If that last sentence made you intensely uncomfortable, know that a truly urgent email is rare. 'I had this client; a lawyer,' says Eyal. 'He couldn't focus because he was constantly being pinged and dinged with urgent stuff, and he said that the urgent stuff was a crucial part of his job.'

Eyal suggested that the lawyer appoint his secretary as 'guardian' of his email, then timebox certain hours of each day for reading and answering them. His secretary was to interrupt if something urgent came in outside of those times. 'For the entire week of this system, the secretary didn't need to interrupt him, even once.'

It's an urgency myth that we collude in. Really, we know that 99.9 per cent of emails – and messages in general – just aren't.

The foraging effect

In *Dopamine Nation*, Dr Anna Lembke theorised that smartphone scrolling and tapping is so addictive because it reminds us of the repetitious grind of farming and foraging. '[They're] cleverly exploiting ancient habits of repetitive motion,' she wrote, 'possibly acquired through centuries of grinding wheat and picking berries.'

This is great news! I'm not sinking my precious evening into Rightmove, OK? I'm basically grinding some wheat. Speaking of which, why am I still obsessed with Rightmove? I have absolutely no intention of moving. My last move was a heinous two-year process involving many collapsed chains, thousands of pounds wasted, two rentals and four house moves in a year. In 2023 I wrote this on Instagram:

'Today we moved into the house we thought would never happen. I could kiss the floor, I might lick a wall, and if you catch me looking at Rightmove within the next decade, please do bat the phone out of my hand.'

Maybe your property drug dispenser is Zillow or Zoopla but if you relate, this tic of looking at houses you have no intention of buying can be traced back to two things. One, it now being frictionless. It used to be bloody hard to look for a house. You had to prowl estate agent offices, *talk to* estate agents, leave clutching a brochure, get into your car and drive to another estate agent . . . repeat. Now the drug supply from dozens of local estate agents is in our pockets.

Two, property leverages our bias for the 'hedonic treadmill'. I wrote a whole book about this (*The Unexpected Joy of the Ordinary*), so I won't dwell on it here, but to summarise: we want what we haven't got, then as soon as we get it, we want the next thing we haven't got. The glow of 'satisfaction with' is swiftly supplanted by 'longing for', whether it's a new house, relationship, job, holiday, gadget, bike or capsule wardrobe.

Hence it being a 'treadmill'. We never reach the end. Wanting to upgrade our caves for a better cave served us very well in hunter-gatherer times, but now it just means we're all like, '*All I want* is a semi-detached!' when we fought tooth and claw for the 'All I want' terrace we're currently in.

We also now have the capability to look *back* at what we had before, particularly when it comes to exes. When you meditate hard on it, it's a really bizarre situation that we're in, needing to remain 'friends' with our ex who was a bit of a tosser, for fear of looking bitter. Even if we do unfollow or defriend, many of us still keep tabs on them. And we can see their new partners, perhaps even what they look like in swimwear. It's a major headfuck, and none of us are psychologically equipped to deal.

Myself, I block all of my exes, whether it ended amicably or not, to avoid said headfuck, and I highly recommend it. I tell them when we split: 'No offence, but I will block you. I don't think it's healthy to look backwards. After all, we're not going that way.'

The reel world

Reels are a whole 'nother level. You can tell yourself it's just like watching telly, but it's not. 'TV-bingeing is almost a *quaint* problem when compared to scrolling through shorts on TikTok or Instagram,' says Dr Korb.

'Even with junk TV, you could still make the argument that you learned something, or did some emotional processing. TV does have redeeming qualities. Whereas scrolling through cute, enraging or funny 60-second skits is like sending nudes on dating apps. Ultimately unsatisfying and meaningless.' He's not a fan, as you can tell.

They may be short, but the impact is big. 'The shorts spark a little flash of dopamine, but it doesn't lead anywhere,' he says, 'given there's not even a deeper story to pay attention to. So, to replace that empty feeling, you just end up needing more dopamine.'

What Dr Korb is saying reminds me of what cocaine felt like: a super-short high followed by an almost instant craving. I only did cocaine a dozen-ish times in my 20s and early 30s but, within seconds, I felt the ache for more, the drug having gouged a hole inside me that could only be filled by more cocaine.

On that note, the craving for cocaine hits so fast because of the dopamine spike, after which our dopamine level is dragged far below baseline. I learned all of this from *Dopamine Nation,* which also revealed that, for a rat in the box, cocaine 'increases that basal output of dopamine' by 225 per cent. Sex is 100 per cent. The plunge after a line is profound, which is why we immediately want more.

This is why those cocaine-fuelled nights so often ended with a group of us sitting around a mirrored tray with rolled-up twenties until 5am, calling dealers for more, talking too loudly about ourselves. Cocaine scared me more than alcohol did, ironically.

Back to TikTok. This will seem counter-intuitive but, if you're addicted to TikTok, you might fare better if you tell yourself that you're not addicted to TikTok. A study of 5,000 people unearthed this quirk; success in staying off socials was predicted if users described themselves as 'not addicted', even if they logged in just as much (or more) than their 'addicted' counterparts.

Weird, but true. The language we choose can become a self-fulfilling prophecy.

How they blow up your phone-free Sunday

It's by design that you now need your phone to do almost anything. Trying to have a phone-free work afternoon by leaving your phone turned off and downstairs?

Good luck with that, poppet. Because even if you have chosen email for your two-step verification rather than phone, here's some new twattery; needing access to the 'authenticator app'. *Deep sigh* – goes and gets phone.

You now need your phone as well as your laptop for everything from tax management, to making any sort of payment, to accessing a little-used email address. It makes digital detoxing nearly impossible. Trying to go for a phone-free stroll in the countryside? Cute! You'll find you can't pay for parking, and that you need to scan a QR code to order a coffee from the cafe. Oh, and you can't have any music either because iPods are obsolete.

All of this means our phones are always in our hands, an extension of our body, an irrefutable necessity in order to navigate modern life. I genuinely don't know how people with dumbphones manage.

The tech companies are always going to pivot in this way, says Eyal. 'It's a cat and mouse game, and it always will be,' he says, with us the prey, and them the hunter. 'But the deeper truth is this: people are becoming more affluent and, as they do, they become more important to market to.'

The rebalance of the radical

Radicals of the Techlash would say that it's no coincidence that persuasive technology labs use agricultural terms such as data farming and attention harvesting. We're the livestock now, our data the corn for sale.

'Policymakers don't feel as motivated to regulate the phone stuff,' says Professor Schüll. 'Even though it's *clearly* affecting us. But it's not a substance. It doesn't make you pass out. Gambling has always been a focus because of the money. I'm always saying with phones, "but look at the *time*". People are always talking about the "attention economy" and, in my mind, time and attention are the same thing.'

Tristan Harris is stark in his appraisal of the ruthless time grab. He told the BBC that just as a whale is worth more dead than it is alive, or a tree worth more as planks, we are 'worth more as dead slabs of human timber'.

Obviously app-creators don't want to kill us, but they do want to colonise our time. Your typical British adult now spends 3 hours, 21 minutes on their phones every day. (That's a *good* day for me.) Time is arguably our most precious resource – and also now our biggest expenditure.

All of this is true. But what is also true is that phones do great things. Not all screen time is created equal. I *love* redesigning a photo with a few taps on Snapseed, or stopping mid-shop to tap out a sentence my mind has just written into Notes. I prop my phone against the tiles to follow recipes, and it's how I discovered the best poke bowl dressing ever. I listen to invigorating audiobooks to liven up long drives. I live for jumping around on a beach to 'Messy' by Lola Young, shouting the lyrics into the wind while my bemused dog looks on, asking me to throw the ball already.

All of these beautiful things are c/o my phone. Let's not demonise what can also be gorgeous.

To conclude, I want to extrapolate on something Aza Raskin said about it being his 'dubious honour' to be credited with inventing the infinite scroll. He lamented the fact that it then 'got used not to help you, but to *hold* you'.

Help, rather than *hold*. It struck me as the skeleton key.

As with all addictions, phone overuse is person + thing. The only power reclaimable sits within 'person'. Knowing about the mind control helps us rail against it, for sure, but unless we *do* something about it, we're in a sinkhole. They're never going to stop making apps hookier, or pivoting to find new ways to keep our phones in our hands.

We need to start using our phones to help us, rather than hold us.

Dear little phone addict,

I want to talk about something close to my heart, as a reformed doomscroller.

The reason doomscrolling is so hard to stop is that there's always something urgent and potentially world-ending on the roster. It's an infinite apocalyptic scroll.

There's a worldwide pandemic allegedly started by a bat in a Chinese market, or World War III could be about to start because of land-grab wars between [insert superpower] and [insert oppressed nation], or nuclear submarines in a faraway land are doing something sinister, or somebody whose approach to foreign policy is akin to a drunk and obstreperous uncle lumbering about at a wedding has been elected (or re-elected).

It's not my intention to belittle the grave seriousness of all of the above. All of the above was – and is – gravely serious, and has involved – or could involve – the loss of many lives.

My point is, there's always something. There always *will* be something. There always has been something. Our tendency to think that right now is an outlier in history, that what came before was less urgent and less significant, is called Travis Syndrome.

And if there's nothing newly urgent, the news feed falls back on the consistently urgent matter of climate change (which I'm not applying Travis Syndrome to, FYI), which will almost certainly spell the end of humankind.

The impending apocalypse is good for their business, while our fear is currency for more clicks. We feel like knowing it all makes us good and responsible citizens, when it actually does sod all to actually implement change. The knowing feels like doing, but it's not.

The other bait they use is microcosmic and pertains directly to us, uncannily so, because they've been inside our browsing histories, or have scanned our messages that aren't end-to-end encrypted.

It's of the ilk of 'this could change your world'. In my feed, I get neuroscientific advancements, articles on the perimenopause, first-persons on neurodivergence, fitness discoveries, life-extending hacks, property porn, animal psychology. My news feed knows me better than some of my family do.

We also get fed the flipside based on our datasets, in the shape of 'this could be the end of your world': spiking mortgage rates, surging food prices, warnings about needing a £500K pension pot, fears for the mental health of children, rising pet thefts.

Even 'incognito' or 'private browsing' modes aren't entirely private, given they leave trails of data outside of our devices. Google was sued in 2020 in a class action for tracking millions of users in these so-called private modes. It has since agreed to settle (plaintiffs were seeking $500 each, totalling $5 billion), has updated its privacy policy to make it clearer and confirmed it would delete billions of people's 'private' browsing records.

Know that you're being played. You are a harp, and they are plucking on your strings. Also know that we're not supposed to be informed on the minute details of every terrible event in the world.

Over and over, regular news checks have been shown to be calamitous for our mental health. Out of therapists surveyed, 99.6 per cent believe news consumption negatively impacts mental health.

Looking away isn't the answer either. Obviously we need to know about it, in order to do something about it. I subscribe to Apple News still to keep roughly abreast, checking in a few times a week, but the rest of what I used to spend on subscriptions to several news outlets is now directed to overseas aid efforts, homeless charities and animal/child welfare.

My way is not *the* way, I would never claim that, and if your knowledge is powering your activism I will give you a standing ovation. But otherwise, ask yourself what your being all-knowing is really changing. Probably only your own mental health.

Love,
Cath x

PHONE MICRO TACTICS

Experiment with vibrational signatures
If you constantly have your phone on vibrate, this tip comes from Tristan Harris.

He talks about the 'ambiguous vibration sound' Burke alluded to earlier. This is a problem. Aza Raskin adds that vibrational ambiguity acts like 'cognitive lingerie', because it 'stimulates emotional arousal'.

They suggest personalising vibration signatures for more important items, like a text from your partner or friends, differentiating it from SMS spam.

Most smartphones carry this option, including iPhone, Samsung Galaxy and Google handsets. Look for 'vibration' within settings.

Make your own iPod with an old phone
I love to have music on while I work, mainly to make my dog feel like he's in a spa, rather than have him barking at everybody inside our postcode. But this meant my phone was in the same room, or just outside. So, when I upgraded from an iPhone 8 to an 11 (Luddite to the end), I kept my practically worthless 8 logged in to Spotify, with the music downloaded on it. It doesn't do anything else, given I've migrated it all over to my new phone and it has no data, so it's the next best thing to an iPod.

Shun the 'everything is content' state of mind
This sounds fiendishly simple, but some of the best strategies are. If you find yourself in the snafu of an 'everything is content' mindset, thinking that a day out didn't happen unless you post it – just like a falling tree in the forest didn't make a sound – here's what you do: nothing. Don't post. Sit on your hands. Refrain.

A 2015 study of 5,000 people who were asked to stay off socials for 99 days found that those who relapsed were in a psychological trap. A trap of using socials to manage what other people think about them. And this 'thought management' happens via posting. If you don't play the game of roulette by uploading, then you'll quickly lose interest in being in the casino itself.

If you need more than your own resolve, the app One Sec, which we talked about on page 107, could be worth adding to your arsenal.

Educate yourself on what's being tracked

Those who know that their every key stroke and direct message is being tracked on socials also find it easier to use it less, said the same 2015 study.

Remember, if the product's free, then *we're* the product. Our use of it is being sold on. And the way datasets about us are built is via our navigation around – and communications within – these apps.

Start wait training

The ability to sit with the discomfort of not phone-checking can be built like a muscle, says Burke. She coined the brilliant term 'wait training' to capture that it'll feel uncomfortable at first, but lean in; it's only making you stronger.

'Start off with a walk for an hour,' she says. Keep your phone with you, in case of emergencies, but just turn your data off. Then build it up.

'It's about turning your FOMO into JOMO,' she says. Turn your OOO on, or update your WhatsApp status, if it makes it easier. 'With time and repetition, you'll start to get the dopamine from *not* being on your phone. What felt restrictive becomes the reward.'

Remember, dopamine loves completing tasks, even if the task is to *not* do something, like pick up our phones. Our reward system can be a messy hedonist turned irritatingly perky personal trainer if we allow it to reform.

Commit to data-free Sundays

Burke does data-free Sundays. 'I can still use my calendar, look at the clock, take a picture. That's OK as I don't get addicted to any of that. It was data that turned phones into a whole different beast.'

She's right. When we all had cute flips or clamshells, we weren't picking them up 96 times a day (the national average).

Burke encountered some pushback about not receiving texts. 'I just had to repeatedly say, if it's important, you can always call me. If you're running late, just call me.' It led to more – and better – conversations, she says. And a lovely release at the end of the week.

Try the symbolic storehold

Think about the thing you'd like to do more of when you have reduced your phone usage. Now write it below.

I want to spend less time on my phone and more time

………………………………………………………………………

Now, find an item that serves as a symbol for this thing, placing your phone either beneath or inside it. It could be a tub of board wax because you want to go surfing more, or one of those empty boxes shaped like books because you want to write a novel. Needing to retrieve it from this symbolic storehold every time will remind you of the Higher Want you have neglected.

Whenever I decided that I wanted post-8pm to be purely family time, I started placing my phone under a rainbow-coloured seal of my daughter's. And, I kid you not, this simple hack mostly cut my phone use in half, from four hours a day to my desired two.

Practise forced timeboxing

The infinite scroll and autoplayed 'up next' are the digital equivalents of an all-you-can-eat buffet. We consume much more than we intend, then feel like crap.

A Cornell University study on bottomless bowls of tomato soup, which were imperceptibly refilled using hidden tubes, found that people ate 73 per cent more.

As we touched on, one of Eyal's cornerstone tactics is 'timeboxing', where you confine something moreish to a set square of time, such as 'I will only stare at YouTube from 7–8pm tonight.'

If your mastery is yet to catch up with your intention (likely), then a gadget like Brick (currently £45) could be handy. It's a small, square gadget that you tap to disable specified apps; then need to physically re-tap to reactivate them. Leave the Brick at home for a guaranteed social media free afternoon with friends.

CANNABIS

Sticky eight

We're talking about cannabis. The professor pushes his glasses up his nose and his eyes widen.

'One year, I was present in a laboratory when they emptied the amnesty bins from Glastonbury,' says Professor Philip Murphy. He's a psychobiologist on the brink of retirement from Edge Hill University, and has devoted his life's work to the study of cannabis, among other drugs. He's the very image of a distinguished academic, and what AI might pluck out if you said, 'Hey Siri, show me a photo of a male professor.'

And then, the professor tells me something shocking.

We'll come back to that. First, let's get into these bins, literally. I've seen them at festivals. They usually have shouty block lettering saying 'DRUG AMNESTY BIN. No questions asked' and *everyone* walks past them. I would imagine that most of the drugs going into these well-intentioned bins are either a) confiscated during searches, or b) leftovers that carousers don't want to take home to their Middle England parents' house. *No narcotics in the conservatory, dear.*

The contents of these bins are a treasure trove of information about illegal street drugs and they're therefore opened – then analysed – by scientists in toxicology labs.

I know, I know, I don't really think of cannabis as an 'illegal street drug' any more either. Nonetheless, recreational use is still forbidden in the UK.

Socially acceptable *and* illegal

Recreational cannabis is widely accepted among my social circles, in a way that cocaine or MDMA is just not. MDMA is widely used but in a more covert manner with known allies in the loos. Puffing on a vape full of cannabis at a party, however, would be more socially accepted than sparking up a Marlboro

Light. I've been to many birthdays where I've been given a disclaimer about the contents of the brownies.

Medicinal use of cannabis was legalised in the UK in 2018. Helping heat up the pressure cooker for this change was the UN's revelation in 2016 that the UK was the largest exporter of legal cannabis for medicinal purposes, mostly shipped to the US, while simultaneously denying Brits the use of cannabis for medicinal purposes.

Awk-ward.

This understandably prompted cries of hypocrisy, until the UK legalised. Nowadays, upwards of 20,000 Brits have prescriptions for cannabis for epilepsy, chemotherapy side effects, Parkinson's, MS and more.

If you look at a 'legality of cannabis' global map, there are great swathes where recreational use of cannabis and/or medical use of it has been decriminalised – especially in the Western hemisphere. This includes 40 of the 50 American states, all of Canada, and in Europe – Malta, Portugal and Luxembourg. But most of the world map is still red, signalling 'illegal' and legally enforced.

More 'tolerant' nuances that live next door to decriminalisation are seen in the Czech Republic, Switzerland, Belgium, Austria and (most of) Spain. Nuances abound but, usually in these countries, possession of a small amount of cannabis is seen as a misdemeanour or similar, sometimes carrying a small fine.

Most people don't know that the Netherlands is merely 'tolerant' of recreational cannabis use, despite Amsterdam being the global capital of cannabis tourism. It's technically still illegal, with only certain licensed 'coffee shops' permitted to sell it. You can't smoke on the streets; you could get a hefty fine.

In a landmark move, Germany has become the first major European player to fully legalise. Adults can own up to three cannabis plants per household. There are even 'cannabis clubs' with tiered subscription fees dependent on your desired monthly usage, much like ClassPass, but instead of getting ripped, you get baked.

Cannabis as the innocuous fun guy

In films, cannabis is personified as harmless, merely making users giggle and/or lasciviously enjoy nachos.

Collectively and culturally, cannabis is officially No Big Deal, and we could all play cliché bingo while movie-watching for:

- 'I have a prescription for that!' while the police officer rolls their eyes and ignores the bong they just saw.
- The 'cool parent' sharing a joint with their teenage kid rather than confiscating it.
- The uptight character who smokes a spliff and is then looser, cooler, funnier.

But, cannabis isn't actually innocuous. Maybe in the 1970s it was, when my father started growing – and smoking – cannabis plants in our attic. One of my earliest memories is seeing him tend to his plants up there, underneath fluorescent lights.

These days, evidence from amnesty bins and seizures have revealed that the average strength of THC (the psychoactive ingredient that produces the 'high') in cannabis has increased a shocking amount: up to tenfold.

'In the sixties, average THC levels were two per cent,' says Professor Murphy. 'But nowadays, with selective breeding, the average THC is more like 15 to 20 per cent.'

Skunk, kush and hash are the highest-offending varieties, often being over 20 per cent THC, with brick weed usually bringing up the rear, usually well below 10 per cent. 'Then you have the synthetic cannabinoids, which are much stronger again,' he says. 'This means that, in the past few decades alone, cannabis has become a much more potent and dependence-producing drug.'

Some dabs or oils can even go as high as 90 per cent, says Yale Medicine – a psychosis-inducing level of high. 'Dabbing' is not just a dodgy dance move; it's a scary drug trend.

Also recent and scary, the CBD content is simultaneously dropping, said a King's College London report. And given CBD generally has an anti-psychotic effect, this is worrisome. In 2008, the ballpark THC to CBD ratio was 1:1. Now it's more like 3:1.

The theory that THC and CBD should come as a pair, both medically and recreationally, is called 'the entourage effect'. In the 2000s, this synergy was shown to reduce unwanted effects of THC reported by those taking medicinal marijuana, like hunger ('gimme those Doritos'), sedation ('I think the sofa's trying to eat me', I once said while stoned) or anxiety (your classic 'whitey' – British slang for feeling ill or paranoid after smoking weed).

We still don't know exactly what ratio works best, and many academics say the blanket assumption of the 'entourage effect' hides holes where research should be. One study on edibles found that, rather than CBD softening the negative effects of THC, it actually dramatised them.

Critics of the entourage effect claim that marketeers of medicinal cannabis (a ~~booming~~ blooming market) are using this as a marketing buzz term, when we actually need more research on the nuances, and quickly.

Plus, unless you live someplace where you can buy legal product, all of this chat about ratios doesn't help you a fat lot. Unless you're skilled in the arts of the dark web, you generally buy what your dealer has. You have no idea what strength it is and that's that. Indica strains traditionally have more CBD, and sativa usually features more THC but, nowadays, most street cannabis is a hybrid.

Legalisation of cannabis (ideally) demystifies all of that, meaning you finally know what you're buying, which is why everyone is closely watching Germany, to see how its full decriminalisation unfolds.

Even my dad, a lifelong stoner, quit weed in the last five years of his life, given the strength of product. 'The modern stuff is too strong,' he complained. 'I just want to get lightly stoned, I don't want to drop into a THC hole.'

Cannabis is highly addictive

The urban myth goes that you can't get addicted to cannabis. So, isn't it odd that almost all of us know people who are/were addicted to cannabis? Curious, that.

'Many of the guys I grew up with are chronically consuming marijuana,' Dr Clayton Hickey told me. 'We think it doesn't have addictive properties because we're not putting our thumb on the button in quite the same way as with drugs such as cocaine or heroin. But it's still heavily addictive.'

Yale Medicine says that one in ten who use cannabis will go on to become addicted, which is about the same as guesstimates with alcohol (although with alcohol the true figure is now believed to be much higher, so maybe it is with cannabis too).

Professor Murphy says that, in his decades of research, he's come across many who admit to being dependent on cannabis. He's worked with hundreds of participants on studies, asking for a seven-day wash-out period before the study.

'We've had no problems asking people to quit alcohol for seven days, ordinarily,' he says, 'but with cannabis, we've usually had to content ourselves with two days.' Habitual users can't do longer, he says, 'because cannabis *is* dependence-producing.'

End of.

Myself, I've dated at least three people who were addicted to cannabis. Wake and bakers. Perhaps there's something about me that makes people want to get stoned. And given how many people I dated in the '90s and '00s, I will take that as an anecdotal dataset of around 10 per cent.

Back in *real* research land, a colossal study of 500,000 people found that the biggest rise in cannabis use in the US is not among teens. The US Centers for Disease Control and Prevention (CDC) reported that teen use of weed has actually *decreased* by six per cent since 2013. The biggest upswing in recent years has been seen among Americans with a college degree, while those with a family income of $75,000 or more have also seen a steeper-than-average increase in use.

Those with ADHD are more attracted to it, says neuroscientist Dr Judith Grisel, a former user herself. 'There's a strong relationship between ADHD and cannabis, in the same way that there's a relationship between anxious people and alcohol, or pain-prone people and opioids.'

She cites the hyper-focus linked to ADHD. 'You can focus very well indeed – if you care – but those with ADHD find it hard to care about stuff that's mundane or tedious,' she says. 'With cannabis, what was mundane or tedious now feels perfectly wonderful, rich and interesting.'

Doing the dishes, playing with a child, baking cookies or even just the carpet texture become ultra-enhanced, she says. 'Everything's suddenly rich and salient and interesting.' But habitual or chronic use then dampens that.

Let's take on another myth: 'cannabis is a gateway drug'. Most of us grew up being told this. Yet cannabis use hasn't been proven to lead to anything else other than: maybe more cannabis. And/or an oversized portion of pasta + *Tomb Raider*.

But, seriously, this has never been proven. After initially labelling cannabis as a gateway drug in 2010, then US President Joe Biden even walked back his stance in 2019, saying: 'I don't think it is a gateway drug. There's no evidence I've seen to suggest that.'

What does cannabis do to our brains?

Cannabis helps us forget, essentially, which is part of the reason people like it.

'Memory returns to normal with abstinence,' writes Dr Grinspoon, the author of a book about cannabis called *Seeing Through the Smoke*.

Professor Murphy disagrees. 'I don't think we've got a firm handle on that yet, ie, whether stopping means memory impairments are restored.'

Probably the scariest study I saw looked at 1,000 New Zealand teens, testing their IQs at 18 and again at 38, cross-referencing those results with cannabis use. Occasional and habitual users (habitual defined as 4x per week) held true IQ-wise, but the chronically addicted lost eight IQ points in those 20 years. Ordinarily, your IQ remains robust over your lifetime.

Much like opioids, we like cannabis so much because it hacks into – and supercharges – an already existing painkilling and bliss-giving system in the brain.

'All of us have tiny cannabis-like molecules floating around in our brains,' writes Dr Grinspoon, for *Harvard Health*. 'The cannabis plant, which humans have been using for about 5,000 years, essentially works its effect by hijacking this ancient cellular machinery.'

The endocannabinoid system (ECS) plays a crucial role in things like learning, memory, hunger and sleep, says Dr Grinspoon. 'One of the main side effects of high dosages of recreational cannabis use is the temporary disruption of short-term memory.'

Endogenous cannabinoids are the naturally produced molecules produced by the ECS; the first of these discovered – anandamide – was named after the Sanskrit term for 'bliss'. Exogenous cannabinoids are artificial inputs. 'When you take an exogenous cannabinoid like THC, you're disrupting the natural order of that system,' says Professor Murphy.

I ask Professor Murphy if we have a natural pharmacy in our brains that THC mimics. 'Oh yes,' he says. And by using drugs that artificially plunder that, are we messing with that natural pharmacy? 'We do mess with it,' he says.

'I tell students that our ECS did not evolve for us to get stoned,' says Professor Murphy. 'It evolved to serve important psychological and bodily functions.' And the use of cannabis carves out the desire for more. If we'd never used it, we would never crave it. Our body would be entirely satisfied with the natural pharmacy our brain automatically provides.

Many experts use the metaphor of an orchestra for the ECS, with the naturally occurring endogenous cannabinoids as the musicians. Extending that metaphor, whenever you introduce an exogenous cannabinoid into that delicate balance, it's a little like driving a car into the orchestra section with a banging sound system.

And with genetically engineered sativa plants producing THC that's tenfold higher than it should be? That in-car sound system just became a nightclub sound system, pulled along in a trailer. BOOM.

The higher the THC, the more withdrawal

This then has a knock-on effect on withdrawal. 'The higher the THC, the higher the likelihood of withdrawal,' says Professor Murphy. 'And the severity of the withdrawal.' This is profoundly important, given if we didn't ever feel withdrawal, we probably wouldn't *ever* overconsume.

All of this is making me think that the Germans truly have the right idea. At least their high-earners/college graduates/both (the *true* growing users of cannabis, it seems) are growing their own un-genetically engineered, bona-fide cannabis sativa plants. Knowing what they'll get, rather than a mystery pouch of who-knows-what from 'dodgy Steve'. Knowing that they're vaping a mellow two per cent THC rather than a scary 20 per cent. Knowing that the CBD ratio will be what nature intended, rather than the CBD manipulated out.

'Dealers will still sell the high THC mind-bending, psychosis-inducing shit,' my partner pointed out to me. 'Even if they legalise and we all then grow cannabis in our house, they'll sell it.'

It's true, they probably will. And there will be a niche demand for it; just as many houses in Ireland have a forbidden bottle of 80 per cent proof poitín (an Irish version of moonshine) somewhere in the cupboards, in case of an 'I need to get drunk really fucking quickly' emergency. (Not sure what that emergency would look like, but I can report that when you drink poitín, you get drunk from the feet up.)

But most of the cannabis users, including you, dear reader, would probably love to know exactly what it is they're smoking, vaping or eating.

It's high time it's legalised, in my opinion. Pun intended. For the sake of our brains.

Dear little cannabis addict,

I've never enjoyed cannabis. I've tried to, dozens of times, egged on by the aforementioned partners who loved it. But I was prone to those 'whiteys'.

Dr Grisel tells me why this happened. 'It enhances what's already going on,' she says. 'So if you're already anxious . . .' Makes sense. That's why alcohol was my drug. It sedated my anxiety.

The only things I've enjoyed doing while stoned are: eating and snogging. It made the snogging more languid, sensuous somehow. And it made the eating of anything more delicious. I remember it turning average food into what tasted like a Michelin-starred meal.

I was curious as to the other effects I've never experienced, so I asked some friends/friends-of-friends who are – or were – habitual smokers/eaters/vapers of cannabis. 'What do you like about it?' Here's what they said.

Likes

- 'That slight disconnect from reality, but how you can do it on a week day and still function, unlike alcohol.'
- 'The ritual of rolling. Getting it perfectly coned. Putting some pre-rolls in those cute tins for festivals.'
- 'Discussing the nuances with other enthusiasts; are you a weed or hash person, are you indica or sativa, what are the highs like for you. It's almost like being a wine connoisseur, but it's not legal.'
- 'The sex. Your senses feel heightened; it's like you can get out of your head and into your body.'
- 'Doodling, photography. It feels like it opens the creative brain. I think about parallel universes a lot.'

- 'The community of playing traffic lights with friends (a smoking game), and the shared language of knowing who's a beginner because they don't observe the three-toke pass.'
- 'Doing chores while stoned. It feels like cheating the system, vacuuming while high.'
- 'I'm less obnoxious stoned than I am when I drink.'
- 'Being in nature, like going biking along a river when I'm only slightly high.'
- 'It helps with period pain.'

I also asked them: 'What do you *not* like about it?'

Dislikes

- 'The paranoia that someone will knock on the door, or ask me to adult in an emergency, and I won't be able to deal because I'm high.'
- 'Stoneovers while driving, knowing my reaction times are slightly slower.'
- 'It keeps me insular, sitting in dark rooms, gaming, getting takeaways. But then I go out into the sunshine and I'm like – fuck. This is lovely too. I miss this.'
- 'I've worked with some people who have schizophrenia so, for me, the risk of psychosis is terrifying.'
- 'Diarrhoea. Weed used to have the same welcome effect that coffee does, in unstoppering me, but it went too far.'
- 'That tinge of paranoia, where you're wondering if everyone is talking about me, laughing about me. When it stops having the desired effect of dampening that down and only heightens it.'
- 'The constant worry of "is a neighbour going to report us?"'

- 'I get into dark cycles of intrusive, repetitive thoughts. It's so insular an experience that it creates this echo chamber of "don't think of a pink elephant on a bicycle". All I can think of is the pink elephant on a bicycle.'
- 'I hate the inequalities around the policing of it. Where Black men are arrested and charged more frequently for possession.'
- 'The disconnect from reality. Once, I thought I was killing it at this split-screen game. Then someone was like, "Amy, what are you doing?" Turns out my character was just jumping in a corner, repeatedly shooting into the air. It was the other player who was killing it.'
- 'Now that you can vape it in an odourless, even smokeless way, that removed too many obstacles for me. I'd started doing it during lunchtime at work.'
- 'The cravings.'

Interestingly, most of the friends – and friends-of-friends – surveyed no longer smoke. Some have moved to edibles, but the lion's share had quit altogether. Nonetheless, most seemed fond of weed. 'Fond' seems like a strange choice, but it's the only word that fits. Even if the person had broken up with weed, it seemed to be amicable rather than acrimonious.

This is usually not the case with alcohol or cigarettes. 'I like weed, but I don't do it any more' was the defining sentiment.

The word 'insular' came up over and over, so I asked Dr Grisel about it. 'I was just reading a paper with some students about that,' she says. 'It showed that using cannabis undermines "theory of mind", so it makes us more insular in that way.'

Theory of mind is the ability to understand that others have thoughts, beliefs and desires that may differ from our own. It's the skill of placing yourself in another's shoes, essentially.

Now, I want to ask the same two questions of you:

1. What do you like about weed?
2. What do you not like about it?

If you're trying to moderate your cannabis use, it might be an idea to concentrate hard on your answer to those two – seemingly elementary – questions. Because they contain important clues.

The latter is what you want to have less of, obviously. But the more you successfully moderate, the more you will forget what you *don't* like about it.

This is why moderation cycles often create a loop-the-loop of reduce-increase-reduce-increase. Our minds are incredibly good at selective forgetting to get us closer again to a little addiction, as if it's an ill-advised ex. 'It wasn't that bad!' it'll say. 'The sex was great!'

So be prepared for that. Outwit the 'selective forget' in advance, and while the 'what I don't like' is immediate and powerful, get it down somehow; recording a video of yourself, writing your little addiction a letter and sealing it in an envelope, telling a friend, whacking it on a vision board, choreographing a dance themed around 'if I'm still smoking in five years' time'; whatever it is that you need to lock it in.

With regards to what you like about it, all I can tell you is what I know from being 12 years alcohol-free. You need to find something else – or many things – that give you the same pleasure. For me, my drinking hadn't been fun for a long time. That needs emphasising. The problems had totally obscured the fun, on the fun/problems paradigm. But when it was still fun, here were the experiences I wanted to hang on to and recreate. And how I now do so, without alcohol.

ALCOHOL-FUELLED FUN	ALCOHOL-FREE FUN
That feeling of rushing on to a dance floor with my friends. To jump around and shout to our favourite Arctic Monkeys anthem.	Running unlocks this same musical abandon for me. It's why, mid-run, I can often be found pogo-ing around a lonely beach singing along to 'Dramamine' by the Middle Kids.
The cosiness of a glass of red, warming me from the inside out, beside a crackling fire in an olde worlde pub.	The cosiness of cuddling my dog, Arlo, while I'm under a heated blanket, beside a scented candle in my tiny terrace.
The connection of a life-righting chat with a friend, our feet tucked under us, our hearts swung wide open, the alcohol dismantling our inhibitions.	The connection of a life-righting chat with a friend while picking our way through a mossy forest, our inhibitions lowered by true intimacy and trust.

My point is, if you're determined to do so, you can find ways of getting to the same emotional place. It'll just require a different route. Usually a slower one, as per the 'slow dopamine' activities we will discuss on page 182.

Maybe you crave the rested but still sleepy feeling of weed. Get more afternoon naps in on weekends (all the parents laugh drily). Or you notice a similar mental stillness after a swim. Join your local pool, or buy a Dryrobe for after a sea dip. Invest in your new thing. Grand investment gestures work.

Or maybe the only other time you feel like you lose yourself is when you're immersed in a novel. Do I have to say it? Don't make me say it.

It might be that the precise same thing isn't achievable. My alcohol-free fun does feel different to alcohol-fuelled fun. It's obviously purer and less edgy, rather than the abandon of the delinquent lash.

But if you seek, you'll find something close. And potentially, something better.

Love,
Cath x

CANNABIS MICRO TACTICS

Deploy cue-hiding

Cues are powerful. 'Environmental cues capture our attention, trigger a craving response and are something very difficult for us to ignore,' says Dr Hickey. 'We call this "incentive salience".'

Cannabis and its bandmates of king-size rolling papers et al are usually hidden in a wooden box someplace, but you'd be surprised at how much the lighter on the side, the coaster featuring the famous sativa leaf, the chair you use in the garden, or the dark chocolate propped in the cupboard (if you're a baker) can trigger the cue-craving cascade. Hide them as much as possible.

Use some essential oils

Don't roll your eyes. I felt that ;-) Smell is arguably the biggest cue for cannabis use. 'Smell is a very potent cue to consume,' says Professor Murphy. 'Often as humans, given we're so visually dependent, we overlook how much power our other senses can have.'

Even if you can't consciously smell cannabis, your bloodhound nose will be picking up on that linger in your living room – or even garden. Mask it with scent – worn or diffused – for fewer cravings.

Try reading a novel for a 'theory of mind' boost

I ask Dr Grisel whether 'theory of mind', which we talked about earlier, can be re-bolstered by reading fiction, particularly first person, where we're essentially looking out through the eyes of the main character. 'I don't know for sure but I think it's a terrific idea,' she says. 'ToM is about our self not being at the centre, so it would probably work.'

Lift weights instead of a spliff

A single weight-lifting session has the power to activate your endocannabinoid system naturally. As usual, it's tough to study this on humans, so most of what we know comes from animal studies. Scientists had rats do the equivalent of a leg press (a paw press), to discover the link. Some experts claim that just 15 minutes of lifting a day is enough.

If you hate weights, cardio works too. The fabled 'runner's high' – previously attributed purely to endorphins – is now thought to be because of endocannabinoids.

Use a cookie jail

If you just shuddered with horror at this suggestion and want to remain 'master of your own bake' (Let me have it, c'mon), then here's an idea. Think of those indestructible kitchen safes, the ones with the timers, that people previously used for cookies and are now using for their phones. Most people aren't aware that you can lock things away in them for up to 10 days. Perfect for a spot of kush you're saving for the weekend, but don't want to be tempted by on a Tuesday.

The most renowned brand is K Safe, and you can pick one up for around £50. It seems like a lot of money to lay out but, if it works in downsizing your use, it could pay for itself pretty quickly.

Go low and slow with edibles

Edibles *seem* like a softer option than smoking, but because it's harder to judge the potency, and it takes much longer for the high to arrive, you can more easily find yourself in a whitey. 'Low and slow' is for the best, whether for space cake, gummies or brownies. Start slow, then wait two hours before having more, so you can be sure it has fully kicked in.

In case you're new to this, be sure to keep leftover edibles – and cannabis – out of the orbit of not just kids, but also pets.

ULTRA-PROCESSED FOOD

Sticky eight

In order to understand the predicament we now find ourselves in with food, we have to go back, way back. Metaphorically, our brains still have a honey axe in their hands. Given the chance, they want to crack open that beehive, fight off the angry bees and then gorge on honey until they feel sick. 'Everybody finds honey meaningful,' says neuroscientist Dr Judith Grisel, author of *Never Enough*. Not that every modern human *still* likes honey. 'But, evolutionarily speaking, those who didn't find it meaningful wouldn't have survived.'

In fact, *not* being an overeating honey monster could have meant death. 'If a Stone Age woman came across a tree groaning with figs, the most sensible thing to do was to eat as many of them as she could on the spot, before the local baboon band picked the tree bare,' Yuval Noah Harari wrote in *Sapiens: A Brief History of Humankind*.

Sounds like me when I find a forgotten box of chocolates in the cupboard. (Who am I trying to kid, I never forget about boxes of chocolates in the cupboard.)

'The instinct to gorge on high-calorie food was hardwired into our genes,' Harari wrote. 'Today, we may be living in high-rise apartments with overstuffed refrigerators, but our DNA still thinks we're in the savannah. That's what makes some of us spoon down an entire tub of Ben & Jerry's when we find one in the freezer, and wash it down with a jumbo Coke. This "gorging gene" theory is widely accepted.'

We evolved for rarity and seeking, not delivery services of crisps and ice cream within a half hour. 'If you look at the ancestral diet, it was really low carb naturally,' says evolutionary expert Dr Andrew Thomas. 'Tubers were really hard to dig up and break down. We only really even started eating wheat 10,000 years ago and we are naturally very drawn to it given it's calorie-dense.' Wheat is in bread, pasta, baked goods, cereals.

'In fact, we are drawn to anything calorie-dense,' Dr Thomas adds, a shrug in his voice. It's not personal, it's just evolution. Your brain is just doing its job by telling you to eat as much of it as you can. 'Your brain has evolved to do that for good reason,' says neuroscientist Dr Alex Korb. 'Our environment used to put a natural cap on it because we couldn't eat as much as we wanted again and again. We still have the same brains, and food companies are exploiting that, by offering us a way to have it again and again.'

This 'eat as much as you can' bias was already powerful way before ultra-processed *anything*. I'm sure our grandparents often found themselves on an unplanned second round of homemade jam on bakery-baked bread. But with clever taste engineering on a massive scale, the lever these foods pull within us has become supersized.

What is ultra-processed food?

Ultra-processed food (let's call it UPF, for brevity's sake) has only recently entered our lexicon. The first time I heard of it was in 2023 from Dr Chris van Tulleken's excellent book, *Ultra-Processed People: Why do we all eat stuff that isn't food… and why can't we stop?*, and he probably took great inspiration from those who went before, particularly the work of former US FDA commissioner Dr David A Kessler, who served under Presidents Bush and Clinton, devoting his life's work to exposing the Frankenfoods that make us compulsively overeat.*

UPF is so voluminous a category that, unless food looks like it did when grown or raised in nature (think frozen peas, chicken, cans of butter beans, eggs, fish, a cut of unprocessed red meat), then it's probably UPF. If it comes in a packet, has a long shelf life and isn't a bag of unseasoned cashews, it's almost certainly UPF. *Great.* 'My personal rule of thumb' writes van Tulleken, 'is that if I'm struggling with whether to call a food a UPF, then it probably is a UPF.'

Dr Kessler's book, *Food or Fiction: the truth about the ultraprocessed foods making America sick,* includes a long list of problematic UPFs: pizza, milkshakes, hamburgers, fries, most types of bread, biscuits, puddings, cereals, pastries, crisps, cakes, granola bars, crackers, sweets, ice cream. Other UPFs

---

* Much of the information in this chapter has sprung from the tireless research of Dr David A Kessler in *Food or Fiction*, and Dr Chris van Tulleken in *Ultra-Processed People*. All of Kessler's and van Tulleken's quotes come from these books. If your interest is piqued by this chapter's shallow-dive into this topic, which is restricted by room, I encourage you to check these two books out for a deep dive.

include ready meals and chocolate; even sanctimonious high-cocoa dark chocolate.

Unfortunately, all of the above could be a laundry list of my diet in the past couple of weeks, while I've been finishing up this book. When I'm in 'survival mode' like in times of high stress, UPF is the auto-choice. Ironically, a mostly UPF diet should really be called 'anti-survival mode', since Kessler and van Tulleken take pains to point out that these foods, when overconsumed, can and do kill us. *Also great.*

Both doctors have previous with overeating. It's often the case that those lifting the lid are *also* those who found themselves trapped under the lid. Probably because to get through the colossal task of writing a book, there has to be a propeller of what Gretchen Rubin calls 'me-search'.

Dr van Tulleken openly declares that his relationship with UPF was an addiction, describing bingeing cheap takeaways to the point that he vomited, although he resists defining it as disordered eating. Dr Kessler opens *Food or Fiction* with disarming honesty: 'I'm a doctor with a lifetime of experience in the field of nutrition and health, but for most of my life I have been trapped in a body that I could neither control nor understand. Food was my nemesis.'

Kessler writes of eating to feel better, finding a suspended reality of 'zoned-out bliss', then coming back to Earth, crumbs on his shirt, only to plan his next meal or snack.

Our other expert in this chapter, Shahroo Izadi, also has previous with food. She told Steven Bartlett on his *Diary of a CEO* podcast that she was 'using food as a drug' and ate to the extent that she was '126 kilos, and it eventually culminated in secretly getting a gastric band fitted. I started working in addiction treatment, and I started realising that I was going about this the wrong way,' she said. 'I wasn't meant to be making my body smaller. I was meant to understand why I didn't like myself enough to take the same advice I'd give someone else.'

Since her struggle, she's published three books on food psychology and has dedicated her life's work as a psychologist to her 'kindness method', which is all about creating a landscape of kindness towards our body, meaning we're more likely to then want to give it healthy fuel. She rails against the diet industry, and her most recent book is *How Diets Make Us Fat.*

So, why are all these experts so upset about ultra-processed foods? 'I learned that the multibillion-dollar processed food industry has discovered how to engineer foods to trigger an endless eating loop,' writes Dr Kessler. 'In other words, foods designed to make us overeat.'

He goes on to say that food in general isn't addictive, but UPF is, and that this is well-evidenced. I mean, it's common sense, isn't it? Pretty much nobody is out there overeating carrots, but they are overeating cake. I don't struggle to stop eating pumpkin seeds, but I do struggle with sweet and salty popcorn.

What is addictive about UPF?

First up, the trap is that it's quick. Right now, as I write, I don't have the time to make a sea bass, rice and asparagus feast from scratch. I don't care if the chef flogging the recipe tells me it'll only take 20 minutes: it'll somehow take me double that and, even though fish, rice and vegetables would actually be my mouth's preference, I don't have time, OK?! I need some fuel, and I need it now, which is why I'm falling onto UPF.

It's the go-to banquet of those with lots of work to do (paid or otherwise), and not enough time. Our diet is usually the first thing to falter when we have a baby, start a big new job or go through something stressful, such as a break-up.

Not only is UPF available quickly, with frozen fries dinging in the air fryer within 10 minutes, it's also easy to eat quickly once it's on your plate. The biological structure of the food has been altered for extra speed and palatability, either so that it's puffed and crunchy, like a stuffed crust or tortillas, or soft and yummy, like gummy bears or a shop-bought trifle.

Van Tulleken calls this structural change 'pre-chewed', while Kessler goes one step further with 'pre-digested'. 'Their molecular structure has been destroyed, essentially making them streams of glucose,' writes Kessler.

We need the chewing, though, he says. We *need* the structure. A plate of actual food takes us much longer to eat, so it signals to the brain that you've eaten. On top of the time aspect, these foods affect our bodies in a different way to whole foods, spiking glucose. In rat studies, Kessler writes that a glucose surge has been shown to command the brain to eat more.

Once the glucose reaches the intestine, it has another powerful reinforcing effect, as the gut also activates the reward circuitry in the brain. 'Indeed, some research indicates that the reward response in the gut may be even stronger than that in the brain,' says Kessler. Simplified, UPF hacks the gut–brain connection, rewarding us twice for eating it.

The food designers make it addictive by design, seeking out the 'bliss point', which is the exact nexus of fat, sugar and salt for moreishness. A whistleblower from the food industry told Kessler, '[We] make it more compelling by adding fat and sugar and salt; the perfect calorific torpedo.'

The holy grail for those tasked with finding the 'bliss point' is this: the moment the consumer finishes their final bite, they want another. And another. 'If we go to a Michelin-starred restaurant, once we finish our meal we feel satiated and it's wonderful,' says Dr Korb. 'But these processed foods have been designed to deliberately induce cravings for more.'

They leave a gap where a full feeling should be. A gap that you then fill with more of the UPF. *Cha-ching.*

Van Tulleken tried out a mostly UPF diet for a month, having his body and brain monitored before and after by scientists at UCL. He gained 6kg and felt dreadful. But what was extra-interesting is that tests afterwards discovered that his 'appetite hormones were totally deranged,' he wrote. 'The hormone that signals fullness barely responded to a large meal, while the hunger hormone was sky high just moments after eating.'

The paradox is that, even though UPF is ultra-calorific, it makes us hungrier. Van Tulleken is just one dude, obviously, but many studies back this finding up, including one cited by Kessler from the National Institutes of Health. They gave participants either an unprocessed diet or an ultra-processed one for two weeks, then switched them over.

Two pounds were lost or gained in that fortnight, depending on the diet. You can guess which was which. The UPF group ate 500 more calories a day, so it's hardly surprising. But the hormones were the most compelling difference. 'Among those eating unprocessed food, levels of the appetite-suppressing hormone PYY increased, while the hunger-signalling hormone ghrelin decreased,' Kessler wrote.

After just two tiny weeks, the unprocessed diet had the power to literally change hormone levels, making the people less hungry. Their diet also looked a hell of a lot more appetising, with the likes of scrambled egg and homemade hash brown, a lunch of chicken breast and salad, and a dinner of stir fry and basmati rice, all served with lots of fruit or veg.

I feel like we've got enough evidence now. UPF is wildly addictive. It's deliberately designed to be quickly edible – its mouthfeel hyperpalatable – then it creates a glucose volleyball spike, telling our brains to eat more, and it's twice-rewarding in both the brain and the gut-brain. Most of all, it's specifically engineered to hit the 'again' bliss point with that exact confection of fat, sugar and salt.

'I think the perfect example of a food that really hacks into this is a doughnut,' says Dr Thomas. 'More diets have been spoiled by the free office doughnut than any other item. It's the perfect mix of everything that was scarce in ancestral environments – fried in fat, high calorie, lots of sugar – and they throw salt in there too, especially with salted caramel.'

The question now is, what do we do about it? We all know it'll probably involve a handful of nuts and some apple slices. Let's accept our fate, shall we? But our experts also have far smarter tricks up their sleeves.

The guilt catch-22

The guiltier you feel, the more you'll overeat. 'If you stop telling yourself that "ice cream is my guilty pleasure", you'll actually find it easier to moderate,' says Dr Korb. Lean into the pleasure part, minimising the afterburn of shame.

'Whenever you get into that brain loop of, "I shouldn't be eating this, it's so bad for me, I need to stop", your brain won't associate ice cream with negative feelings,' he explains. 'It will learn that eating the ice cream is the way to avoid those feelings.' We think the guilt loop inhibits our consumption, but it actually inflames it.

Self-flagellation is also called out by Kessler as 'one of the traps of overeating' given it powers further overeating. 'This is not to say you shouldn't care,' he writes. 'You should care deeply.' But as the recovery saying goes, progress, not perfection. None of us are error-free human bots. The path to change is almost always a series of loop-the-loops, rather than a straight line.

Self-empowerment and self-kindness throughout the loops are where Izadi's behavioural design work comes in. As an interviewee she is frank, fearless and witty, making me laugh out loud. It's easy to see why Steven Bartlett praised her 'no bullshit' approach.

Her first piece of gold is to design for your current self, not an imaginary future self. I constantly fall into this magical thinking, believing that on Monday I'll be a different person to who I was on Friday, or that when I finish the book, I'll suddenly develop an insatiable appetite for decorating and DIY.

'I used to design for an imaginary version of me that wanted to wake up at 6am,' Izadi says. She even resorted to sleeping in her gym gear. 'Nowadays, I do wake up at 6am, ironically, but that's because I designed the gradual changes *around* the fact I'm not a morning person.'

The next step is finding the 'why', she says. The 'should' isn't the key to unlocking it, but the 'why' is. 'I have clients who say they can't be an intuitive eater because, intuitively, they want to go to KFC,' she says. Trying to force yourself to want change because you should want to be healthy is a fool's errand. 'Why do you want to do the thing?' she enquires. 'Is it to feel less tired when you're hanging out with your child?'

Making it a pledge to yourself, rather than other people, is pivotal too. This echoes big addiction recovery, which always maintains that you can only get sober for yourself. 'Specify what the pledge is; maybe it's cutting out UPF 80 per cent of the time. Then prove to yourself that you can do what you said you're going to,' she says.

Grand plans of never eating fried chicken again are destined to fail, as are total overhaul approaches. So, pick your battles, she suggests. 'I know that if I didn't put milk in my coffee each morning, I'd be better off,' she says. 'But the thanklessness and sadness that this brings to the start of my day will mean that, by the end of it, I'm ordering pizza.'

Clients will ask her, 'Should I start the day with lemony water rather than coffee?' 'And I say no – how about you just focus on not ordering the pizza?' In 12-step philosophy, this 'pick the biggest first' ethos is captured in the slogan, 'pick the addiction that will kill you first'.

Urge-surfing requires a board, to make things as easy for yourself as possible, so you can gain speed. 'Make things frictionless,' Izadi suggests. 'If the appeal of UPF is that it's quick, there and comforting, find a substitute food to grab that fits this same criteria,' rather than assuming you'll somehow magically stop being spontaneously hungry, or want to make an omelette first thing. 'Design for your worst day,' she says.

Cues predict what we'll pick up, says Dr Grisel. 'Like Pavlovian dogs, we salivate at the bell,' she says. 'Whether it's the pack of smokes in our pocket, the smell of the coffee beans or the biscuits on the counter.' Whichever of our senses registers that bell, we're going to react. 'You're going to walk past that counter with the biscuits on it 50 times in a day. Stick them in the cabinet,' she says.

For snacks, you're going to want to aim for what Izadi calls the 'sweet potato of life'. 'As with sweet potatoes, some of these foods have been demonised by diet culture, such as the nuts for saturated fat or dates for sugar, but the question is: do they make you want more?' says Izadi.

Do they leave a gap, like UPF does, or do they sate you? The closer you get to nature, the more you'll find you feel a non-gap after eating, a satiated closed loop, given that the bliss point is installed when the food is processed beyond its natural form.

Like all addiction experts I've spoken with, Izadi rubbishes the idea of an addictive personality. 'That's not evidence-based,' she says, matter of factly. 'But what I am is "addiction vulnerable". I exist in the extremes, and that's cool, I'm not going to be moderate, median or sensible. I've started this hectic spin class, and I'm already planning to be an instructor,' she laughs. 'I can't just do a little bit of something.' She leverages that rebel mindset, just like I do, going all in on that tendency to 'go hard or go home'.

Many of her clients are similarly radical. Izadi tells me about a client who had a white board. 'On it, he'd written down his daily goals. Forty five minutes on the Peloton, cook a meal from scratch every day, do five job applications . . . He was baffled as to why he wasn't doing it. "It's all possible, so why can't I master this?" he was asking me.' Izadi realised it was about creating an environment set up for success, prior to mastery. Together, they worked out that if he gets up and puts the Lycra on first thing, he will get on the Peloton at some point. Second, he figured out that if he cuts an onion in half, he will indeed cook. Third, if he opens the Indeed job-seeking website, he'll get drawn in. The very first step, rather than the whole caboodle, was what set the changes in motion.

Everyone has a 'point of no return' behaviourally, says Izadi. 'Don't tell me that it's getting to the gym because, for me, it's not,' she laughs. 'I could get to the gym and leave again. It's *after* I pick up the first weight – then I know I won't leave. So I just have to get myself to pick it up.' Foodwise, it might be that if you eat a banana, you won't eat a chocolate bar, she says, but knowing where your 'no return' line is, is everything.

But the headlines say UPF is fine?!

In the wake of *Ultra-Processed People's* 2023 publication, which reshaped national opinion on these products, the UPF industry pushed back, using all the same tactics from the playbook of Big Tobacco back in the day, or Big Alcohol right now (page 38).

What was their strategy? *Doubt.* They stirred some into the pot, and very effective it was too.

A rash of 'Is ultra-processed food really that bad for us?' style headlines hit, even in reputable publications such as *New Scientist* and *The Times*. In a recently added Afterword, van Tulleken exposed that the source of all this *doubt* could be traced back to a press conference where four of the five scientists presenting had conflicts of interest, having previously been funded by the likes of McDonald's and Mars. *The Guardian* picked up on these conflicts (generally it does, and this is where I get my news) but nobody else appeared to.

We live in a world where clinical studies funded by The Coca-Cola Company et al, are still published in medical journals. If the results are unfavourable to Coca-Cola, they are sometimes contractually entitled to quash the study and consign the inconvenient data to a data graveyard. Ba-bye meanie data.

Meanwhile, UPF manufacturers help fund the British Nutrition Foundation. It's not even a secret – it's right there on BNF's website. Coca-Cola alone has donated over a million dollars that we know of. The BNF's Healthy Eating Week was sponsored by the likes of Kellogg's, General Mills (Old El Paso, Nature Valley, et al) and, you guessed it, Coca-Cola.

Yes, *fantastic* that all of this money for healthy eating initiatives and research is coming from the industry itself, but that also *so bloody obviously* opens it up to corruption. There must be a way of taking the money and keeping the resulting research separate. UK Government, I dare you, please show us that you have some common sense and are not deliberately complicit in all of this.

As with anything that is woefully underregulated, we need to keep our wits about us, only trusting scientists and organisations *not* paid by industry, until the regulation finally kicks in, if it ever does. I'll also be hoping that journalists will start following the money up river, before they report on 'objective' findings, even if it kills their clickbait story.

'I don't study to know more, but to ignore less.'

Juana Inés de la Cruz

Dear little ultra-processed food addict,

I cannot be trusted to be alone with biscuits.

Yesterday I arrived at a lovely writing cabin to finish the book and I found a free packet of crumbly honey biscuits in the gift hamper.

'Oh yes,' I said, falling upon them like a seagull on chips.

'Oh no,' said the little voice inside me that knows better.

The first day, I managed to only eat three. OK, four. Denial is an onion.

The second day, I ate the rest of the packet. Which was about eight.

I tell Izadi about my biscuits issue. My partner has it too, which is why we've banned them from the house. Every now and then we'll buy the purple-and-gold 'fancy biscuits' from Tesco, 'for the guests' we have coming. The guests might eat four. Then we demolish the rest in just two or three days.

The biscuits are for us really. Not the guests. It's collaborative self-deception.

'Can I ask you a question?' she says, when I tell her about the banned biscuits.

'Sure,' I respond.

'Are the biscuits ever not a problem?'

Of course. There are times when I can resist them, and also do. It's not like I'm decimating every packet of biscuits that comes into our house upon entry, like Cookie Monster.

Her fiercely elemental question unlocks something in me. I realise that I do actually have power over biscuits. This is one of the great things about little addictions – our free will is not yet compromised by the proportion of the addiction.

For the next two weeks I do keep biscuits in the house and I do stick to my desired usage of three per day. Then I realise something. I don't want to do this.

I'd much rather spend my self-allocated 'one per day' treat allowance on ice cream or a slab of afternoon cake. The biscuits aren't as important to me.

****

Brief sidebar to explain the treat allowance. When I was 40, I got that free NHS health test that they do.

When the nurse called with my results, I was smug. I was fully prepared to ace these test results, being a non-smoking, non-drinking daily exerciser.

'Umm, so, I remember you said you like cake and biscuits?' she said.

What? This wasn't going as planned.

'Yes I do,' I said, 'Is there a problem?'

'Well, you have borderline high cholesterol. No need for statins right now, doctor says . . . But maybe cut down on those sweet treats.'

****

I realise that I just don't want biscuits in the house. I know they hit my bliss point, no sniggering at the back, and I don't even want to risk a six-biscuit day. Earlier, I joked about chugging a whole tub of ice cream, but the truth is, I rarely overconsume cake or ice cream. I eat both regularly, but can stop easily enough.

And, with that, my decision is made. My 'I *can't* have biscuits in the house' has become 'I *don't* have biscuits in the house.' I can have biscuits; I just don't want to. And as we already know from page 47, behavioural science shows that 'I don't' rather than 'I can't' is a much bigger predictor of success.

I no longer feel sad about my biscuit-less house. Just as with my alcohol-free or smokeless life, I don't feel like it's been forced upon me. I've chosen it.

These meaningful sidesteps are so powerful. Just make one little word different, and the decision feels smoother, differently structured, easier to swallow. A little like UPF.

Love,
Cath x

ULTRA-PROCESSED FOOD MICRO TACTICS

Know your flash times
We all have times when we're more vulnerable. For many, it's the afternoon slump or late at night. 'The smart version of yourself can think of ways to interrupt your autopilot pattern,' Izadi says. Knowing about the flash times is half the battle.

Create new heuristics
Kessler suggests creating new heuristics; things we do habitually, without thought. Say a bread basket gets put on your table in a restaurant and you automatically tear off a chunk to butter it. A new heuristic might be: 'When I sit down in a restaurant, I will immediately tell the server not to bring me bread,' he writes. Others might include walking straight past the sweets, chocolates and crisps aisle during a supermarket shop. Or stashing chewing gum in your car, instead of Haribo.

Reframe the meaning
As with many other substances, the gap between our belief and the reality is often large. 'When I eat UPF during the day, the fuzzy mind and lethargy is palpable,' says Izadi.

It might be that you notice sugary pastries make you feel fractious rather than happy. And that a protein breakfast places you in a much better frame of mind.

You could even *rename*. I discovered this for myself on a business trip. Opening the cupboard, there sat a smorgasbord of my favourite treats, as if assembled by an AI spy. The crisps were ridged, flavoursome and posh. I wanted them so badly, despite the £2 mark-up. But it was 10pm. Instead, I said 'heartburn' and closed the wardrobe.

Do it in a row

Repetition creates new neural pathways, which become more entrenched over time, as per the Hebbian theory of 'what fires together wires together'. Izadi recommends stringing together the longest streak you can, for extra soldering. 'Things get easier when you do them in a row,' she says.

This might mean that mid-week looks one way, while the weekend looks different. A loved one of mine quit mid-week desserts by using 'in a row' dusted with a shake of identity change, by saying, 'I no longer eat desserts, other than at the weekend.'

Context is everything

'In some contexts, you'll want to keep the UPF,' Izadi says. 'Like when you're watching a movie with friends. Whereas by yourself, it might feel more shame-based.' Van Tulleken agrees with this context nuance. 'You may recognise more vulnerable moments and foods,' he writes, 'so that eating a UPF sandwich for lunch with a friend is not going to prompt a binge, whereas eating crisps at home alone while hungry may be more likely to.'

Capitalise on unit bias

Studies have found that we see one portion as one unit, whether it's a kids' can of Sprite, or a Big Gulp, or a 6- or 12-inch Subway sandwich. It's called 'unit bias' and we can use it to work for us, rather than against.

If I buy a chocolate bar, I'll eat the chocolate bar, so now I go for those Kinder treats shaped like hippos, or mini bags of chocolate buttons. (Give 'family size' or 'grab bags' of anything a hard swerve, unless you have the discipline to decant.)

The bars that come in twos or fours work also, says Izadi – think a Bounty or Twix – especially if you're wanting to practise your delayed gratification. She suggests eating three fingers of KitKat and then stopping, simply to prove to yourself that you can.

Inspired by my psychotherapist friend Sam, I also now scoop my ice cream into cones. It automatically limits how much I eat, and means a tub of Häagen-Dazs (not ultra-processed, FYI, look at the ingredients) can last six sittings. You might confine your M & M habit to the 'unit' of an egg cup, or your Kettle Chips to your smallest bowl.

Making a do/don't host list

I previously called this the 'can/can't' host list, and then had a word with myself about not instantly forgetting the very same lessons I've just learned about 'can't' vs 'don't'.

Maybe, like me, you know not to host giant bags of flamin' hot crisps, given you'll end up with a chinful of Cheetos dust from using the packet like a nose bag. Just me? Or maybe, for you, it's those processed hot dogs that will expire after the apocalypse has taken the Earth, and insects rule, which you always eat three of.

You're an adult. You already know what your flashpoint foods are. Keeping them out of the house and only eating them in public means the 'Hawthorne effect' can kick in (when we feel watched, we make better choices).

PORN

Sticky eight

We covered the 'evolutionary mismatch' earlier (see page 27), where our brains haven't caught up with the modern landscape and porn is probably the very best example of this.

Ancient impulses + overabundant modern stimuli = problems.

Our main expert here is Dr Andrew Thomas, an evolutionary psychologist at Swansea University, who has also treated several porn-addicted clients as a therapist, so there is probably no better fit.

'Porn as a stimuli taps into our mating psychology in such a fundamental way,' he says, 'because, up until fairly recently, if we saw a naked person, it was in the context of "sex is imminent".'

And so that stimuli commands our *total* attention.

The obstacles between us and porn have dissolved into nothing, in just a few decades. 'A hundred years ago you would have needed to go to a brothel to see naked people who weren't your partner,' says Dr Thomas. 'Then, 20-odd years ago you would have needed to go to the woods to find the buried *Playboy* everyone knew about.'

(The *what?* I didn't know about this. Suddenly, all the ripped-out porn I saw in woodlands in the '80s and '90s makes a whole lot of sense.)

Professor Clayton Hickey commented on this speedy access shift too. 'In the nineties, porn would have been on the top-shelf at the corner store,' he said. 'It would have been a big deal to reach up and pull that out.'

'And now those obstacles have disintegrated?' I asked.

'Exactly,' he said. 'Now there are none.'

Psychotherapist Hilda Burke and I went a step further while talking about this, imagining that the death of top-shelf porn magazines was probably the cause of the large-scale decline of the physical magazine industry (I still think this is a solid theory, alongside The Internet).

'People often sandwiched the porn in between two other mags, when they went up to pay,' Burke observed. This reminds me of when I was addicted to alcohol. In the shop I would often buy something else too, as an adjunct. Oh, I was buying this fabric conditioner, you see, and I *just so happen* to have slung a bottle of wine into the basket. (Buying unnecessary adjuncts is a sure sign an addiction is enlarging from 'little', FYI. Nobody cared that I was buying wine, or how much, but I felt like they did.)

Even when porn infiltrated TV via cable and Sky channels, there was the inhibitor of needing to sign up to a subscription, which was both financially prohibitive and visible to the rest of your household, even if you were the bill-paying adult.

The internet changed all that, obviously, with its fire-hose of free porn, and then the smartphone changed it all *again*, meaning nobody had to risk a family PC being proliferated by telltale pop-ups of chicks carrying snakes, à la '00s Britney, except naked.

'Nowadays, you have 13-year-olds with Pornhub in their pockets,' says addiction neuroscientist Dr Judith Grisel, a hint of world-weariness in her voice. Indeed, a US report found that seven in ten 13–17-year-olds have watched porn, compared to four in ten in 2005.

I'm actually surprised this figure is so low, aren't you? I most certainly would have watched porn when I was a hornball 14-year-old, had it been available. As it was, I had to content myself with borrowing Beth from one-street-over's *Playgirl*, with its flaccid penises lying on thighs.

I didn't feel how I expected to feel upon seeing my first adult penises. Maybe because they were all fast asleep.

Porn as a supernormal stimuli

What *is* shocking, however, is that over half of these samesuch teens had already watched online porn by the time they were 13.

Thing is, kids have been raiding their parents' porn stash since the dawn of printed porn. Which is incredibly weird when you think about it (using your dad's porn? Yikes), but it happens.

Yet online (and potentially hardcore) porn is a very different creature from that cache of probably vanilla magazines and videos masterfully hidden in the bottom of your parents' wardrobe, where ~~no kid~~ every kid will think to look.

Everyone now knows about the 'fake calculator' app, a keepsake of parentally policed teens, where once they enter a secret password, they can open a vault of porn. And what's inside is ever-spicier, sometimes extreme. *That's* the worrying thing.

This is why it's very welcome news that the UK government has just (since my conversation with Dr Grisel) changed the law. Now, Ofcom legislation has been introduced whereby there are fierce age checks for accessing porn sites, providing credit card details, ID documents like passports and sometimes even live video. Porn sites that don't comply are fined up to £18m (or 10 per cent of their revenue, whichever is greater).

Considering that an Ofcom study discovered that three per cent of 8–9-year-olds in Britain accessed a porn site in the past month (how terrifying is that?). I personally think this fine should be higher.

A bottomless scroll of supernormal stimuli

But what about adults? We also have a limitless wall of naked people, doing things to each other that range from the mild to the unspeakable, available for zero monies and viewing in private windows, which are tracked by data-gatherers so they can build a scarily accurate profile to sell things to us, but cannot be tracked by our loved ones.

A rampant sex drive is, of course, utterly expected in an adolescent (which is why we need to restrict what they can access), and a keen sex drive is also utterly healthy in an adult. 'Wanting to see attractive naked people is as natural as wanting to breathe, eat and drink water,' says Dr Thomas. You won't find any sex-drive-shaming here.

However, porn creators artificially hack this natural urge by turning porn into 'supernormal stimuli', says behavioural scientist Patrick Fagan. 'Supernormal stimuli amplifies features you would never find naturally, but it's natural that we respond to it more,' he says.

'A bird will automatically give more food to a cuckoo hatchling left in its nest because the cuckoo has a bigger beak than its own chicks,' he says. Knowing this, cuckoo mothers leave their eggs in the nests of other birds, called 'hosts'.

'Similarly, brands will work out what these "stimuli" are and put them on crack, supersizing them,' says Fagan, 'just as Disney takes cuteness stimuli – exemplified by big heads and big eyes – and exaggerates it'.

'Adult content creators do the exact same thing,' he adds. We become the unsuspecting hosts, feeding supersized stimuli our attention. Think of breast and butt implants. Some male adult entertainers self-inject drugs like Caverject directly into the penis to get hard, or even subject themselves to penile implants, with a small device hidden in the scrotum to press for erections on demand.

'The act of watching porn is also literally "supernormal",' agrees Dr Thomas, 'because, even though it creates a biological response by physically turning us on, it's artificial stimuli on a flat-screen that we can't reach out and touch.' Nothing about the content or experience is natural, nor have we evolved to deal with it, and so our brains just don't know what to do.

Naked people usually moderate *themselves* by getting dressed and leaving our bedrooms. Meanwhile, porn never leaves. It's always in your pocket, begging you to look for a thrill during a quiet moment. Even in the toilets at work.

'Look at me,' it whispers. 'Turn me on.'

Porn use isn't personal

Like most women, I've discovered a partner's covert porn use, which felt like an intensely personal attack; a commentary upon my enoughness, or lack thereof.

I'll never forget walking down the street with one partner, who nearly did himself a *Carry On*-style injury to check out a large-breasted blonde wearing a low-cut top. When we got home, I said I wanted to watch *Come Dine With Me* (aww, the 2000s), while he said he wanted to work. I popped into the bedroom to grab something and found him furiously masturbating, a large-breasted blonde bouncing around on his work laptop.

It feels like 'you're choosing them instead of me,' when a partner looks at porn, and by extension, 'so, I'm clearly not enough for you'. Indeed, back in 2016, a third of engaged or married women saw porn use as a straight-up infidelity.

Our views of porn have softened since then, with a *GQ* survey finding that 22 per cent of British women now regularly use porn too (among younger women, this doubles). Men who regularly used porn in the same survey stood at 61 per cent; a figure that tends to hold true across data.

Mind you, women are academically known to under-report their use of porn – and men tend to over-report – due to a 'social desirability bias' where we gauge what people expect us to say, and then just *say* it. Who knows, among younger cohorts the gender ratio could be 1:1 on porn use.

The only place in the world – that I could find – where female porn-watching outweighs male is the Philippines. Filipino women *really* like Japanese porn, it seems. Publicly 'out' female figures who've used porn include Cameron Diaz (likes how discreet hotels are in billing it), Lily Allen (just likes it, full stop) and Amy Poehler (likes it how she likes her comedy – professionally done and by women enjoying themselves).

What's saddening is the aftermath seen in these six-in-ten men, from the *GQ* survey: what they report as a porn 'hangover'. More than half of them said they felt self-conscious about their bodies or sexual performance after viewing porn, while 42 per cent reported guilt or self-loathing. It sounds a lot like the aftermath of a food binge. And I couldn't find any evidence of women reporting the same wretchedness, other than Billie Eilish, who has said watching porn from the age of 11 'destroyed her brain' and gave her nightmares.

We'll come back to the possible reasons for that lopsidedness in a moment; experts trace it back to something called the 'porn gap'.

Porn as a facsimile for a relationship

It's an unsubstantiated myth that porn inflames sexual appetite, says Dr Thomas. 'It's a fairytale. There's no evidence, even though it's a deeply engrained societal belief, that an average human could watch a lot of porn and develop a hypersexual appetite.'

High porn use is driven by high sex drive, not the other way around, he says. The sex drive is the input, not the output.

Hypersexual traits – an obsession with sex – tend to be genetic. 'It's highly heritable, actually,' he says. 'If you have a parent who was hypersexual, you're likely to be too. The brother or sister of a hypersexual twin will usually grow up to be hypersexual even if raised by sexually reserved parents.'

People want a simple answer – take away the porn – to a complex problem, he says.

'Occasional use can be a healthy part of someone's sex life,' he says. 'But I've treated clients who are watching it for hours a day, and downloading terrabytes of it on to hard drives.'

The bottomless browse becomes counterproductive, much as the infinite scroll of dating apps mean we spend days scrolling and hardly any time actually dating. 'Men I've treated will spend hours and hours looking for the perfect video.'

Psychologists call it 'the paradox of choice'. Again and again, studies have shown this paradox. 'Those who have too much choice are less satisfied with their eventual choice,' explains Dr Thomas.

It can also lead to 'choice paralysis' where we're so bewildered by the dizzying array that we don't choose at all. This makes me think of many evenings where I spent an hour looking for the 'perfect' film and then just went to bed, having not watched anything but trailers.

Another urban myth is that frequent porn use desensitises people from enjoying real sex. 'Porn doesn't desensitise,' Dr Thomas says. 'What it does do, however, is *disincentivise*. Namely, the creation of authentic relationships.' Particularly for men.

'It provides a facsimile of one of the rewards of a relationship,' Dr Thomas says. And like a fax*, it's a faded, substandard version; certainly not like the original. 'It's a consolation prize,' he says, 'Not the star prize.'

But the net result he's seen is this: many men hooked on porn then ask themselves, 'Why would I go into "hard mode" and risk failures and setbacks, in an attempt to win the star prize . . . when I can just get the consolation prize over and over again?'

When porn use grows horns

There's a surprising sign that a little porn addiction has upscaled. And it's not what you might expect. It's when porn use *stops* being about sex, reckons psychotherapist Hilda Burke.

'When it becomes less about the sexual release and more about the stress release,' she says. This is the tipping point, because it's no longer about the orgasm. 'It's about the feeling beyond the orgasm. Like how people may use a substance – a line of cocaine, or a glass of wine – as a gateway.'

* To younger readers who might not know, a fax is a copy of something that appears elsewhere, via a fax machine.

This resonates deeply. When I was drinking, I wasn't drinking to have a drink, per se, I was drinking to get to the emotional state on the other side. 'When it becomes the main form of emotional regulation, that's when porn becomes problematic,' says Burke. Traditionally, she says, this stress release is most appealing to men. 'Oftentimes men won't share if they're stressed. With porn, they can take care of it all by themselves without needing to be vulnerable, or talk to someone.'

Like gambling, it's easily hidden. 'Nobody's going to smell porn on your breath, or see gambling in your pupils,' she says. Moving out from that space of covert stress release requires this: finding other ways to self-soothe. 'There are many other ways to get that release,' she says. 'It's all about finding them.'

I'm going to leave you with one thought, which is not of admonishment but of awareness. As with fast fashion, if we're not paying the true cost of something, often someone else is. Using free walls of porn makes it impossible to differentiate what is ethical porn and what is not; which actors truly consented and which did not. Many actors do it for complex reasons, like addiction, or as a result of coercive control.

If you want your porn with a clean bill of conscience, I've included some places to go in the 'micro tactics'.

Dear little porn addict,

I'd love to say that porn is not a bedfellow of relationship disquiet but, traditionally, the bulk of studies do show a link. When I was planning this chapter out, I even jotted down 'Not necessarily a sign of relationship discontent – research?' but what I found was the opposite.

However, it's not as simple as 'porn is bad for relationships'. Whether it's the cause or effect of relationship strain is unclear. It could be that the uncovering of the porn use has created the discontent, rather than the discontent pre-dating it.

More recent studies have attempted to tease this chronological tangle apart, with many speculating that 'the porn gap' is the cause. The 'porn gap' is where, in hetero set-ups, the man watches more porn than the woman, and the woman is not happy about it.

One 2023 study of 217 couples (both hetero and same-sex) found something incredibly interesting. When porn use was solo and *unknown* by the partner, relational satisfaction was only impacted on the *day* of the porn use. Coupled contentment over the year remained robust, for both parties.

The researchers speculated that this day-of dip was probably due to hiding the porn use, or maybe a disagreement had sparked the porn use, rather than it being a case of 'Now I've seen this preternaturally hot porn star wearing a unicorn horn, I am less satisfied with super-ordinary you.'

It was only when porn use was solo and *known about* (presumably by a disgruntled partner) that the longer-term satisfaction over the year – for both parties – took a sucker punch. This suggests that the porn-user is not less happy in their relationship overall, other than on the day of, unless their porn use is known about. Therefore, porn use itself is not a symptom of deeper disquiet, but the consequences of it being known of, are. This indicates that it's our partner's reaction to porn use that creates the year-on-year satisfactional drift shown in other historic studies, like continents gradually edging apart. How fascinating is that?

I mean, *that* finding would seem to suggest that porn use is best kept covert, which bucks closely held Western 'tell the truth, always' relationship values. Maybe the takeaway is this instead: don't ask if you won't like the answer. Turn a blind eye rather than hoking around in each other's internet histories or policing each other's masturbation choices.

I mean, I'm not about to give up my one moderately sized vibrator, no matter how threatened my partner feels by it (he doesn't). Why would I? It's nothing to do with him, it's zero reflection on my sex life with him and I've owned it for . . . a scary amount of years actually. Um. I should probably replace it.

Another more recent study by Kohut et al found 'consistent evidence that partners who watch pornography together report higher relationship and sexual satisfaction than partners who do not'.

It's up to you to decide what all of this means for you. Your takeaways may be very different from mine. But I do know that these revelations have changed how I think about porn forever.

Love,
Cath x

PORN MICRO TACTICS

Find ethical sources of porn

You will usually have to pay for ethical porn, since actors are definitely paid. JoyBear is a good one for professionally produced porn featuring strong female roles, and was one of the ethical OGs, firing up in 2003. Afterglow is great for ethical porn too.

See Make Love Not Porn or Bright Desire for real couples; on these platforms, couples willingly submit real videos and take half of the profit (this largely removes the supernormal aspect too). Or go to PinkLabel for inclusive ethical porn.

Know that OnlyFans is particularly addictive

Dr Thomas warns of the super-stickiness of OnlyFans. 'It changes the usual dynamic of porn from this person you've never seen before and can never meet,' he says, 'to someone who probably chats to their user base, creating the perceived opportunity that you might one day meet them.' And, therefore, have sex with them. 'It feels like building an actual relationship,' he says, when it's merely a transaction.

While we're here, Professor Natasha Schüll cautions against the emerging hybrids of gambling and porn, given it spearheads both. 'Like the roulette games on porn sites where clothing is removed.'

De-pathologise your use

As we talked about earlier on page 27, the retrospective 'guilt paradox' reduces the pleasure, which hikes up the craving for more, and feels like something ironic that Alanis Morissette might sing about (mind you, most of the things she cited were merely inconvenient).

So, try out this thought experiment: ban phrases like 'bad habit' from your head when you think of your porn use. Of course you like it; we all like to feel titillated, turned on, juicy. The unexpected twist of de-pathologising might be that you want it less.

WiFi limitation

You may *not* be a parent, but the parental controls on your WiFi can be used as adult controls too. For a full two years, I lived in a flat with no access to porn, but had no clue, given I'd never tried to access it. It was only once my boyfriend-of-the-time moved in that this parental blockade was discovered. 'Are you trying to stop me looking at other boobs?' he asked me. No, I was not, but I found it worrying that he saw these boobs as disembodied.

You can temporarily lift these parental controls at certain times if you do want to have the choice of access between, say 10 and 11pm. This is called 'timeboxing', which we talked about on page 127, and is a great moderation hack. It'll mean you can't possibly look for the 'perfect' video, scrolling forever, and will make your porn use much more '90s style.

The side-door hacks

One for when you're trying to refrain. We talked about the 'side door' of interoception earlier; tuning back into our senses and away from the craving. 'If you want a supercharge, just finding five things you can see, or a couple of smells, is an effective hack,' says Sally Hopkins, a recovery mentor at Delamere rehab.

'You can pare it down even further by reaching for a catalyst; using a sharp essential oil such as peppermint, or eating something sweet,' she adds. This tactic feels *basic*, and isn't unlike distracting a child who wants an ice cream with a toy, but if it works – and recovery experts say it does – then who are we to argue?

Find an honest corner

We'll talk on page 258 about why radical honesty is so important when it comes to downregulating compulsive behaviours. Science says it's so, as does the icon of dopamine, Dr Anna Lembke. But, for now, I'll say this. Porn use is very common, as we've established, but, given it's socially sanctioned, overuse can be driven underground, which can only make it darker, more toxic and harder to bring back up to the light.

It could be transformative to have a corner of the world where you can be totally honest about your use, how you feel about it and the impact. Light has a way of making shame recede, which – in turn – makes people feel empowered, rather than stuck.

You may find this radically honest corner by anonymously starting a Reddit thread, dipping into a group on Facebook using an alias or even hitting a SLAA meeting (the Sex and Love version of the 12-steps. You don't have to be a 'big' addict to hit a meeting, and you can go once or twice and then stop; there are no rules).

THE DOPAMINE-HUNTERS

'Dopamine is probably the most famous neurotransmitter in the brain. It has a long history, and a lot of baggage.'

Neuroscientist Dr Kent Berridge

Neuroscientists weren't culturally sexy until recently. I doubt any of us could have even named a neuroscientist until a few years ago, unless you worked in academia, or you're a geek like me. Nowadays, we have neuroscientists holding the sway of celebrities, with millions of followers, ranging from the obvious heavyweight Andrew Huberman and new kid on the block TJ Power, through to Lara Boyd whose TED talk grossed 43 million views, or Tara Swart who goes viral on TikTok with items like 'The reason neuroscientists don't watch the news.'

Neurotransmitters weren't hot topics either. None of us were talking about dopamine at length over a lunch, but now it's part of our daily chat currency. 'Did you hear about Bean? He knits socks and scarves while we detox from our cheap phone dopamine.'

'Dopamine-fasting' programs now sell out, chefs peddle books that claim to recalibrate your reward system and there are thousands of pictures online of 'dopamine tattoos' (a hexagon with two welcoming arms and a zigzagging tail. Feels apt). We all sing along to 'Dopamine' by Franc Moody.

We know by now that dopamine *is* hypnotic, and shapes our behaviour, but we still don't fully understand it, given it's frequently misrepresented as something which makes us happy. 'Dopamine dressing' is about wearing bright colours to spark joy, while 'dopamine homeware' is all smiley faces on spoons. If only I had a tenner for every time I've seen dopamine referred to as the 'pleasure chemical' while researching this book.

As one of my experts said to me, off the record, while I was packing up my stuff:

'Please don't write that dopamine is about us liking stuff.'

'I won't, I know it's not,' I said.

'I see that far too often,' he added, looking weary.

Meanwhile, Dr Clayton Hickey, a neuroscientist and world-class expert in dopamine from the CHBH (Centre for Human Brain Health) at the University of Birmingham, said it *on* the record.

'The worst thing I see in the press is "Oh, yes, you enjoy scrolling your phone because dopamine's released". It's not the way it works,' he said. 'I don't want to see that in your book.'

He's playful, but also serious. I laugh and agree.

Dopamine drives us to repeat a behaviour, and it is agreed to be the lifeblood of the reward system, but it's *not* the neurotransmitter of pleasure. As Dr Korb told us, it's the 'wanting molecule'. The companions that hopefully come alongside it – oxytocin, serotonin, cannabinoids – are what provide the pleasure.

Many years ago now, neuroscientist Dr Marc Lewis told me that 'dopamine is the fuel of desire, not fun'. Reading his book *The Biology of Desire* is how I first got a real grip on what dopamine means, and what addiction truly is. This grip was strengthened by Dr Anna Lembke's *Dopamine Nation*, which millions read, and meant I could finally start talking about dopamine over lunches.

Most of us now understand that dopamine is the fuel of all addiction, which makes sense, given addiction is all about wanting.

'Dopamine is used to measure the addictive potential of any behaviour or drug,' Lembke wrote in *Dopamine Nation*. 'The more dopamine released in the brain's reward pathway . . . and the faster it releases dopamine, the more addictive the drug.'

As we'll learn, fast-release dopamine leaves a gap, rather than filling it. 'Slow dopamine' doesn't create the same gap. We'll get into that more deeply, but let's start by tackling some of the many misconceptions.

MYTH 1: DOPAMINE IS ABOUT LIKING

Liking is different to wanting. Wanting is different to liking. You can want things you don't like. I immediately think of my experiences with a couple of exes. Or my current tic for wanting to watch terrible films about giant prehistoric sharks that terrorise a medical facility full of plucky staff, where one staff member is always a traitor.

Dopamine wasn't even discovered as a neurotransmitter until 1957, making it as young as many Baby Boomers. It was believed that dopamine was a pleasure-chasing lush. But a few decades ago, our understanding of it shifted tectonically, thanks to the work of Dr Kent Berridge and Dr Terry Robinson.

Brace yourselves, animal-lovers, as these experiments are not kind to rats. As Dr Hickey tells me, almost everything we know about dopamine is from animal research. 'This neuro system is tiny; we're talking a couple of cubic millimetres in rats.' He shows me my dopamine receptors on my fMRI (more on this on page 249), which amount to around a cubic centimetre. It's fascinating that something so small can create so much longing.

'Our techniques are really limited in how we can access that in awake, healthy, behaving humans,' he says. 'You can do a little bit using MRI, but if you really want to know, you have to get invasive.'

In their landmark 1989 study, Berridge and Robinson injected a neurotoxin into rats' brains, depleting them of dopamine. Then they offered the dopamine-depleted rats sugary treats, which they would normally rush towards. The rats just sat there, totally uninterested in the food. They would have starved to death. But when the researchers dropped the sugar into the rats' mouths, they found something unexpected: the rats still *liked* it. They just no longer *wanted* it enough to move a few centimetres to get it. The pleasure was still there, but the motivation to obtain it was not.

Wanting and liking can be separate from one another, therefore, which is why those addicted continue to want, even when the liking is long gone.

'Take doomscrolling,' Dr Hickey says. 'Your reward system may have learned it in a context where it provided enjoyment. Back then, it was reinforced in. But now, you no longer like it, you're no longer having fun, but you still want it, so you have a tough time stopping.'

MYTH 2: DOPAMINE IS BAD

Dopamine evolved into existence for a very good reason. If we don't want something, we don't seek it out, so without dopamine we wouldn't seek shelter, food, sex, safety. Our species would have foundered in one generation, without dopamine. In fact, all life forms would have.

'Dopamine was the very first molecule to evolve into our reward system,' says Dr Axel Bouchon, a molecular neuroscientist. He calls dopamine the 'motivation molecule'. 'It's a general superstar because, without motivation, nothing happens.' Insects only have two behavioural molecules, he tells me. One of them is dopamine. 'Lower mammals are completely happy with four,' he says. We have six of note, which we'll return to.

Dopamine is the headline-maker, though. It grabs our brain's attention when something is news-worthy, says neuroscientist Dr Judith Grisel, author of *Never Enough*.

'It tells us that something is hot or interesting or intriguing or tasty or sexy,' she says. 'Dopamine is really the part of the brain that signals meaning, and drops news. Which could also be bad news, by the way.'

Dopamine is also a puzzle-solver when our brain receives a reward it didn't expect. 'In evolutionary terms, an unexpected reward is a really big deal for you as an organism,' says Dr Hickey. 'Something good happened, and now you have to figure out how to get it again. "How did I end up in this fantastic place?" Dopamine is that pervasive brain signal, and it goes everywhere, across big chunks of the brain.'

So, dopamine is a motivational, news-dropping, puzzle-solving kook. Sounds like the equivalent of a smug early riser who writes a blog a day, takes the time to do ice baths and swears by Sudoku.

Dopamine itself is not the problem. When it's pointed in the right direction, and has its vital companions of feelgood molecules such as serotonin and oxytocin, it can create all sorts of beauty. 'A beautiful family

Christmas, for example,' says Dr Bouchon. 'Or it can motivate you to run a marathon.'

'A parent's love for their child comes out of the reinforcement loop it provides,' Dr Hickey adds. 'It's not always a negative outcome.'

So, if dopamine gets us wanting, then up, moving, striving and doing . . . is dopamine the reason I'm writing this chapter on dopamine? I ask him.

'Yes, exactly,' he says.

Dr Alex Korb equates dopamine to money. 'It's like asking, "is money good or bad?"' he explains. 'Well, it all depends on what you spend it on. Dopamine is a tool that your brain uses to get you to do things. The nature of those things depends on whether you point it towards your long-term wellbeing or not.'

MYTH 3: DOPAMINE IS JUST ABOUT 'QUICK HITS'

Dopamine is no dummy – when it's pointed at the right stuff. 'For a fundamental neuro system that is based deep in your brain, where the oldest parts live, it's also very smart,' says Dr Hickey.

In terms of why it evolved, most of all, dopamine is a huge part of how we learn. 'There are other ways of learning that can occur,' he says, 'but when it comes to reinforcement learning, dopamine is critically involved. That type of learning involves phasic responsivity.' 'Phasic' is also the fast type, creating 'the spikes that, when they happen, happen big,' he explains.

When the 'something fantastic' happened, the phasic dopamine response will have cast around your environment to learn why and how it occurred. You notice environmental cues that led to the unexpected reward. These cues then drive your future behaviour, because dopamine has made it likely that you will respond to the cue in a particular way.

'We call this process "incentive salience",' says Dr Hickey. 'Once dopaminergic learning has occurred about these cues, they capture your attention and become very difficult for you to ignore.'

And this is where the problems roll in. 'Hijack' has become a clichéd word when it comes to clickbait articles about dopamine, but my experts use it too.

'Dopamine can get us to do things that are good for us,' Dr Alex Korb told me. 'But that same neural circuitry can be – and is often – hijacked to make us want and do things that aren't in our best interests.'

Dr Hickey demonstrates a cue, by making the sound of a champagne cork. I'm transported back to early recovery, when the 'pop' of a bottle being opened would trigger an involuntary surge of wanting – *hi, dopamine.* I didn't like alcohol any more, but it doesn't mean I didn't want it. Or, more accurately, my dopaminergic learning system wanted it. Recovery for me was about waiting out the want, listening to the dislike instead, until I'd taught my reward system to no longer want it. Now, you could lock me in a vineyard for a weekend and I wouldn't want to drink.

Dopamine learns incrementally. 'The really cool thing about dopamine is that the phasic response gets pushed back as you learn,' says Dr Hickey. The cues become a daisy chain of back-propagation. At the start, it might just be two or three cues, or daisies, that prompt a want, but with much repetition over years, that daisy chain of reinforced learning can become huge.

This can be in a good way. For instance, I've done so much running over the past decade that I now associate everything from a lone sock (my sophisticated in-bra phone holder) to the Left Bank in Paris with my form of physical therapy. A picture of the Seine sparks an urge to want to run alongside it again.

But this clever daisy chain backfires when we take intensely addictive substances, or do highly sticky things. 'At first, a heroin user will learn to associate the syringe with the heroin use, then it's the spoon, then it's a particular location,' says Dr Hickey. 'Dopamine follows that path all the way back.' The cues are added and added, becoming triggers. A lighter might become a trigger too, as well as particular people or getting money from the local cashpoint. Eventually that becomes just any flame, any cashpoint. You can see how it proliferates, extending so that 'want' is everywhere.

Unexpected things can become cues. For someone addicted to methamphetamine (crystal meth), says Dr Hickey, a light bulb can be a trigger. 'If you've smoked meth off an improvised pipe made of a broken light bulb, light bulbs are going to become salient.'

'Overall, it's easier to change your lifestyle and not have a lot of methamphetamine use around you any more,' he says. 'Unless everyone you know and love is also doing meth, which can be the case. But alcohol is really tough always, because it's everywhere, all the time.'

I guess light bulbs are too, but with alcohol there's the smell (a potent cue we underestimate, see pages 34 and 142), sounds of clinks and glugs, supermarket aisles, advertisements, sports sponsorship, clapboards outside pubs saying, 'No great love story ever started with someone eating a salad.' Not to mention other people who urge you to continue drinking.

This is also true of vaping, given the constant physical cues (the shops, the marketing), social nudges ('coming outside?'), and the smell and sounds the units produce (blueberry storm cloud, *vvvvvssssshhhh*).

I would extend that to cannabis too, despite it being illegal. In Brighton, near where I live, you'll constantly spot torn rolling paper packets in bins from smokers making roaches, see sativa leaf merch in shops or catch a plume of hash smoke as you walk past.

Those with process addictions (see page 15) don't get off the hook either. Every advert break seems to feature a gambling app now, whether it's for bet-building or a 'shake to win' gimmick. Gamers probably have some really omnipresent items in their daisy chain, from a certain chair at home to their phone itself. Whereas with shopping – do I need to even say it?

The power of cues means that, when you start to edit them out of the environment, whether culturally or individually, people find it easier to quit. Like when cigarettes were hidden out of sight in shops.

'This is why they've now gotten rid of all marketing on cigarette packets,' says Dr Hickey. That means no sexy logos, no eye-catching colours, no fancy font even. Cigarette packaging is now plain brown, the brand's name in a standardised font, with graphic health warnings – and pictures thereof – as the only imagery.

MYTH 4: PEOPLE GET ADDICTED TO DOPAMINE

It's not the dopamine they're hooked on. It's what the dopamine has learned to want. As we'll loop back to, the dopamine-deficient don't seek out spiky, fast dopamine because they're short on it. They seek it because they're more prone to its spiky phasic learning.

Dopamine's role in learning, and subsequent starring role in addiction, is why addiction is now largely defined as intense learning, but with an undesirable outcome. Dr Julia Lewis, an addiction psychiatrist, told me that if you took the biology alone, addiction is best described as 'abnormal learning'. I've heard 'maladaptive learning' too.

Dr Grisel took exception to it being prefaced with a negative, as did Dr Marc Lewis, who described it as a 'cognitive adaptation', given the brain is just doing what it was designed to. The brain isn't being 'bad', per se, even though the outcome is.

'Your brain doesn't know whether it's developing a new skill or whether it's about to be a bad habit,' neuroscientist Stephanie Borgland once told *Vox*.

'Addiction is most accurately described as a learning hyper ability,' says Dr Grisel. 'It's a perfect example of how terrific the brain is at learning, even though it's learned a self-destructive habit. We learn things more quickly when they're potent and meaningful. And to the brain, drugs are inherently meaningful.'

Consider this reveal of Dr Lembke's, which, for me, was probably the most shocking part of *Dopamine Nation*. 'For a rat in a box,' she wrote, 'chocolate increases the basal output of dopamine in the brain by 55 per cent, sex by 100 per cent, nicotine by 150 per cent and cocaine by 225 per cent.' Meth, meanwhile, increases it by 1,000 per cent.

Sex, at 100 per cent above baseline, is an urge which is absolutely vital for the survival of our species. So, once you consider that artificially created drugs hack a dopamine spike *higher than sex*, you start to understand the problem. You may argue that cannabis is natural, but we talked on page 134 about how it's been manipulated. Cocaine may originate in the coca leaf, but it has been significantly chemically engineered.

'The reward response to these drugs is *so* huge,' says Dr Hickey, 'that you're really overloading this learning system, which is a really critical part of human cognition. I don't think there *is* a more critical part of cognition, actually. Then you get these incredibly strong cue-related phenomena in addiction.'

'If you're taking cocaine, it's wildly influential over you, because your brain never evolved to be in that circumstance, so it has no control over it,' he says. 'A thousand years ago, there was no opportunity to stimulate that system in the same way.'

MYTH 5: WE NEED TO PHASE DOPAMINE OUT

'Dopamine-fasting' as a concept has been misconstrued by many.

'The dopamine system is also responsible for some of the most fundamentally positive experiences in our life,' says Dr Hickey. 'Situations and drugs can manipulate the system in ways that are not great, but it is also deeply involved in the things that allow you to be a whole, happy human being.'

The idea of dopamine-fasting was popularised by Lembke's 2021 *Dopamine Nation*, and it was presented elegantly, in the context of one source of dopamine being phased out, usually that of a big addiction, in order to provide data. Data both to the client about what life is like without their main *thing*, and to Dr Lembke about whether this was the source of most of her client's problems, or masking a co-occurring condition beneath.

But now, people are trying to fast from all 'dopamine hits', which makes no sense. 'You can't "fast" from a naturally-occurring brain chemical,' wrote critic Dr Peter Grinspoon in *Harvard Health Publishing*.

The psychiatrist who coined the term 'dopamine fast', Dr Cameron Sepah, backpedalled on it himself to *The New York Times* in 2019, saying that it was a headline only, not a realistic lifestyle choice. '[It] is just a mechanism that explains how addictions can become reinforced, and makes for a catchy title. The title's not to be taken literally.'

Dr Sepah suggested 'stimulation fast' as an alternative title, to capture overstimulating activities including drugs, gaming, gambling or porn (basically, all of the 'sticky eight' in this book).

'When we overstimulate with dopamine, we do make ourselves less sensitive,' says Dr Grisel. This sounds like a good thing, but it's not. 'It means you need more, an extra cup, an extra swipe, to feel the same satisfaction. In young people who are still forming their dopamine system, this overstimulation could maybe even dampen the sensitivity permanently. Almost like losing a certain frequency of sound, which you then can't detect later.'

She's in favour of fasting, saying, 'I think monks probably enjoy life more than people who are stimulated all the time. The problem is, though, do you reset things only to go overboard again?' Not many of us are going to fast to monastic levels and stay there.

This over/underdoing it seems to be a trend, writes Dr Grinspoon. 'Unfortunately, legions of people have misinterpreted the science, as well as the entire concept of a dopamine-fast. People are viewing dopamine as if it was heroin or cocaine, and are fasting in the sense of giving themselves a 'tolerance break' so that the pleasures of whatever they are depriving themselves of – food, sex, human contact – will be more intense or vivid when consumed again, believing that depleted dopamine stores will have replenished themselves. Sadly, it doesn't work that way at all.'

I asked Lembke about the widespread binge-purge-binge-purge misinterpretation, where people see it as a way to reset the pleasure an activity or substance brings them.

'This is a real danger of fasting of any kind,' she wrote to me. 'It happened to me when I went back to reading romance novels after a month away. Sometimes called the abstinence violation effect. You see it in rats too, and I believe that's all in the book. It still doesn't defeat the point. Some people will benefit from a dopamine-fast, others will not. You don't know until you've tried it, and the experience alone provides a wealth of data to inform next steps.'

Unhealthy binge-purge cycle aside, I have the utmost respect for Dr Lembke's work, but don't think that 'dopamine-fasting' is the right term for how society has interpreted Lembke's idea. I think it was apt to begin with, in the original context of *one* type of fast dopamine, but we now need a name that's not a misnomer, if it's more of an overarching life overhaul.

We can fast from one stream of dopamine, or a few, but we can't fast from *all* dopamine. That's not only impossible, it's also undesirable. Because, as we've covered, dopamine is how we get up in the morning, why we strive, why we work, why we eat, why we see people. There's no life without dopamine. For us non-academics, I think it's an important distinction to make. The acute irony is, without dopamine, a dopamine-fast would never even occur.

That's why, in this book, we'll talk about 'dopamine-shifting' instead of fasting. Not as catchy, but a lot more accurate.

With little addictions, given we may be editing down several forms of fast dopamine, we should aim to replace that overstimulation with slow dopamine. This may have happened naturally, regardless, but if you do it consciously, you'll feel much better.

The dopamine shift

What exactly is fast dopamine? The 'sticky eight' of this book were all mentioned to *The New York Times* by Dr Sepah. Dr Grisel and I identified these eight – together – as the most addictive substances and processes. TJ Power agrees with these too in *The DOSE Effect,* calling them 'quick dopamine' (although he doesn't include gaming and funnels overall phone use down to 'social media'). The rest of the items in this book are also fast (excluding people-pleasing, procrastination and judgement & gossip, which are more behavioural), just less so.

You'll often see fast dopamine referred to as 'cheap dopamine'. That's a misnomer too, as it's the most expensive sort. Anyone who knows what they're talking about will use a different term. Dr Alex Korb refers to the nuance as 'short-term' or 'long-term' dopamine, while TJ Power uses 'quick' or 'slow'.

The reason fast dopamine is so expensive is the subsequent price tag. 'As the laws of physics explain,' TJ Power writes in *The DOSE Effect*, 'what goes up, must come down. Your brain and body are always seeking something called "homeostasis", which simply means balance. With this in mind, when dopamine levels increase incredibly fast . . . the brain thinks, "Wow, how are my dopamine levels so high?" In order to achieve homeostasis, or balance, the dopamine then has to quickly drop an equal amount below our baseline level in order to rebalance, making you feel even worse than before.'

In short, fast dopamine gives us a spiky surge, followed by a crashing low, which makes us feel terrible. We often seek to anaesthetise this discomforting deficit by reaching for more of the – or another – source of fast dopamine. Eventually, the reward system becomes burned out. With big addictions, this leads to something called 'anhedonia', which Dr Anna Lembke defines as 'the inability to enjoy pleasure of any kind.'

I've read that anhedonia usually hits around the same time that we think we need our drug or process in order to live. Indeed, I remember alcohol feeling as vital to me as oxygen. 'Human brains can confuse the need for a drug for survival,' Dr Lembke says neatly.

To get away from this spike-crash cycle, we need to dopamine-shift. By reaching for things that trigger a slow release of dopamine instead, which here we'll shorten as 'slow dopamine'.

When I ask Dr Lembke for specific examples of these, she tells me to refer to her *Dopamine Nation Workbook* for them, so I'll repeat some of those 'slow dopamine' sources here.

> **Slow dopamine:** Being in nature, washing the car, spending time with animals, meditating, cooking, saying we're sorry, exercising in moderation, writing thank-you notes, talking to a stranger, reading a book, making music, walking or cycling instead of driving, caring for children, decluttering, reaching out to old friends or relatives, telling the truth, ice-water plunges and gardening.

You'll notice that all of these require some sort of delayed gratification (sorting your wardrobe, having the guts to talk to random people, planting seeds), physical sacrifice (cold water! Tired legs) or mental grit (sustained concentration, or asking for forgiveness), which is part of why they work. Dr Lembke writes that when we lean into a little bit of pain, it amplifies the pleasure, leveraging the science of 'hormesis'.

But, most of all, these sources don't place us on the dopamine roller coaster.

While doing them, 'our dopamine levels rise slowly over the latter half of the activity,' she writes, 'and remain elevated for hours afterward before going back down to baseline, without ever going below baseline.'

Above baseline is where you want to stay, mostly or entirely.

The self-control daisy chain

Self-control, c/o dopamine, can be *the* thing that creates the massive daisy chain of learning. Daisies are probably too fragile a metaphor for something so powerful, but let's go with it.

To illustrate this, Dr Hickey uses the example of my writing books to demonstrate, given this is my sixth one. 'The back-propagation here is the control,' he says. 'You've had to control yourself again and again, and the reward of producing a book has reinforced that control.' Your brain learns that self-control eventually leads to an ultimate reward. Just as my brain once learned to associate the wine bottle – the pop of a cork – then any restaurant – then any drink being poured – then any glass – with having alcohol. It's the same system of back-propagation learning; it's just re-angled towards a more healthy pursuit.

'You learn to break the million things you have to do to write a book into sub goals,' he says. 'The longer your task is, the more delayed the gratification is, and the more difficult it is for the reward signal to back-propagate.'

I have to say, my reward system is enjoying all of this praise. *Again, again,* it chants. *Look at all the 'giant shark' films I didn't watch!* it says.

He has some words that speak to my shark film habit. 'There are so many things that we do, where we think "Oh shit, why am I doing this?"' he says. 'We think, "I know better than this. I know it's not going to cause me any pleasure." But you've learned a response. The only way to get away from that response is to start to establish control over it. And that control is going to be reinforced by the positive outcome, so it gets easier.'

We learn a different type of daisy chain. One of delay and restraint leading up to a supersized reward.

Those with a naturally lower baseline

Many of us have a lower 'tonic' rate of dopamine. This is our baseline dopamine, which we can't change without pharmacological intervention.

Plenty of clinical evidence links ADHD and autism with dopamine dysfunction. Whether this means a lower basal tone remains to be uncovered, but some experts speculate that it might. Other conditions, such as restless leg syndrome or depression, have also been linked to low dopamine.

Whether the source of lower baseline dopamine is neurodivergence or not, it's not as simple as low tone = fast phasic dopamine-seeking, although it does often manifest that way.

'Just saying "you're short on dopamine so you need to find more . . ." it's not really that,' says Dr Grisel. 'It's that if you have a low signature tonic rate and you get a big rise via a burst of phasic dopamine, you're more sensitive to those stimuli. The phasic dopamine will be more meaningful to you because of that bigger gap between the two. This can lead to more risk-taking, more novelty-seeking and a person possibly more prone to addiction.'

Dr Hickey agrees. 'With higher tonic dopamine rates, they get less firing of the cells in response to environmental stimuli,' he says. In layperson speak, they're less distracted by cues to consume, whether it's a shop or a cake. 'They learn less, which is some sort of control structure. The higher tonic rate inhibits the exploratory learning response.'

Ergo, those with higher tonic dopamine rates are less likely to 'learn' addiction.

Irrespective of whether it's down to dopamine, we know that there's a massive Venn overlap between neurodivergence and addiction. Adults with ADHD are three times more likely to experience addiction than those without ADHD. Meanwhile, a University of Cambridge study found that, while autistic adults are less likely to use drugs like alcohol or cannabis, when they do, they are *nine times* more likely to use these substances to self-medicate, particularly dampening autism-related symptoms such as sensory overload, or even using/drinking to provide the comfort of routine.

When I ask Dr Lembke about this link, she said, 'Funny you should ask.' Turns out she's received 'quite a few' letters of late about this, about individuals with autism. 'These families are describing out-of-control self-stimulation behaviours that sound a lot like addiction.'

It might be that addiction *is* an attempt at stimming. It's just that, rather than a fidget toy or hair twirling, drugs and processes get picked up instead.

Molecular imbalance is cresting

I'm going to call it now. I think the next big thing in our collective hotness for neuroscience will be molecular balance. This balance-seeking is what TJ Power's book (*The DOSE Effect*, with DOSE standing for dopamine, oxytocin, serotonin and endorphins) dives into, and it's also the backbone of Dr Axel Bouchon's life work, which has manifested in the *Matter Neuroscience* app.

Remember how Dr Bouchon said that insects are sustained by two molecules, lower mammals are all about four and we have six? That.

'Dopamine is the first, then you have testosterone, oxytocin, cannabinoids, serotonin and opioids,' he adds. His work is all about 'what's the qualifier of the dopamine?' Dopamine alone – or even with one other molecule – does not make us feel happy or complete.

He gives the example of us being driven to make more money, or succeed at work, above all else. 'That is only triggering two molecules,' he says. 'Dopamine and serotonin, or motivation and pride/recognition. In a way, this is our economy developing us backwards. We are at the level of ants if we are only winning at work.'

'We are built for the hexagon,' he says, impassioned, and I believe him. That's why he co-created the *Matter Neuroscience* app, to show people how to find the hexagon of hitting all six.

'If you look at my metadata,' he says, 'you'll see that I'm really topped up on family love (oxytocin), given I spend a lot of time with my three daughters, but I have a huge deficit in cannabinoids, which are mainly triggered by friends and pleasure. I have work to do,' he says. But at least he knows where to point himself.

Even if all you do is see the 'want' of the dopamine and delay its gratification, you're already on your way to more molecular balance, Dr Bouchon says. 'The dopamine says, "I want to do this". If you go silent and watch it, you've already brought in some serotonin because you're proud you've resisted it.' If only for a little while.

The rats who try to eat the light

Meanwhile, Dr Hickey is testing ideas from the King of Dopamine, Kent Berridge, using human neuroimaging.

He tells me that the next big thing to break will be all about dopaminergic learning, which – as you'll recall – can lead to addiction. And it involves rats who try to eat lights.

I never thought I'd relate to a rat, given I don't eat from the floor and I don't *love* sewers, but in this context I do.

'What you have is two types of rat in the Skinner Box,' (see page 32 for a refresher) he says. 'The light goes on, the food comes out. After a while, the animal goes nuts just when the light's coming on. Then we see these two different types of behaviours.'

'Goal-tracking' rats, who approach where the food comes out, and 'sign-tracking' rats, who approach the light. You can actually breed rats to favour either.'

'You have these rats trying to eat the light,' he says. 'And they're the ones with the biggest dopamine response to it.' Therefore, their learning is more based on dopamine than the 'goal-tracker' rats, and this learning then drives their behaviour. The light-eaters are the ones who become highly addicted, he says.

'I have a feeling I would try to eat the light,' I say.

'Me too,' he laughs. 'Which is why I'm careful with drugs and alcohol, because it's in my nature and family history, and trying to eat the light is a huge predictor for addiction.'

This twofold dopaminergic learning bias could unlock the mystery as to why some people do a whole bunch of cocaine and never want it again, he says.

'And others do a little bit of cocaine and then want it for the rest of their lives.' Us light-eaters, we're just really, really good at learning via dopamine.

'Actually, it was Terry Robinson who developed a lot of this work,' Dr Hickey says, championing the lesser-sung hero of the pair of Berridge & Robinson. And, as I'm sure you'll agree, it sounds like this 'eat the light' research could lead to a major breakthrough in the addiction world.

Don't regret your sensitivity

I ask Dr Grisel a question I pretty much already know the answer to. Can we change our tonic rate of dopamine?

'I don't think so, no,' she says. 'Can I ask you a question?'

'Please do,' I reply.

'You would want to make it higher, so that you're not as turned on by these stimuli?'

'Exactly,' I say. *Make me less sticky, please.*

I recently found out I'm neurodivergent, and although I'm still processing my exact flavour and have only told about six people, it feels like she somehow intuits this whenever she responds.

'Yes, it's true that, given some of us are more sensitive to these things, it also means we're more prone to addiction,' she says, her heart in her voice. 'But it also means that we're more sensitive to value. Maybe we're sitting ducks – you could make that point. But I do think that this kind of hearing, seeing, feeling sensitivity can be a *good thing*.'

She's right, I think, and so this perspective flip may comfort you, if you too are sticky and/or neurodivergent. The way we learn quickly, our sensitivity to our environment, to people, our ups and downs, our desire to eat the light . . . can mean bad things happen, like we become addicted. But it can also mean that we become society's canaries – hearing and sensing that which passes others by. We experience the greater falls, but also the greater rises.

Personally, now that I really think hard about it . . . I wouldn't change it.

DOPAMINE-SHIFTING CHEAT SHEET

1. Pay attention to how fast vs slow feels

'For a healthy reward system, you're looking for all-round contentment rather than specific over-excitement about one thing,' says addiction psychotherapist Chris Lomas, of Delamere rehab centre.

He says that fast dopamine has a slick of unease to it, comparing it to when we were kids and going to a theme park the next day. 'Those pre-roller-coaster jitters and longing were not necessarily pleasurable,' says Lomas. 'Physiologically, they could even be interpreted as nervousness. The excitement almost makes you feel a little sick.'

'Excitement is great,' he adds, 'but there seems to be a cost to that, and it's a cost that doesn't exist for contentedness. That nervous feeling you get from that type of dopamine is very different to walking on a beach and feeling contented, serene and hopeful.'

2. Be prepared to be a little bored

Whenever you're dopamine-shifting away from the shorter-term, faster fixes, your brain may well buck with boredom.

'The things that sustain us in a certain, steady, long-term way are less interesting to us,' says Dr Korb. Not unlike the job we've had for five years, or the person we've been married to for ten.

3. Picking new 'slows' as a counter

Newness lengthens the dopamine's effects, Dr Bouchon says. 'New things are the best. The surprise effect gives you an extra portion of dopamine. It's like a puzzle where we have to get as many different types of dopamine input into our lives as possible.' Because, once you do, you can't desensitise to it. 'With lots of little dopamine inputs, there's always enough times for the receptors to go back to zero and become sensitive again,' he says. The Matter Neuroscience app that Bouchon co-created seeks to help us do this, among other lovely life-affirming things. The 'fifty tiny cogs' method we talked about on page 92 will also work here.

4. Slow dopamine is device-free

Sorry, poppets. In the 'slow dopamine' activities she lists, Dr Lembke is careful to write 'unplugged', 'unplugged', 'unplugged' over and over next to them. Try walking through a forest only listening to the wind in the trees, or gardening without catching up on a podcast. She didn't define that the reading had to be unplugged, however, so I'm guessing a Kindle is just fine.

5. Redirect dopamine via list-making

'Just before we meet a set goal, we experience a surge of dopamine,' says Lomas, 'which helps us set *even more* goals.' This is why list-writing and ticking works. 'It can be a tremendous upwards spiral, once you get going.' Dr Hickey agrees, suggesting splitting big goals into lots of tiny sub-goals to leverage this.

6. Timebox the 'fasts' into a narrow window

If you want to keep some fasts in a limited way, which you probably do, that's totally cool. Maybe try timeboxing them, though, as per Nir Eyal's behavioural strategy (see page 117). Dr Lembke is also a fan of this tactic, and cites a study on rats (always with the poor rats), which found that when they're given access to cocaine for six hours a day, they'll hammer it so hard they'll eventually kill themselves. Whereas when their use is restricted to a narrow window of one hour a day, their usage remains consistent. They don't increase it day-on-day.

Let's be crystal clear; I'm not endorsing the use of cocaine for one hour a day. God, no. But we can take this timeboxed window-narrowing strategy and use it for other *safe* sources of fast dopamine.

JUDGEMENT & GOSSIP

There's a little ritual I do every morning that I would love to recommend to you all.

I hop out of bed, yawn luxuriously, chop a lemon, flick the kettle on, lay out my yoga mat, don't do any yoga, ignore the lemon, then sit and drink the fattest coffee my AeroPress can make.

After a good half hour of staring into space, I go out into the world to run my dog, and the first thing I do as soon as I see other humans is this: judge one of them.

I can find almost anything to judge. It's really a skill. Maybe they're driving too slowly or too fast – judged. Maybe their two-year-old is clutching a packet of sweets – judged!

This very morning, I saw a smiling man walk towards me. *Oh no*. He was wearing a T-shirt I disapproved of, given its very visible logos. (My logos are also visible, but daintier.) He had a neck tattoo, and even though I also want a neck tattoo (of a pretty swallow) this ink was the wrong sort and on the wrong part of his neck. He had a Rottweiler and, as all Rottweiler owners do, claimed it was a 'sweetheart' when it bounced up to my dog, who is handily scared of all things in the world *except* for other dogs potentially wishing him harm.

I can report that the dog was not a sweetheart. But the man was, and I left our encounter feeling downright cheerful.

Judging ourselves for judging

Obviously, I'm not serious. I dislike how judgemental I am. Who do I think I am, the grand ombudsman of T-shirts, tattoos and dog breeds?

The person I judge the most harshly is myself. I will shake my head, as if I can shake the thought from it. I wonder if I'm going to be one of those people who gets the face I deserve, given my thoughts are not constant sunbeams. Maybe I should get a neck tattoo of a Rottweiler instead, as penance.

Thankfully, psychotherapist Hilda Burke has some comforting words for me. 'I go on retreats and, within the first five minutes, there'll always be someone who really irritates me,' she says. 'Like a tech bro with a man bun and tie dye T-shirt, who's trying to get in touch with his inner spiritual guru.' She'll spend the first few days bristling, only to find that 'that very person is often my favourite person at the end.'

'Our ego doesn't like it when we're wrong, but our hearts like it,' she says. (Mawww. I love that. Put that on a tie-dye T-shirt and sell it to the man with the bun.)

We all have inherent biases, Burke says. 'Someone carrying a bottle of water and a plastic bag might activate your planet anxiety. Or someone with a lot of Botox, reading someone commercial we wouldn't read.'

The hack, she says, is to try to restrict our judgements to actual behaviours, rather than outward trappings. Looking beyond clothes, accents, piercings, jobs – whatever it may be that's giving us unfair pause – and seeing what they *do* instead. 'If they've slammed a door in your face rather than held it, then fair enough,' she says. 'But do get curious as to why you've taken such an instant dislike, as it'll usually reveal something interesting about yourself.'

As usual, judgement evolved for excellent reasons. 'Being judgemental is just an extension of making judgement calls,' Burke says. 'And judgement calls were essential. *They're friendly, they're threatening, that's poisonous, that's health-giving* . . . Where it becomes mutated in the modern day, however, is when we engage in collective pile-ons – trial by social media, when people weigh in without having all the facts.'

I'll never forget reading Professor Paul Dolan's take on judgement, in his book *Happy Ever After: A radical approach to living well.* It was a sentence that rearranged my brain, forever impacting how I do life. He said that doling out judgement carries a compulsively addictive neuroscientific reward. 'There are now a range of brain-imaging studies,' he wrote, 'to show that we feel pleasure when we can punish those who do not conform to what we expect of them.' I immediately thought of a car horn.

The inaccurate pinking of gossip

Gossip is unfairly gendered. We often think of a gossip as a curtain-twitcher who berates number 48's flowerbeds as a 'disgrace' (I live at number 48 and my flower beds *are* a disgrace) or her younger trope, the 'U OK babes?' commenter who then sets up a WhatsApp splinter group called 'Debbie is not OK'.

This is nonsense. Men gossip just as much, found a University of California study, which attached audio recorders to 500 people. Both genders spent on average 52 minutes a day talking about people who weren't present, the study found.

'I love a gossip,' says psychotherapist Josh Fletcher, author of *And How Does That Make You Feel?* A gossip is generally 'here's why we're better than them' disguised in a chat about others' personal lives, which is why he believes we like it.

'We all enjoy feeling superior to others, and this is reflected in the British media's cycle of building people up, then tearing them down,' says Fletcher. We are keen voyeurs to this spectacle of love-bomb/devalue, particularly when it involves preternaturally gorgeous or talented celebrities. 'Because we then feel reassured that they're only human too,' he says.

This sanctioned bloodsport of the Western press is undeniable; think of the millions who read the *MailOnline*'s Sidebar of Shame (I'll happily out myself as a former reader). We're the hunt; celebrities are the fox.

Nowadays we've lost the '90s-style red circles around cellulite or zoomed-in signs of hair transplants, but the take-down is still there; it's just sewn into euphemisms such as 'steps out in a daring dress', subtexted in commentary about a 'very quick' rebound, or imbued in the editorial choice to print the very worst pictures their long-lens paparazzo took.

The court of gossip

Before courts doled out sentences, or people were pelted with fruit in stocks (I still can't believe that happened) gossip served a crucial role in hunter-gatherer world; it kept people in line.

There were larger punishments for stealing a goat skin or a partner, but they needed a slap on the wrist for smaller social infractions such as slacking on vegetable-digging duty, or lying about eating the last fig. And judgement and gossip were it.

Language evolved for information swapping, but equally important was gossip. 'Our language evolved as a way of gossiping,' Professor Yuval Noah Harari writes in *Sapiens*. 'It is not enough for individual men and women to know the whereabouts of lions and bison. It's much more important for them to know who in their band hates whom. Who is sleeping with whom. Who is honest and who is a cheat.'

'Social co-operation is our key for survival and reproduction,' he writes, and gossip was how it was achieved, with Harari calling it a 'much-maligned ability, which is in fact essential for co-operation in large numbers.' It's how our bands of a few dozen were able to enlarge to bands of hundreds. 'The gossip theory may sound like a joke, but numerous studies support it,' he concludes.

The tribe needed a shared consciousness of what was right and what was wrong. A shared constellation of meaning. And gossip helped it achieve that.

Common enemy intimacy

Let's talk about the darker side of gossip: venting. Also known as 'bitching', but that implies only females do it (given a bitch is a female dog), so let's not.

The darkest part: the person we choose to vent *to* is often someone also very close to the person we're venting *about*. It's a shady triangle of what experts call 'common enemy intimacy'. The two venters feel drawn closer together, but it's an illusion.

'It feels like you've created an alliance,' says psychotherapist Anna Mathur, author of *The Uncomfortable Truth*. 'But we're fools if we think that, in this set-up, the same isn't happening once our backs are turned.' It frays trust, rather than building true intimacy, because you will then always wonder, will they, or *do they* do the same to me?

Oftentimes, if we're in a triangle of sorts, the person who holds the most power in the triangle can act as a double agent. In my twenties, I was in a friendship trio with two other women. The alpha of our group nicknamed our other friend (who wasn't the brightest crayon in the box, it's true), 'the amoeba'. I laughed along, even though it left a bad taste in my mouth. It made me feel chosen, special, elevated to ascended status (of not being a single-celled organism?! Lofty), given the alpha clearly thought I was smarter than our other friend. I later found out what my nickname was, also chosen by the alpha. 'The amoeba' told me. I won't print it here, but it was infinitely worse.

In the moment of common enemy intimacy (let's call it CEI), we feel an illicit buzz, hence the brain-imaged pleasure we talked of earlier. It's almost next door to a turn-on, but instead of a twitch of the hips, you feel a twitch in your lips. *I shouldn't, but.* 'It can often be veiled as concern,' says Mathur. 'But we all know what we're doing.'

I've wrapped CEI in 'worried about them', for sure, but also 'just to check I'm not overreacting' or 'I don't know what to do, can you help?' You'll know when you've engaged in CEI by how you feel afterwards, says Mathur. 'You'll feel a bit dirty. The conversation wasn't constructive.'

This is also known as the Karpman drama triangle, says Burke, where one person is the victim (the one venting), one is the aggressor (the absent subject of the vent) and the listener is the rescuer. You can collapse this triangle quite easily, she says, by empowering the victim. 'Asking "could you speak up about that to them?", inviting them to make a different choice, or "how does it serve you to still have that person as a friend?" are good ways to break the pattern.'

Even if you've always done things a certain way, you can still choose to do them differently.

The climactic release

Our motives for judgement or gossip towards loved ones aren't evil, although the product can look that way.

Usually, we feel mistreated, or angry, or hurt, and this rant is a release, a climactic discharge, like lightning. Our resentment towards that particular person or thing builds up, up, up – just like storm pressure building – and then, KAZAM! We release it. But not without harm.

There is a third option, beyond talking to the person vs talking about them. It borrows from both Buddhism and traditional recovery philosophies. And that's getting curious as to why this bothers you so much, as Burke suggested. An outsized reaction usually means it pushes on a decades-deep wound. Maybe what they did made you feel unimportant (they ignored my birthday!) and as a result you feel the urge to release that discomfort. But why does feeling unimportant create that climactic build-up within you? That's the real question, which could have the power to soften its growl.

Maybe you were neglected or ignored as a child and, therefore, feeling seen and heard is crucial as an adult. Or maybe you've lied to partners in the past but are now reformed, thus your flash of judgement towards others' lying is more of a reflection on how you feel about your former self, rather than the person it's being directed towards right now. (*Well, hello,* projection.)

I loathe the phrase 'if you spot it, you've got it', but maybe there's some truth underneath it? 'It's become a cliché, but yeah,' says Burke, 'if we're hating on someone, there's usually an element of ourselves that we're hating on too. As attributed to Carl Jung almost a century ago: "Everything that irritates us about others can lead us to an understanding of ourselves".'

Hanlon's Razor also potentially feeds in here. 'Never attribute to malice that which is adequately explained by stupidity,' said Robert J Hanlon. Almost nobody is walking around the world intentionally trying to piss you off. I know, I find that surprising too, but apparently it's true. We're all mostly just blundering about, trying the best we can.

Dear little judgement and gossip addict,

We've now spoken of judgement and gossip with loved ones, but what about acquaintances?

Enter: 'the narcissism of small differences' – a fascinating theory first posited by Sigmund Freud, whereby the setting we meet in determines if we become fast friends or mortal enemies.

We'll take a theoretical case study. Let's call him Brian. So, if you were both teenagers with a Saturday job in a supermarket, you and Brian might become fast friends, due to your shared love of heavy metal and smoking weed.

But if you met on the metalhead scene, perhaps at a gig, and hung out in a larger group of other metalheads, you and Brian might become nemeses. You might judge and run down Brian, and he you.

Maybe because he rates Metallica and you think Iron Maiden rules forever OK, and so you fall out over 'the narcissism of small differences', because in this nuanced niche of the world, your small differences look larger.

This is what happens in groups that bond at university or college and reunite continuously over decades. I constantly see it in the sober world too. I bet this happens in retirement communities. I look forward to meeting my retirement nemesis (come at me, Brenda). And on and on it goes.

If you met in a different world setting, you'd probably really like each other, rather than care that they're uptight about splitting the bill and you're not, or they did AA and you didn't, or they heckle the bingo caller and you don't.

Once we know about this psychological quirk, the minutiae can become a little easier to let go of. I know learning of it helped me.

Love,
Cath x

JUDGEMENT & GOSSIP MICRO TACTICS

Think about what you're consuming

What goes in often comes out. When I was at my absolute *twattiest*, I was consuming a lot of gossip columns. Mostly Lainey, who is admittedly hilarious, but back in the late 2000s, was also vicious. She used to call Jessica Biel 'Stage 5 Clinger', Tom Cruise 'Xenu' as a reference to his Scientology membership, his then wife Katie Holmes 'RoboBride', Ryan Phillippe (of the original *Cruel Intentions*) 'Carb Face' and Ryan Reynolds 'Foundation Face'.

She's reformed now, and these old articles carry a disclaimer of: 'This article was posted during an early period of the site when some of the writing was extremely offensive. Since then, our site has grown and evolved.'

Once I realised this 'input/output' connection, I switched to more right-on sources of mindless comfort reading, such as recovery bloggers and mindbodygreen. And, OK fine, I might have believed in auras and numerology for a minute there, but I also became a much nicer person.

Be prepared for a cost of disengaging

Idle gossip goes dark when secrets about others are shared like currency. When information-gathering about others becomes a way of wielding power. *Did she?!* Or *I can't believe he . . .*

'Disengaging from gossip once lost me a friendship,' says Mathur. 'All she wanted to do was talk about others within the group; that was our dynamic. Once I stopped, and asked her to stop too, our friendship ended. It was painful.' This loss of a shared language can nix any warmth you once shared. There may be a cost, and if you're going to stop, be prepared to pay it.

Notice who are the firestarters

Some vents are necessary, says Mathur, but she adds the caveat: 'Choose well who you offload to.' You want someone who puts a fire blanket on your anger, rather than someone who chucks petrol over it.

'I rant to my best friend about my husband,' she says, 'but she knows and loves him, while also loving me and knowing I'm not perfect.' Mathur says to look for those who feel like a balm, broaden your perspective and ideally will have the guts to challenge you. 'After a healthy vent, you should be nudged along in the narrative, "I know what I'm going to say to them now" or "I know why I feel that way",' she says. Instead of the vent keeping you stuck and making you angrier, it's moved you through.

Strike lightning that does the opposite of harm

Every night I do something called a 'lightning inventory' as part of my gratitude listing, which I once heard about in a 12-step meeting. A lightning inventory is a quick, sharp 'here's where I could have done better today, here's why I think it happened and here's how I'll try to handle it next time'.

This nightly accountability stops me from spiralling off into a judgey rant about someone, or a passive-aggressive gossip, as I own my part when things go sideways.

I also record all the things I did *well* that day, for some self-esteem-warming balance.

Try a 'rage page'

The root of 'resent' is 'feel again' and indeed, sometimes I do feel a resentment over and over again, again, no matter how many times I vent, or try to get underneath it, soften it, earth it.

I've written before about 'fuck you letters', a rageful letter that you never send. This suggestion from a recovery friend proved to be one of the most useful tools I've ever picked up. Now it's evolved to become a 'rage page' that lives on my desktop. It's always empty, because I hammer away furiously into the document and then – I raze it. It's about releasing it, not keeping it.

The 'behave' mantra

This comes from Jerome Fagan, the ex-priest proficient in banter from Delamere rehab. 'Nowadays, whenever I start my car or enter a supermarket, I repeat this one-word mantra: "Behave",' he says. 'It reminds me not to get annoyed if I have to wait at roadworks or in queues at the till, and to not send people negative energy.'

I now use Jerome's mantra and it's mischievously powerful. It feels self-flagellating upon first try but is actually self-care, given we're only ruining our own day by getting wound up.

They're in stories we know not of

The emotional antonym to judgement – and its offshoot, gossip – is empathy. And to summon it, I try to remember that there is so much about people's lives we don't know about. Obviously, this applies to strangers, but also people we know well.

Maybe that road rager is grieving a parent? Maybe your friends who last-minute bailed on your big party just lost a baby and they're not telling people?

Empathy tenderises affront. Fact.

Try this social experiment

Only say good things about other people for one day, even the ones who wind you up the very most. *One little day.* You can do that, I know you can. See how you feel. It's just an experiment, not a lifelong commitment. I'll be over here, trying it too.

DATING, FLIRTING & SEX

I was once so addicted to dating that my friends christened me a 'love monkey', given I would merely swing from partner to partner. I was once the flirtiest flirt in Flirtville, who would often get into misunderstandings, as everyone thought I wanted to shag them. And I once had a lot more sex than is considered polite, but if I had been a man, it would have been just fine.

I discovered in my recovery from drinking the world that I was a bona fide love addict too, which is why I took a full year off dating, flirting, sex and even holding hands – get me to a nunnery – because I needed an intervention, and I staged it on myself. Because everyone else was too chicken to talk to me about it, or thought that I might try to shag them if they did.

During that year off, which I wrote about at length in *The Unexpected Joy of Being Single*, I can sum up my discovery in one word: validation. I realised that the reason I was flirting and dating voraciously was because I was entirely dependent upon external validation. I didn't have any inner source of validation. If you'd opened me up, you would have found emptiness where batteries should have been. That year ended up being mostly about creating that internal power source.

Inside that fun Easter egg was another finding. I also discovered I was hooked on the chase – a hunter for sport rather than sustenance – and *thought* I wanted to get married, but also ran from anyone who actually wanted to marry me, or went cold myself once I converted someone from unsure to sure, because of the 'paradox of choice'. We'll come back to that.

For now, rest assured that whatever you've done in your little dating, flirting or sex addiction, I've probably done worse. As the recovery saying goes, if you've shagged a zebra, somebody has always shagged two.

Dating apps are like fruit machines

We covered a lot of the 'apps are like gambling' ground in the Our Phones chapter from page 108, but dating apps are insanely addictive because they're like fruit machines, where people are the fruit, their desires the sinkhole of randomness we get sucked into. We swipe for more chances to win in the bottomless lucky dip of people.

The reason dating apps are some of the highest-grossing apps of all time is simple. They take a remodelled Skinner box, throw in ultra-variable rewards (page 33), and then mix it up in a cocktail shaker with one of our most powerful primal drivers – our inherent desire for romance and partners to have intercourse with. I would argue that, of all social apps, dating apps are the most addictive – the data certainly suggests so – and my screen time when I was on them (six hours total on a bad day, two of those on dating apps) can attest to it too.

This is why app creators are now finding themselves in the dock, with lawsuits filed against them. A lawsuit filed in California against the likes of Tinder and Hinge claimed that these apps 'employ recognised dopamine-manipulating product features' to turn users into 'gamblers locked in a search for psychological rewards'.

The plaintiffs clearly have a healthy sense of humour, since they filed their lawsuit on Valentine's Day. Match Group has denied the claims and called them 'ridiculous' with 'zero merit'.

Slogans such as 'designed to be deleted' are sweet and all, but the fact remains that the apps wouldn't survive if all of us logged on for a month, found our forever, then logged off for the rest of our lives. That may well have been their intention upon creation of the app – I want to believe it was – but it's not what actually happens.

This is because of the 'paradox of choice'. Coined by psychologist Barry Schwartz, this captures a uniquely modern problem. In a nutshell, an overabundance of choice can lead to final-decision paralysis, as well as dissatisfaction with that which we actually choose. What a lovely double whammy.

There are many studies proving this phenomenon, whether we're choosing jam or jeans, but evolutionary psychologist Dr Andrew Thomas cites one on dating apps themselves. 'When people were given just five dating profiles to pick from, they were more satisfied with their choice than those who had been given 20 profiles to choose from.' Twenty is obviously a tiny amount. So why don't you multiply that dissatisfaction by a few hundredfold and you might have our current predicament.

You may remember that we heard from neuroscientists, as well as Dr Thomas, already (see page 27) about our brain's design being the same as it was when we lived in tight-knit communities of maybe 150 people maximum. Back in those ancestral communities, there might have only been three hotties on the savannah to choose from. Oh, one of them just stole an axe and was socially excommunicated, while the other just got together with Wilma. One, then.

Large towns and cities became lighter fuel for dissatisfaction; now apps are a flamethrower. 'If we're in a supermarket that sells ten different sorts of baked beans, it can send us into choice paralysis,' says Dr Thomas. 'Whereas Stone Age dating was like Lidl. One type. Do you want the beans or not?'

This mismatch is why we can't deal with having hundreds, even thousands, of people to choose from. It freezes our brain into a 'can't compute' glitch, and/or has it constantly scanning around for better options.

In the modern world, dating apps have *become* dating, Dr Thomas says. 'This means that any weakness in the apps has become a weakness in dating overall. Before them, we tended to meet people through friends, so they already came stamped by interpersonal approval. This increased our chances of success, given the filters were innate. If your friend thinks they're decent, they probably are.'

Meeting in person also meant that, even if you weren't a certain height, clothes size or conventionally attractive, being smart or funny could level the playing field.

Now, we're swimming in the shallows, he says. 'When we're given thousands of options, we tend to get pickier, because we have to be. If I plugged 'computer mouse' into Amazon and 10,000 options came up, what would I do? I would filter it down by appearance, size, shape, when it's available. I have to narrow my options somehow.'

We discount people who would have been a great match for ridiculously shallow reasons. Not because we've suddenly become *Shallow Hal*, but because our brain is not calibrated to cope with this artificial amount of options, just as it's not built to be measured around ultra-processed food or cocaine.

We make snap judgements for ease, not necessarily prejudice. 'I used to think I wouldn't date a vegetarian, and now I'm married to one,' says Dr Thomas. 'Turns out it's the least problematic thing ever. We just use two pans. Big deal.'

In fact, he wouldn't have met his wife at all unless he'd lied on his dating profile about his height. 'I said I was six foot, but I'm five foot eleven,' he says. She'd filtered for six foot and over.

This twangs recognition in me. I used to filter for five foot eleven and over too, given I'm five foot eight. Even though most of my partners have been under five eleven, so that makes no sense. My partner is only a little taller than me, and I barely noticed that when we met, let alone it being a dealbreaker. It seems that, in reality, height doesn't bother me, but on the apps it did.

Some dating apps are now building in the equivalent of an 'Amazon's Choice' badge, by charging users to have similar. It works because people need these shortcuts, in the midst of bewildering choice. There are also more conscientious apps that use conversational prompt cards, to discourage superficial dismissals. Let's face it, though. We all look at the pictures first, don't we?

In-house we get appraised too, by the app employees themselves. Tinder has admitted using a 'desirability rating' to rank popular vs unpopular members. Hinge, too, must surely have some sort of internal system for sending you those ideal daily matches, superficial or no. And then there's Beautiful People, which only lets you in if its staff deem you fit enough. It's all pretty ugly, really. Maybe I'll set up an app called Pretty Ugly; start the backlash.

Add to all of this the dopamine traps built in to gamify romantic connection – think super-likes, fireworks, vibrations on match – and you can see how they make us crave more and more. 'You have matched and may now advance to the next level.' It's all too easy to get snarled into 'winning' people, forgetting that the actual goal was to advance to a meaningful relationship and delete the app (if it was).

Interestingly, dating app use is down – dramatically so – in Millennials. In the past decade, average use has plummeted from 100 minutes a day to 51 minutes. I mean, that's still a lot of minutes, and I will just point out that I more than doubled that (two zebras – toldyouso), but average use having halved means something big is afoot.

Millennials are just exhausted by the grind of them, said a *Forbes* poll, which found that 80 per cent of that age group say they're worn out. The more shallow hook-up apps, such as Tinder, are on the decline, and those that attempt to be more about personality and relationships (Bumble, Hinge) are on the rise.

Specify the dream

Minimise the shallows by all means, but also be specific about the dream, says behavioural designer Nir Eyal. He has heard from many readers who've been played or ghosted on apps. 'When you invent the ship, you also invent the shipwreck,' he says magnanimously, quoting philosopher Paul Virilio.

But he does have an anti-wrecking map. 'I've noticed that the people who benefit from these apps are those who use it seriously to find a spouse and don't get deterred from their criteria.'

He's not talking about height or salary, but a vision for the future. 'I had a buddy; I guess you'd call him a tech bro. He spent his years digital nomadding, having a great time, and then decided it was time to find a spouse.'

Eyal tells me that the tech bro started a document on his phone detailing what he wanted with his future partner: to live in New York City, have three kids, have dinner parties every two weeks. Sounds exhausting. And some other women agreed. 'On dates he showed women these goals before they even got started, asking "how does this sound to you?",' Eyal says. 'Half of the time she left. "I'm not for you." Half of the time, she stayed.'

I wouldn't have believed the next part, were it not for Eyal's candour. 'Within 30 days he sits down with this woman and, again, shows her the document. She brings out her phone and shows him her document. Their visions match up. Now they're married and realising them.'

I included this story because it made me reflect upon how often I got distracted by shiny baubles, by outlandish 'what ifs' when I was on the apps. I love the countryside, monogamy, reading and being at home with my dog (I know, I'm a riot). I have dated both, and discovered I am better suited to ex-hedonists, just like myself, rather than current hedonists. (*Never* hedonists? I just don't relate. Weirdos.)

On the apps, it was like I forgot who I am and what I want. I constantly got distracted by 'What if's, grabbing them just because I could. We *never* would have crossed paths in real life. I dated polyamorous travel junkies with man buns and MDMA habits. Weed-smoking musicians who were out five times a week and didn't treat dogs as if they were people. Rock-climbing, hard-drinking lawyers.

I wasn't compatible with these people, but I dated them anyway. It was fun, but it wasn't future-making stuff. Only 11 per cent of Brits met their current long-term partner through an app, said a recent survey. I wonder if this is why.

Stuck in the dopamine trap

'More, again, now please' chants the dopamine, not just incited by the app's design but also by the inherent nature of early dating in general.

You can get hooked on the changeability of the first few months, says neuroscientist Dr Alex Korb, because: dopamine. ('Because: dopamine' could be a catchphrase of this book. I might put it on some T-shirts and mugs.) 'When you're first dating someone, it works like an addiction,' he says. 'If they don't text you back immediately, you feel stress and anxiety.' Much like withdrawal. 'Will they ghost you, or will it lead to heartbreak, or will this change your life?'

The stakes are unnaturally high, which increases the dopamine. 'The high uncertainty leads to high stress but, simultaneously, a high dose of dopamine. Which hijacks all of our attention and focus.'

As usual, this makes sense when you consider the environment in which our brains evolved. 'Imagine you walked past a fruit tree every day and it was always fruit-bearing. You wouldn't fixate on it,' he says. 'But if it's only in season for a week every year, or the fruit is hard to reach, our brain is wired to focus more upon it.'

Changeable things – like newfound romantic suitors – give us much more of a dopamine rush, 'Precisely because we have less control over them,' says Dr Korb. Dopamine drives us to repeat the behaviour, and forms a habit. Date for a while – discard – date for a while – discard.

Then, even when we're coupled, many of us are still keeping an eye on the apps (one terrifying survey showed that almost two-thirds of Tinder users are in a relationship). This is because of the dissatisfaction created by both the hedonic treadmill (satisfaction is fleeting, and then we seek to upgrade, see page 118) and the choice paradox. This push-pull of 'coupled but also still looking' has been called 'stable ambiguity' by relationship psychotherapist Esther Perel.

The secret to not getting stuck on that early days dopamine roller coaster is to find those (ideally slow) dopamine sources another way once you're single again, rather than just rubberbanding straight back on to the apps.

Or, if your fling settles down into a longer-term thing, look for acceptance.

Acceptance that it would be unhealthy for it to continue feeling urgent, heady, exciting and stressful. It's a relationship, not a trip to Thorpe Park.

'It's natural for the brain to calm down after the first few months,' says Dr Korb. 'We think the spark is gone, but that's just what should happen, given those early dopamine spikes are not healthy or sustainable long-term.'

Good long-term relationships do retain *some* dopamine bursts, though, he says. 'Which is how you keep things fresh, by doing new things and surprising each other.'

Otherwise, you might seek it elsewhere. Which brings us neatly to . . .

Flirting when you oughtn't

Flirting shouldn't be a problem if you're single. Go get 'em, tiger. So, I'm going to assume that if you want to downscale your little flirting addiction, it's because you shouldn't be doing it. And if you shouldn't be doing it, it's probably an emotional infidelity, defined as a relationship with someone else, minus the sex.

Many years ago, I was engaged in an emotional infidelity so intense that we may as well have been (emotionally) engaged. We were texting each other every day – sometimes hundreds of times a day – sending selfies, doing long voice notes, emotionally supporting each other through life events. I was even telling him about minutiae – the salad I had for lunch, a funny line in a book I was reading – that I wasn't sharing with my partner.

I'm not proud of it, but it happened. And the way it stopped happening was this. I looked at the things I was getting from this emotional affair that I wasn't getting in my then-relationship. And then I tried to reinstate them in my long-term relationship. It didn't work, but at least I tried.

Often, emotional infidelities spark from flirting at work. 'I think many of these little addictions originate in boredom,' says psychotherapist Hilda Burke. Which is why it's so important to mix it up. 'I work with men incarcerated in Wormwood Scrubs prison, many of whom are struggling with addiction. Oftentimes they relapsed because of a big headline – mother died, partner left – but sometimes it's just that they felt bored. They were on the bus and had nothing to do, and saw a guy they used to buy from.'

This is relevant to you, I promise. 'It's the same with workplace flirtation,' she says. 'Work is boring, offices are boring,' she says. Even if you do have a break-out room with bean bags, a basketball machine and free gumballs, the boredom's gonna getcha. 'In that tedium, we're always looking for ways to break that monotony, for quick dopamine rushes, and a covert flirtation with someone will do.'

Out in the wild, it probably wouldn't happen, she says. 'You wouldn't look twice at them. But you're both enclosed in this tight space, and they're kinda cute, and it's more about needing some excitement than it is about them.'

Millions of us do jobs that aren't stimulating to us, but our brains crave newness, says neuroscientist Dr Axel Bouchon. 'New, surprising things always give us an extra portion of dopamine.'

Meanwhile, our society funnels us into doing the same thing day-in, day-out, for eight whole hours, five days a week. 'We're not built for that,' he says. 'We didn't evolve for that.' Even if you *like* being an accountant, your brain will strain and rebel against the monotony.

This is why we have to create the newness and surprise ourselves, consciously. Otherwise our brains will find it, and it may not lead us down the best path.

People as addictions

I wanted to give a special mention to certain people who become addictive. This is probably the ex who you just can't shake, who you keep contacting even when you delete their number from all the places.

I've been caught in this snafu too. One ex and I managed to date, split, rinse and repeat, over an entire decade, with other partners in between. Until one night, when I tried to resurrect our ill-fated cycle, and he texted back with 'I'm now engaged.'

The massive magnetic pull he had over me was his unpredictability. I never knew what was going to happen – it could be glorious or grim – and, even though there were more lows than highs, it kept me gripped. It was no surprise when I found a copy of a pick-up artist handbook (the community of skincrawlers Neil Strauss famously exposed in *The Game*) in his wardrobe during one 'on' phase.

I talked about pick-up artist tactics with Professor Natasha Schüll. 'They are very similar to poker handbooks; how to bluff, not have tells, keep people guessing. It's teaching how to *be* chance.'

My ex *was* chance. And I couldn't look away. 'The person becomes a puzzle you can't figure out, and you get stuck in the puzzle,' she says. The non-resolution of it is the thing, she says. 'It's the final aspect of the ludic loop,' she says, alluding to her model of how things become addictive. 'Another interval of uncertainty that opens up. Just as with, in a game of poker, there's another hand dealt.'

So, we pick up our cards and go again, trying to dominate chance into order. Maybe this time we'll crack it.

Sex you regret

Sex is great. There'll be no sex-shaming here. If you had a good time, and don't regret it, there is no problem. But, given you want to change your habits, I'm going to assume you regret the sex after the fact. Which could be for myriad reasons – you're in a relationship, you didn't truly want it, it left you feeling grubby, many more besides.

It's stating the obvious, but we're designed to want sex. 'The way that evolution works is, if we can get by using a "quick and dirty rule" for something, then we will,' says Dr Thomas. 'And the "quick and dirty rule" for sex is this: if you have the sex, everything else will take care of itself.'

What? But babies don't take care of themselves? He says that back when we were in these tight communities or tribes, there were always people to look after the babies. 'Family planning is a modern invention, given we no longer have that village,' he says.

'It takes a village' we all say to each other over soft play, but none of us actually have it. Even the lucky ones (so lucky!) with hands-on grandparents. One day a week of help is ***not the same*** as how it would have looked back then. Zero days a week is just not how it's supposed to be.

Babies and modern setbacks aside, that 'quick and dirty rule' remains. 'Our drive to have sex is as inbuilt as the drive to drink water, eat and breathe,' says Dr Thomas. Other mammals never regret sex, but we do, due to the way our brains work. 'On top of that drive, we have this extra level of executive function.' He's talking about the prefrontal cortex, the adult of the brain. 'It's like when the urge to eat a doughnut strikes,' he says. 'You're feeling both "I want it but I also don't want it, for these other reasons". We have to fight the urge to have sex in the same way.'

Often we fight the urge because we're monogamous. Casual hook-up apps capitalise on our 'want to', making it easier to push aside the 'don't want to' higher-level executive reasoning. Some deal in 'ethical non-monogamy', such as Feeld, which caters for the polyamorous crowd and more, but others are clearly for cheating. You'll see more body parts there than faces (I'm thinking Adult Friend Finder et al). Would you like to date this ballsack? Tempting, but I'll pass.

We can also hide WhatsApp conversations altogether now, meaning they only pop up when we specifically search for that user and, even then, aren't accessible without fingerprint or face ID. Of course, privacy is a good thing too, and this feature could be used by an abused wife plotting a getaway, or a teenager being hit by his dad. But for the little sex addicts, this means that real-life consequences are circumnavigated, so animalistic urges can abound. They can eat the damn doughnut and not be found out.

This is a problem when you're trying to resist it, given apps and features like this make cheating so much easier. A behaviour that used to be socially minimised is now technologically enabled.

Our short-term selves

I'm guessing that, for little sex addicts, our short-term selves are in charge, while our long-term selves take a back seat. I ask psychotherapist Hilda Burke if that's about the size of it? 'Yes, exactly,' she says. 'It feels good right now, so let's do it.'

But what about when you're single and your regret springs from elsewhere? 'Here, it's usually because we told ourselves we just wanted to have pleasure and an orgasm, but then, afterward, a side agenda makes itself known, which wasn't previously conscious.'

So, we're in denial about what was actually driving the sex? 'Yes,' she says. 'We told ourselves it was just a casual bit of fun, and it was agreed as such, but when we don't get that tick of validation afterwards, the secret side agenda pushes its way out. Then we feel shit or used because they don't call.'

Or, maybe it's the other way around. Maybe *you* agreed a no-strings liaison and it's them who are now trying to turn it into a whole thing, culminating in a Sicily wedding with harpists. Which is now prodding you into feeling guilty. If that's the case, and your communication was clear about you not wanting anything other than a shag, you have nothing to feel guilty about, my friend. You did your bit.

I feel mildly ridiculous that such a vast topic has been covered in 5,000 words. I could write 50,000 words. But, needs must. This book can't be an encyclopaedic collection of several books, because nobody would take *that* on holiday. And then I wouldn't get a chance to ruin everyone's holidays with all of my moderation chat.

Dear little sex addict,

I had to choose one of the three, and you're the one I've chosen.

Having sex we regret isn't always the result of a stashed side agenda. Sometimes our body just seems to want it, and so we do it, and we don't secretly want a relationship with them, but we regret it anyway. Confusing.

Here's what could be going on. Our bodies might have wanted it for reasons other than sex. It could be a misdirected case of 'skin hunger'.

Maybe you're in a predicament right now. There's a person in your bed, or on your sofa, or in your sex dungeon – no judgement – who is expecting you to have sex with them.

It's unlikely, because why would you be reading this book when coitus is imminent. But let's imagine. And let's also imagine the possibility that the thing you crave, that got you into this exact situation, is not a craving for sex itself, but an urge to feel a human body lying alongside yours.

We've already covered how deep the ancestral hardwiring of sex goes. But alongside that urge is a craving for human touch, and the two can get jumbled up in our interoception.

'Skin hunger' – also known as touch deprivation – is defined by experts as a longing for human touch. As with most things, our desire for touch is a spectrum, with some wanting zero and others wanting a lot.

In most hospitals now, newborn babies are placed directly on to bare skin, given it starts the bonding process, cascading oxytocin in. Oxytocin makes us feel glowy, relaxed and blissed-out.

But, like Goldilocks, we're looking for just right. We also get 'touched out', especially through parenting. I used to want much more human touch than I got, trying to smoosh myself up against partners during the night, while they tried to get away via the *Friends*-famed hug and roll, but now that I'm a mother, I want a lot, *lot* less.

A crucial thing about skin hunger, by the way. It's fed by non-sexual human contact. Which means that you don't need to have sex to sate it. Feeding it can look like a massage, a tender adjustment from a yoga teacher or a long hug from a friend.

If we're single or in a coupled sex drought, skin hunger can strike. Unless we're on regular touching terms with our friends and family (rare), this urge can then be misinterpreted as a longing for sex. We want someone to hold our hand, lightly spoon us, or stroke our hair while we watch a film. None of those things has to be within a sexual relationship. I did all of these things with my daughter today. Yet, if it's adult-to-adult, it tends to only happen in a relationship – or sexual – setting.

And so, in order to get to the spooning, the thing we really want, but which we can't obtain platonically, we often end up in a sexual clinch. Our body's calling the shots, but we mishear it.

I've been there. As a thirsty (in both definitions of the word) twentysomething, my favourite late-night activity wasn't reading in candlelit baths as magazines kept telling me I ought to do; it was illicitly smoking out of my flatshare window at midnight, while drunk texting people I had the hots for.

I would often drop my phone in panic if someone replied, flipping it face down, having felt suddenly and uncomfortably seen. I so infrequently got replies to my batshit hornball texts after midnight that it was like throwing a tennis ball into a black hole. When the black hole threw my tennis ball back, it scared the shit out of me.

The alcohol played a part, obviously. If only when we were drunk or high we craved that which is good for us, rather than bad for us. That way, instead of coming into the kitchen after a big night to find the remnants of a midnight MacDonald's, we might find the aftermath of a buddha bowl.

'*Jesus.* Where did all of these cucumber shavings come from?!'

If you'd hoovered all of the alcohol out of my system, I may well have realised the nuance at play. I didn't want to go to bed alone, but I didn't want to sleep with them either. Unless they were up for watching *Good Will Hunting*, tracing circles on my back, and then literally going to sleep.

For me, the thing making me scattergun text was not the sex. I know that now. If I'd been able to find a massage therapist at 1am – one that didn't try to give me a happy ending – I would have done.

This is all just my experience. Maybe yours is different, and you know for sure that your horniness is separate to your skin hunger, and you're going to throw down this letter in disgust and go back into your sex dungeon with your bland safe word (avocado) and have a fine time. Good for you.

But I thought it was worth mentioning. Before this mishear has you undressed, when all you really wanted was a hug.

Love,
Cath x

DATING, FLIRTING & SEX MICRO TACTICS

Make your side agendas conscious

This comes from Hilda Burke, and it works on a few levels. Aside from peeling back the layers of denial around why we want to have sex, it could also expose why we're flirting or having a full-blown emotional affair. Do we *really* want to blow up our relationship and get with this person instead? If so, go for it. That's how some lifelong relationships start. If not, then what is this side hustle bringing you that you're not getting from your main? Bring it up to the light and then figure out what to do with it.

Date nights with a twist

You can arrest the dopamine decline by following Dr Bouchon's lead. Remember that newness in a relationship doesn't have to come from a new relationship. 'The biggest positive change I've made in the past year is date nights with my partner,' he said. These aren't just any date nights. 'It's not just dinner or theatre. We put in a real effort and take turns to plan something new, special, exciting and surprising.'

(I feel sure this tip means my partner and I are finally going to have to do an escape room, rather than just lying at home under our dog watching all 300 seasons of *Bosch*.)

Try weighted blankets

Hear me out before you denounce this as woo(lly) woo. The bonus is you might not need to enlist actual people to appease your skin hunger. Many experts believe a weighted blanket can mimic the feeling of a bear hug. In fact, weighted blankets were once something that therapists prescribed. It's only lately that they've become a privately purchased trend.

The 'if they read it' test
A hallmark of being in an emotional infidelity is hiding messages (and yes, archiving counts). If your partner would be unhappy if they read your message chain, then, yeah, you know the rest. It's time for a shrinking of this little addiction.

Know about the 'halo effect'
When we see an attractive face, we tend to assign other positives to that person too, according to the research of Joseph Walther. The photo deck on the app only enhances this halo. There's a photo of them with their mum, aww, so they must be kind to family. A snap of them with a baby (nephew! they stress), so they must want kids. No, no, and indeed, no. They haven't earned your good opinion yet, and the rest are unfounded assumptions.

Apps that cut the choice down
Matches drop off Bumble within 24 hours if neither of you have conversed. Hinge serves you a new match each day, to try to prevent endless scrolling, and will stop you from messaging someone new if you've left too many people on read (eight is the limit). Breeze is for people tired of days of messaging beforehand; they send you 20 profiles they think you'll like twice a day, not allowing you to chat in-app at all. Instead, if you match, they charge you £9.50 for them to arrange a date instead.

PEOPLE-PLEASING

I remember the first time I realised people-pleasing is fear.

I'd previously read about it being about control. Controlling other's perceptions of us. Making sure others don't think poorly of us. And that's true. But it doesn't take us all the way. It felt like the key that fitted but wouldn't turn.

I was on Instagram in psychotherapist Anna Mathur's feed when I found the key-turn: 'People-pleasing is not love,' she said. 'It is fear wearing love's clothes.'

It opened a door in my head. And here's what I found inside.

My compulsive people-pleasing *has* been about managing other's opinions of me, but what has driven that has been fear of being disapproved of and, ultimately, cast out. I spoke to Mathur about this, and she said: 'People-pleasing *is* about controlling other's perceptions of us, but beneath the control is something more vulnerable and childlike.'

From year dot, many of us are conditioned into people-pleasing. 'We've been told that the more you give away, and the more depleted you are, the more loving you are,' says Mathur, author of *The Uncomfortable Truth*. 'We then get burnt out and resentful. Which makes us snappy, irritable and, ironically, less able to love.'

The fear at people-pleasing's core is that of being cast out of a tribe – a family, a friendship group, a work pack, a workplace. This runs incredibly deep because, at one point, being in or out was a question of survival. People-displeasing could literally kill you.

'You're 100 per cent right,' says Dr Andrew Thomas, an evolutionary psychologist at Swansea University. 'Familial or community exclusion would have been a little death sentence in the ancestral environment.'

Even just 100 years ago, somebody who was cast out from their family didn't face great hopes of thriving, or even surviving, due to a threadbare welfare system. This is why family provokes the most powerful urge to please. 'It's primitive,' says Mathur, 'and it feels like real jeopardy if you start to refrain, because once upon a time it *did* mean real jeopardy.'

The fear of family-displeasing has been calibrated over hundreds of thousands of years. 'We are primed to develop fears towards things that were consistently a threat for humans,' says Dr Thomas. 'Our fear of heights comes online alongside a cliff face, but not at 35,000 feet up in an aeroplane.' And these primed fears run deep, he adds. 'Many people in the UK have phobias towards snakes, a real ancestral threat, despite the fact that in the modern day UK, we only have one form of adder that poses any threat, and fatalities from that species are very rare.'

We're even wired to *feel* physical pain when we're socially excluded, given how ancestrally important inclusion was. 'There have been these interesting experiments where people are on a PC playing *Cyberball* with two other players,' says Dr Thomas. 'When two players start to exclude one, the brain imaging shows that, in the excluded person, the pain centres of the brain light up.'

Are women more inclined to people-please?

The cliché goes that women do it, and not men. And, definitely, females born pre-2000 have often been subject to rampant 'good girl' conditioning: put others first, look pretty, be fragrant, don't take up too much space please. When we break from these expectations, historically we have been punished.

But men have been conditioned to people-please too, just in different ways to women. They've been taught not to 'kill the buzz' and down a damn pint already, followed by a Jägermeister. To agree to lift heavy things to spare others' backs, to talk about sports when they don't give a flying fuck about sports, to have sex they don't want, even. Right?

I put all of this to psychotherapist Joshua Fletcher, author of *And How Does That Make You Feel?* He tells me I'm wrong, in the politest way possible. 'I don't think younger men feel all of that toxic masculinity pressure,' he says. 'But I do know that I'm just as likely to get a male people-pleasing client as a female. And, socially, I see it all the time; chums all around an alpha telling him he's great, even though he's acting like a dick.'

Fletcher is quick to tell me that the psychotherapists' term for people-pleasing is 'fawn'. Mathur gets this in sharpish too. 'Most of us know about fight, flight or freeze, but "fawn" is rarely talked about,' she says. Both tell me that 'fawn' is the largely unknown fourth sibling of that survival mode family, which make up the four Fs.

But where does a propensity to fawn come from? It can be an emotionally abusive relationship, workplace or school experience. 'For me, it goes back to being bullied,' says Fletcher. 'I was threatened every single day at school so, as an adult, I felt the urge to fawn every time I met someone new or bigger than me.'

The 'fawn' response can also be traced back to familial dynamics. 'A cause I see often is an emotionally unstable parent who withdrew love if you upset them,' he says. The kid learns to prioritise the feelings of others over their own, he explains. This sets us up for a lifetime of high alert for the bad moods of others. 'We scan people's faces, are sensitive to tones in emails, obsess in the shower over social interactions we've just had. Did I offend them, did I speak too much, or too little, do they like me?'

Are they *pleased*, ultimately.

The constant threat-assessment is at its core a search for safety, he says. If the other person is OK, you can feel OK, so you'll forever try to attain everyone else being OK . . . so that you can be OK.

Ad infinitum, forever and ever Amen. *So* relaxing.

Displeasing family

When family are displeased, we feel a desperate need to get them back on side, says Mathur. She flags the physical distress it causes. 'It activates our reactive, emotional limbic system, which we then feel in our gut, in shortness of breath, in tense muscles.'

When we start to resist family-pleasing, Mathur says it can lead to real discomfort, in both body and mind (which sounds a lot like withdrawal from a drug). The urge to apologise when a family member is displeased, whether it's warranted or not, is almost irresistible. 'It can feel absolutely terrifying to ride it out,' she says.

But when we apologise in fawn state, it pulls us out of alignment with ourselves, which leads to resentment. 'Fawn gets us rewarded,' says Mathur. 'It serves others. But it often means we have to steamroll our own boundaries and pretend they're not there, just to repair that connection. Apologising out of fear of abandonment is very different to apologising when you genuinely think you're wrong.'

Sometimes the connection becomes irreparable if we don't fawn, which is very sad indeed. 'It's rarely talked about, but when you stop people-pleasing and start to hold your "no", sometimes you can lose even a parent or partner,' says

Mathur. Sometimes they cannot accept – or continue with – your 'no'. They've become so dependent on your yeses, that your no is anathema.

I've been there myself with family, and holding my 'no' felt existentially threatening and unnatural. But it was also necessary. It had been necessary for decades, in fact. It had just taken me that long to work up the courage.

We ought to be able to say 'no' to those we love, even if they are blood relatives, and *still* be loved.

The overbooking knock-on

Let's zoom out now, beyond your inner circle. A dead giveaway you're a people-pleaser is that when you look at your calendar for the next month, your heart wants to cry. Because there are many things in there – parties, meetings, favours, whatever – that you don't actually want to do. And that you don't have time to do. And you feel fucking knackered just looking at it.

Most of us are now eminently contactable, not only by everyone we've ever been to school with, or worked with, or met at a BBQ one time, but also by complete strangers. Nowadays, our DMs and work emails tend to be overcrowded with people asking to see us, asking for favours, or simply asking 'What you been up to?' when we haven't seen them for a decade, so to answer would take approximately four hours.

'We are pack animals and need to feel accepted,' says Mathur. 'But a generation ago, our parents would have only been trying to please a tight circle of family, friends and work contacts.'

This expansion of our circle is breaking our people-pleasing operating system, says Mathur, given we are now trying to please and placate hundreds – even thousands – of humans contacting us, rather than a couple of dozen at most. Mathur encourages me to imagine what my social and work demands might look like if I didn't have Instagram, WhatsApp or an email anyone can access.

The answer is: pretty manageable. Very, actually.

'We're now trying to feel accepted by people we've never even met,' she says, 'and when we inevitably fail to do so, given we just don't have the capacity to maintain that number of connections, we feel less and less safe.'

'Safe' seems like a strange word, but when you consider how emotionally activated we feel when we get a follow-up 'Hello?' chaser, from a loved one or stranger (personally, I feel scared I've been rude, morally attacked and, therefore, yes, unsafe), then it makes sense.

Calming the fawn

Whenever I read about people-pleasing being fear, the first instance that sprang to my mind was this one. I spent many years working on women's magazines. Believe me, *The Devil Wears Prada* was not only accurate, it was an understatement. The cliques, entitled bosses, backstabbing . . . all very real.

I was once called a 'useless c*nt!' by a boss, while she swept through the office like Ursula the Sea Witch in sequins, then slammed her corner office door so hard my teeth chattered.

This isn't an attempt to prove the cliché that predominantly female workplaces are bitchy. Nope. What was also real was the exact opposite to that viper's den trope; the lifelong loyalties forged, the bosses who hid my failings, the women talking each other up rather than putting each other down.

Anyway, at a different magazine from the useless c*nt one, I was sitting at my boss's desk, having a meeting, when I glanced at her screen and saw an email I'd just written sitting in her inbox. Only, I hadn't sent that email to my boss. It was an email I'd just sent to another colleague who I thought was my friend. My 'friend' had emailed me saying 'Are you OK? You seem blue.' And I had voiced my dissatisfaction with a work situation. My response was very private, very personal, very for-her-eyes-only. This 'friend' had then forwarded my email directly on to my boss.

The email was entitled 'Just call me Judas.'

It was like a dagger in the throat. They all secretly hate me, don't they?! And yes, yes they did.

I started to pay attention to the shared glances when I walked into a room, the whispered conversations, the emails tapped out while I was talking, the swoosh of an email arriving in the other's inbox, conspiratorial peals of laughter as I walked away. For months – years, even – afterward, I became smaller, quieter, more agreeable; a human who'd had a personality transplant, in order to make myself acceptable. Because, I told myself, I can never go through that again.

This blood-freezing experience, of *the people are displeased*, and I'm not paranoid, it's actually real, is universally felt in some shape, and it's why we're all so afraid to experience it again. It's why we placate, smoothe, please, shrink, fawn.

'The fawn response is created by the amygdala,' says Fletcher. 'Shaped like an almond, and one of the oldest, fastest and dumbest parts of our brain.' It's responsible for anxiety, as well as the four Fs, which – if they ever became a sibling band – would probably make fawn be the roadie.

Fletcher says that the only way to rewire the amygdala, and to teach it to behave differently in future, is while it's activated. 'It's like a clamshell. It needs to be open for you to get inside.'

This means *during* the anxiety. 'And if you're continuing to go along with your amygdala's fawn mode urge, by laughing at jokes you don't find funny, agreeing with things you don't agree with, saying yes when you mean no, you're teaching your amygdala that it needs to continue to fawn,' he says.

The amygdala, if you recall, is part of the striatum, which Dr Korb compared to a dog. It does what you train it to do, truly it does, via repetition.

This reminds me of a dog-training hack I learned recently. My dog, our hypervigilant head of security, raises the alarm if a leaf falls to the floor outside. When he barks, we tend to repeatedly ask him to desist, by telling him off. But all we're doing is reinforcing his behaviour. 'They're alarmed too!' he thinks. 'The peril is real!'

Once we changed tack and started staying calm when he barked instead, touching him gently on his side, saying 'thank you, but it's all good,' he stopped barking. It felt like magic, but it was just logic.

We need to give our amygdala the same story. A 'thanks, but it's all good' story. Giving our fawn permission to leave.

Caveat: don't say no to everything

It's about moderation, not abstinence. 'Sometimes, once people start saying "no", particularly if they've been wearing the "good" hat for decades, they can get a bit high from it, and go too far,' says Mathur. She likens it to a kid who's just learned to walk, tries to go too fast and falls over. 'That's when you need to slow down.'

I really relate to this. When I first started people-displeasing there was initial deep, deep discomfort, followed by a stage where I experienced a thrill of euphoria every time I batted something back with a 'no'. I became trigger-happy with my 'no's. I definitely had to walk it back.

Mathur encourages us to remember that healthy relationships require sacrifice, on both sides, at times. 'Sometimes we do things we don't want to do,' she says. 'And that's important. We get up at 4am to fetch them from the airport, and we get no airspace whatsoever when it's all about their break-up.'

Sometimes the natural ebb and flow means we give a lot more than we get. And that's OK. It's about thinking of ourselves like a cake, cut into eight slices, she says. 'We can still generously give away wedges of cake. We just need to keep enough back to sustain ourselves.'

Burn out is what often comes *before* the resolve to cease people-pleasing. 'When we burn out, we've routinely been giving the entire cake away, day by day,' says Mathur, 'leaving only crumbs for ourselves.' We need to hold back a few slices, she urges.

I love this metaphor, but I also now really want cake. *Hi, little cake addiction.*

Dear little people-pleasing addict,

I want to tell you a story.

It's about a woman who, as she was approaching the milestone age of 40, realised she had people-pleased her entire life . . . and, worst of all, the people didn't even seem pleased.

- She'd said yes to entire years-long friendships because she didn't want the other person to be disappointed, and the other person wanted to be her friend. Even though when she first met them, her body said 'no thanks'.
- She'd been on holidays she didn't want to go on, because other people wanted her to go on them.
- She'd bought outfits other people wanted her to wear.
- Gone on dates with people other people wanted her to date.
- Not dated people because other people didn't want her to.
- Answered phone calls at 10pm when she wanted to do anything but, and was getting ready for bed.
- Said yes to doing so many favours for others that she had an entire folder on her desktop marked FAVOURS, and didn't have time to do her own workload.
- Worked for free. Many times.
- Burned out twice, manifested in physically vomiting, having to cancel two holidays (that she wanted to go on) and being unable to function even slightly as a human.

This person was me. And the thing that made me realise I chronically needed change, and I needed it now, was when I was learning to drive aged 39 (I wouldn't pass until my third attempt aged 42).

Here's what happened.

'Why are you looking in your rearview mirror all the time?' my driving instructor asked me; a zen legend of Buddhist-monk proportions called Norman.

Me: 'Because they're up my arse, they want to get past.'

Norman: 'So what, let them.'

'They look angry,' I said.

'Let them!'

(Mel Robbins, big love to you, but Norman got there first with the 'let them' theory.)

I continue to glance in my rearview mirror every few seconds.

'Why are you looking at them rather than the road?' Norman said, his zen momentarily cracking. 'Concentrate on the road; they can do what they want. If they go into the back of us it'll be their fault, not yours.'

I would rush into roundabouts before I was truly comfortable, if a queue was forming behind me. I would drop parking spaces like a frightened kid giving another kid its lunch. I would allow people to bully me from the overtaking lane on the motorway, even when I was legitimately overtaking, because they wanted to speed. I drove at 50mph down serpentine country lanes I didn't know, because the person behind me wanted to go faster.

I had to change. And I did change.

Here's what happened, ultimately.

- Fewer friends
- Less family favour
- Fewer messages in my inbox and WhatsApp

That sounds like a bad thing, right? But it's not. Because as a result, I now have:

- Fewer friends – who I love more
- Time for myself

- More peace of mind
- Less resentment
- More money
- More nights in

Once you stop people-pleasing, some people will be really bloody displeased, and may well call you 'selfish' or say 'you've changed', either to your face or behind your back.

These are probably those who benefited from your people-pleasing the most. Who you had to get into the most uncomfortable shapes for. And that's OK. They're not your people.

In the words often attributed to Dr. Seuss:

'Be who you are and say what you feel, because those who mind don't matter, and those who matter don't mind.'

Talking of Dr. Seuss, he added the 'Dr.' as a wry nod to the fact his father wanted him to become a doctor. Instead, he decided to publish and illustrate 60 children's books. Generations of children would have lost out, had Dr. Seuss people-pleased his way into the realm of medicine.

Your life is yours. Not theirs. They have their own life. Take yours back.

And then, in the words of Norman the driving instructor: *let them.* Let them have whatever reaction they damn well please.

Love,
Cath x

PEOPLE-PLEASING MICRO TACTICS

Train away the fawn

Repetition is the key, says Fletcher, when giving your fawn permission to leave. 'The more you're brave enough to speak your mind, or crack a joke you felt scared to crack, or say "no", the more your amygdala will realise the fawn response isn't needed after all.'

Avoid the daylight robbery from loved ones

Our top-tier relationships suffer when we've people-pleased ourselves to depletion all day, says Mathur. 'We've spent our limited social capacity on low-level interactions. After a day like this, a friend will ask, "Do you want to go out for dinner?" and we'll be like "no!" because we've spent all day DMing on socials trying to gain the acceptance of strangers, or on WhatsApp in lower-level interactions. It truly robs from our most important relationships.'

Being careful of where we expend our energy is the key.

Data-gather for the ratios

Once you start saying no, says Mathur, you'll gather important data. 'Your palms are sweating, you're clenching your butt cheeks and every bit of you wants to apologise, but then they say "That's OK" and move on.'

If you data-gather enough, then Mathur says you'll realise the people who push back on your 'no' and try to break it are actually in the minority. 'The realisation therefore lands that, when people disrespect your boundary, it's more about them than you,' she adds.

Resist the knee-jerk apology

In Britain, we apologise for everything. People bumping into us, involuntarily bodily functions like sneezing, not hearing something someone said, being in a space someone else wants to use, asking somebody to do their job . . . even just *standing* somewhere. We apologise for existing. This is why the average Brit apologises 3,285 times a year.

It will feel radical and egregiously rude, but start trying to not apologise for existing. *Especially* try not apologising for someone else's infraction. And slowly, but surely – subtly, but firmly – you may feel emboldened to also stop apologising for having plans already, not wanting to do something you've expressed no interest in doing and not having time to do an unsolicited favour.

Adopt a pause

Have you ever noticed how the healthiest people in your life, when you invite them to something, will say 'Let me check and get back to you'? Well, that was never me. I would check my diary that exact moment and say yes or no. 'Adopting a pause,' says Mathur, 'even if you know that you're free, means you can look at the whole week and figure out if you'll have the energy.'

The 'if it were today' tactic

Time does a curious thing, whereby the further away something is, the more likely we are to schedule it in, thinking that future us might be up for hosting that event, doing a skydive or a weekend glamping, even though current us wouldn't be. Mathur suggests this hack to crack open our true willingness: 'If that thing were happening today or tomorrow, would I say yes?'

SHOPPING

The best and brightest among us have had shopping addictions. Even addiction experts themselves are far from immune.

The iconic Dr Gabor Maté, trauma expert and author of *When The Body Says No*, grew hooked on buying classical music, spending thousands on CDs in a single spree, hiding the spoils. When his wife asked him, repeatedly, whether he'd been 'obsessing and buying?' he revealed:

'I look directly at my life partner of 39 years and I lie.'

Meanwhile Dr Anna Lembke, addiction therapist and author of *Dopamine Nation*, became obsessed with buying romantasy, forsaking sleep, socialising and family time to devour the latest drop on her Kindle. *Twilight* served as a gateway drug to fairy, witch and werewolf erotica.

Both of these doctors are probably geniuses, hyperaware of the hallmarks of addiction, and, therefore, serve as walking, talking cautionary tales that show that all of us can fall prey to this, regardless of IQ or education.

What's extra-interesting about these addictions is the unexpected nature; operatic symphonies and spicy stories seem innocuous enough, so appear unlikely to grow teeth and claws, and yet the behaviours around them were just as corrosive to their familial relationships as a traditional 'big' addictions might be.

Me? Shopping addiction and I have been regular bedfellows. Never so much that I ended up penniless, but enough to be occasionally toothy.

My first real shopping binge was after getting my paws on my first ever credit card in 1999, issued automatically with my student account (or has my denial woven that convenient tale? Who knows). This starter tricycle for two decades of wheel-spinning debt had a limit of £150; I remember thinking that was *riches*. Feeling like I was re-enacting *Pretty Woman* without the sex work, I took it directly to a branch of Intimissimi and bought five sets of candy-coloured lingerie.

I was engaging in magical thinking that lacy knickers would get my boyfriend at the time to propose, then build me a house with 'blue shutters and a room overlooking the river so I can paint' (bonus points if you know the movie), or at the very least not dump me. My magical thinking was c/o 19 years of hardcore Victoria's Secret-sponsored conditioning that, if you're sexy, pleasing and fragrant enough, you'll get rewarded with the ultimate treasure of an engagement ring.

A fine example of how, when we're shopping, we're frequently not seeking the thing itself, but rather the thing we think the purchase will secure for us. The thing beneath the thing. Commitment c/o underwear.

It took me four years to pay this credit card off, given my long-term financial nous was non-existent back then (teach APR rates in schools, already), and I only managed the piddly minimum payments, plus I got slapped with a bunch of late payment charges at £12 a pop. By the time the underwear disintegrated, it had lasted two years longer than the relationship, and had actually cost me triple the price tag, at £450. I may as well have bought knickers made with cashmere and gold thread.

Undeterred, I have continued to shop *just* out of my price range, even though I now earn a decent whack. The TK Maxx sprees of my mid-30s, when I was making just £18,000 as a freelance writer, have become COS and Selfridges turns in my mid-40s, now that I earn circa the same as my age. It's as if I am determined to get rid of all my spare money. Hate money, how can I make sure it all goes away? *Throws it into the air*

It's not that I hate money, of course. It's just that the instant high from shopping is much more persuasive than the slow burn of saving.

Nowadays, I would characterise my little shopping addiction as fourfold:

1. Slouchy athleisure, because I hate to be uncomfortable, and no longer care if you fancy me, but also want to look like I am prepared for parkour 24/7.
2. Vinted binges on tiny clothes and shoes for my daughter, during which I tell myself I am an eco-hero, given I am buying pre-loved rather than new, despite the carbon footprint of 25 separate deliveries trundling towards me from 25 of the furthest corners of the UK.
3. Interiors items – think solid mango furniture and paint named after mouse fur – because I finally bought a little mid-terrace house aged 43, and now need it to look like Soho House in order to feel adequate.
4. Books. More than one human could ever read in a lifetime. I find buying them comforting, soul-affirming, joyful; but then my towering to-be-read pile gives me anxiety of the likes of stress dreams about eternally losing a race.

I don't know one human – not one! – who doesn't have some sort of Shakespearean tragic flaw when it comes to shopping. We all do mad shit in order to hunt and gather new stuff.

It might be getting the latest iPhone, even though there's nothing wrong with the handset we've owned for two tiny years, which we acquire via 'free' upgrade, meaning the handset costs us hundreds more than buying it outright. Or, we hoard a skyline of designer fragrances, all almost flipping well full, but then can't resist the latest one advertised by Taylor Swift, who fell through an enchanted mirror into a chandelier-filled forest to sell it to us, so it would be rude not to. Or we sign up to a totally unreasonable 29.9% APR to spread the cost of a new fixie bike, when we already have a nearly new fixie bike. Collecting crystals, oracle cards and essential oils is another common one, given these spiritual items carry promises of future-telling, life changing and emotional bliss. And who wouldn't want a piece of that?

The primal drivers behind this

So, why do we overconsume? Why do we buy more than we need – or spend slightly more than we can afford?

A scientific study published in 2023 (studies always have such fun names, and this one is *The behavioural crisis driving ecological overshoot*) posits that the landscape of little shopping addictions may be modern, but the impulses powering them are ancient, calling out 'the innate suite of human behaviours that were once adaptive in early hominid evolution, but have now been exploited to serve the global industrial economy'.

This is a dry, academic way of saying that the behaviours that once saved our cave-dwelling skins are now caffeinating our credit card habits. The authors of the study call this 'suite' out as mainly:

- Hoarding and defending resources
- Pleasure-seeking and pain-avoiding
- Displaying dominance via ornamentation
- Gaining romantic approval c/o beauty

Whenever you're buying almost anything, you are secretly being driven by one of these ancestral urges. Once you identify which one it is, you're in with a chance of dismantling it.

Maybe you think you deserve a treat after a clusterfuck of a week at work. The urge to burn £50 on a Deliveroo lands. You identify that the thing beneath the urge is: pleasure-seeking. It's not so much about the food as the reward for being a super-worker. 'When you've done enough' as the (masterful) Uber Eats slogan goes.

How can you seek the same pleasure, the same feeling of having a treat, without being £50 poorer? It might be that picking up one of those £12 meal deals, where you get a main, side and drink, is enough to give the same buzz.

Or you might tell yourself that you *need* a Ninja air fryer. But once you dig beneath that apparent need, you find that it's because your brother is coming to visit and he's been bragging about his model, and you feel the need to compete. You can drop out of that imaginary race for dominance and buy the cheaper one recommended by *Which?*

'The evolutionary drive to acquire resources is by no means exclusive to the human animal,' the study points out. But unlike squirrels who can only find so many nuts to bury (known as 'caching'), we have access to unlimited gatherable baubles.

There are parallels, though. When we're buying clothes, fragrances or beauty items to make ourselves sexier, we're not unlike the male satin bowerbird, which exclusively collects blue items (berries, bottle tops, shells, feathers) and then sits among its blue treasure, expectant and horny, waiting to attract a mate. It even grinds up blue things to make a pigment to colour its nest. Now *that's* commitment.

Ancestral hunting and foraging

Traditional gender roles also drive our shopping behaviours. Way back when, men would have predominantly been the hunters of big game, rightly or wrongly. Hunter stalks animal, kills animal and carries it home, pronto. Meanwhile the gatherers – mainly women with babies in slings or small children at foot – would have operated in groups, browsing at length from food patch to food patch, micro-analysing colour and quality, with an intricate knowledge of seasons and harvests.

Women would have hunted too, evolutionary psychologist Dr Andrew Thomas told me, and they were actually the main providers of food. 'The more consistent calories would have come from women in these societies, mainly via foraging, but also from hunting rabbits and birds.'

The gendered pinking of 'shop till you drop' clichés are grating. Men – some of whom are the most discerning consumers out there – are meanwhile stereotyped as clueless grunts grabbing the nearest jumper and lurching from the shop. And yet the expert chatter about these tendencies is everywhere, when you dig into the evolutionary roots of shopping behaviour.

One study theorised that this hunter/gatherer assignment is why women tend (emphasis on *tend*) to see shopping as recreational and social, seeking out as much information as possible prior to buying, and will even pursue opportunities to shop on holiday, given that it represents a brand new harvest to peruse. (I don't relate to any of this. Maybe I would have been off on my own with a slingshot for the birds.) This same study says that men tend (again, emphasis on tend) to be less interested in shopping in general, less attuned to nuances like colour, or to linger once they've achieved their goal. They point out that women are less likely to be colour-blind and are proven to be 'more sensitive to pinks, reds and yellows than men', which is thought to be linked to the need to identify ripening fruits and vegetables, back when they were mainly the gatherers.

This is all super fascinating – as well as irritatingly binary – but we need some tangible tools.

The anti-buying lever

We know from a groundbreaking 2007 Stanford University study, that there is a particular process in the brain when we decide whether or not to buy an item. The study leaders linked shoppers up to an fMRI (for the earthlings among us: a brain-scanner) to analyse what exactly happened in the brain.

When assessing an item for purchase, this is the process:

1. When looking at the item, a shopper's nucleus accumbens activates first, a mid-brain section known for appraisal.

2. Next up, the medial prefrontal cortex gets involved, which is associated with sophisticated executive functioning.
3. If the shopper decides not to buy, the insula – a region known for negative arousal, disgust and loss aversion – lights up. (Experts refer to this reaction as the 'pain of payment'.)

'Excessive prices activated the insula,' the study said. This is why fast fashion is catnip for shoppers. The insula is less likely to be activated, given it's so dang cheap.

Fighting against the allure of that is the recent exposure as to *why* it's so cheap, with companies such as Shein, Temu and Zara being hauled into the dock for damning ethnical issues (at times literally in the dock, with a Shein lawyer notoriously refusing to answer a committee on where exactly they source their cotton).

The lack of insula activation could also be why buy-one-get-one-free deals and 'free' gifts to bigger spenders are so tantalising. I can think of several occasions I've bought an extra beauty item I entirely did not need, to get a free goody bag of tiny toiletries I entirely did not want . . . which I may end up re-gifting to someone I partially do not like.

Using a credit card is thought to activate the insula less, or not at all. Brian Knutson, the neuroscientist who led the Stanford study, theorised: 'Maybe [a shopper's] insula isn't engaged when they're using credit cards.' The study says that the abstract nature of credit, coupled with delayed payment, may 'anaesthetise' the intervention of the insula. Other studies back this up, including one from the Massachusetts Institute of Technology, finding that using credit cards places financial costs 'out of mind'.

In other words, credit – whether via an overdraft, 'buy now, pay later' or trad credit card – disrupts a necessary seesaw, in that the pleasure of a purchase is usually counterbalanced by the painful thought of immediately needing to pay for it. Without that requisite seesaw, wahey! Let's buy the world. Who wants a pony? I'm buying.

But the insula's intervention ordinarily *is* good news. It means that we can use this as a lever to turn the urge to shop off. So, if you want to stop buying fast fashion, the swiftest way to activate your insula might be via moral outrage, by learning about underpaid – or child – labour via documentaries. Or your button to press for outrage might be illegal deforestation or land grabs, also strongly linked to fast fashion.

Becoming a subscriber of ethicalconsumer.org is also a good way to de-muddy the waters. They score over 40k brands – from fashion and food through to confectionary and tech – on their ethics.

Another way to activate your insula might be to imagine the long-term consequences of this little addiction to shopping. Myself, I have no pension. Yup, zero retirement savings whatsoever. This is my useful way to prod the insula.

Right now, my nucleus accumbens is trying to tell me I cannot live without a £399 onyx coffee table, which I definitely cannot afford and definitely do not need. As my insula is not staging an appropriate intervention, I can use my pension-less lever like so:

I imagine myself having to downsize from my far-from-upsized 2.5 bedroom mid-terrace when I hit retirement, because I was a financial fuckwit and spent all my bloody money on onyx coffee tables, even though I don't know what onyx is. I picture having to go and live in a studio flat with my gorgeous onyx table, and a pot of instant noodles sitting upon it given that's all I can afford for dinner.

Yeah, no, I don't want that table any more. I want a pension, thanks.

See? I mean, insula activation is not a fun game, I grant you. I can think of fantasies I'd much rather have and none of them involve me eating Pot Noodles as a pensioner. But it does work.

Your way of activating your insula might be this: because you didn't start an ISA for your child – due to your penchant for Ray-Bans that you keep losing – you imagine them living on the greased pole of renting until their mid-forties, where they just get poorer and poorer despite how much they earn, and they then denigrate you to their therapist who they can't really afford to pay for, but have to go to because they're so depressed. Fun!

Or it might be that you figure out that your daily cellophaned sandwich, which could easily be made at home, adds up to £960 a year, which could pay for a magnificent fortnight in a Welsh cottage.

Coming back to my retirement self-envisioning, this tactic is backed up by science. A fascinating 2011 study exposed participants to age-progressed versions of themselves via virtual reality. They found that those who saw the rendering of their future self then allocated more than *double* of an imaginary windfall to retirement savings. They also committed to saving nearly two per cent more of their future pay for retirement.

We're going to talk about the wily ways retailers manipulate you into spending what you don't intend at much greater length on pages 241 to 246, but for now, I have a letter for you.

Dear little shopping addict,

I need to tell you about a little-known bias that – once I named it and understood it – shook my little shopping addiction loose.

I'm a binge shopper. I often apologise to fitting room attendants wondering how to deal with me trying to take 11 items in, or overstretched till staff raising their eyebrows at the amount of stationery items they now have to ring up.

I tell myself that since I don't really enjoy shopping (lies), when I *do* do it, I 'go hard or go home', as if I'm a pro sportsperson. This adds a layer of athleticism to my overspending, as if I've sweated so hard I have to change out my top mid-match (not actually unheard of on an Olympian shopping day). Somebody give me a medal and pay me to jump around a skate park in branded leggings.

Those with a little addiction to shopping are rarely consuming one or two items. It's usually a binge, where once you start, you go until you drop.

This bias is called the Diderot Effect. Essentially, our new stuff makes our old stuff look unworthy, like a supermodel standing next to an earthling, and so we spend more in an effort to 'complete' our now mismatched living room, or wonky work wardrobe, or lopsided vinyl collection.

This bias is named after a French philosopher who described the effect in his essay called 'Regrets For My Old Dressing Gown', which is a pompously comic masterpiece.

'My old robe was one with the other rags that surrounded me,' Diderot wrote. 'A straw chair, a wooden table, a rug from Bergamo*, a wood plank that held up a few books, a few smoky prints without frames . . . All is now discordant.'

---

* Bergamo is a sexy walled city in Italy, which makes me think Diderot was prone to a humblebrag.

He was the master of his old dressing gown; now he's become a slave of the new. His acquisition of this dressing gown then leads to him nearly bankrupting himself and forgetting his family exist, given it rolls into him buying new artwork, a writing desk, a large mirror, a gold-plated clock and a leather chair . . . all to match his singular new 'precious garment'.

Meanwhile, in deepest Sussex in 2024, my partner and I decided that since our home office resembles that room in *Harry Potter* where they put all the random crap that they don't know what else to do with (the 'Room of Requirement'), we should tart ours up. Or at least simply make it less likely that we accidentally die in there.

Of course, I told myself that this office refurb was an essential prequel to my writing of this book, that I simply could not start work until I have a gleaming home office with hanging plants and colour co-ordinated bookshelves, and 'This must be the place' flying up the wall in neon, even though the coolness of neon signs and colour-blocked shelves died in Hackney sometime in the late 2010s.

Turns out I am the human embodiment of the Diderot Effect. I set out to buy three things: a new desk, chair and paint colour. But once I started . . . I realised the new desk would show up our brassy £9 lamp. That the sleek Swedish chair would make our carpet look like knitted beige pubes. And that the 'cooking apple green' paint would sit smug and pretty next to our dirty and unpretty concertina blinds.

Everything had to go. Everything had to be new. I intended to spend £700 and spent £1,500.

And so I have never related to a fellow consumer more than this French 18th-century philosopher. If Diderot and I lived in the same century and hit the super-mall of Bluewater, I feel sure we would give them a bumper profits day, and then rebuild our strength with burgers and milkshakes, surrounded by our cityscape of glossy bags.

'Evil instinct of the convenient!' he might cry after our milkshakes, shaking his fist at Uniqlo beside us, and then I might try to fist bump him, but he leaves me hanging because they don't know about fist bumps in 18th-century France – and besides, we're both deep into midlife so should know better. And then Diderot falls to the floor muttering, 'My friends, fear the touch of wealth. Let my example teach you a lesson,' rocking in the foetal position.

Then I'll ask him if he wants to do a quick lap of Lululemon before we leave because the sale's on and nobody in their right mind buys Lululemon full price, and he'll agree because we're both little addicts.

Here's the denial that sits within the Diderot Effect. I fool myself that this upload of new items will be the upload that finally completes my office or winter wardrobe or living room. Maybe you do the same, telling yourself that this set of kettlebells will be the crowning detail of your home gymware, or that this set of Japanese knives is the pièce de résistance of your cooking kit.

But it never ends. The buying of stuff. There's always more box-fresh stuff to buy, that you tell yourself you can't live without, that you claim to need, but let's face it, nine times out of ten you just want.

Knowing about all of this is half of the battle won. Applying your intelligence – your discernment – to your own biases and deeply entrenched drives, plus knowing about the retailers' ploys, sensory wiles and charm tactics – that knowledge gives you the edge in the tussle of your limited money vs the many people who want to take it from you.

Love,
Cath x

SHOPPING MICRO TACTICS

Interoceptive body hack

We talked about interoception at length on page 83, and studies have shown that it can turn the insula *on* and, therefore, turn the urge to buy *off*.

You could hack this via a change of temperature by stepping outside the shop briefly or downing a glass of water when you've just filled an online basket. For those into medieval-style self-flagellation, researchers say that pinching your arm will do nicely.

The record collection tactic

The only shopping habit I have, for which I have failed to turn the insula on, is book-buying. Whether it's wilful defiance or not, I cannot bring myself to be disgusted. Given that the stress caused by my book-buying is purely mental (the to-be-read pile) and not financial, I've found this hack that works. I now think of my book collection as a record collection, rather than a chronological to-do list. I'll pick *that* one up when I'm in the mood for it, just as I would pick up a Khruangbin vinyl. It's helped, enormously.

Cancel the word 'budget'

Language matters, when reminding yourself of what you want to spend. Even writing the word 'budget' makes me want to upturn a table, race out of the door to an outlet store and overspend wildly. There has never been a more staid word, and I feel like it lives in a briefcase delivered by John Major. I like the phrase 'spending boundary' because it makes me feel empowered, but if you're allergic to wokespeak, (unlike me) maybe try 'ceiling' or 'limit'. These feel much more voluntary and self-imposed.

Capitalise on the 'butt brush' effect

No, this is not a weird item sold by sex shops. It is the name of a shopping bias, named by retail researchers. Compelling evidence shows we're less likely to linger in packed shops where people might brush up against us, particularly from behind.

If you have a spending ceiling, you could leverage this by deliberately going shopping for essentials at the busiest times. Your butt may well be so offended that it grabs what you actually need and powers you out of the shop before you can buy anything else.

If you don't need it, don't touch it

Shoppers feel more attached to items they have touched, a UCLA study found. This is why brands often provide a 'touch window' on items like toys or packaged underwear. This even extends to us preferring online items that are being touched by other humans in the images, which is why hands are often seen holding products in marketing images. Think before you pick it up.

If you want to stay objective, use your laptop

Behavioural scientist Patrick Fagan says that the 'touch it, buy it' bias even applies with touchscreens. 'A study found that we also feel more attached to an item that we "touch" by scrolling on a touch screen,' he says. This means that we exert greater control when shopping using a good old-fashioned laptop or monitor.

Beware of 'free' things that aren't free

As we've covered, I am a total sucker for 'free' delivery thresholds or 'free gifts' or 'spend £100 to get 15 per cent off'. It's like my IQ drops 30 points, and I immediately cast around to spend £23 more in order to not pay £2.50 on shipping. If you're the same, get wise to this tactic. You're playing into their expert hands. They are nefarious geniuses, with their free-but-not-free switcheroo. Thankfully, you are clever too.

Seeing 'future you'

Remember that study which showed how seeing an age-progressed future us can lead to us doubling our retirement savings? Most of us don't have the VR tech to hang out with a pensioner version of ourselves, but we can easily see an age-progressed picture for free via an app. I accessed an imagined image of 70-year-old me via a free week's trial on the YouCam Makeup app (in 'AI styles' and 'AI ageing'). As with all apps, you must cancel *instantly* after obtaining the image, to avoid bonkers yearly subscription charges (YouCam Makeup is £79.99 a year). Cancel via Apple Account – Subscriptions if you have an iPhone.

THE SECRETS RETAILERS DON'T WANT YOU TO KNOW

Retailers are more manipulative than you can possibly imagine.

And why wouldn't they be? Their survival depends upon your spend. Many employ psychological gurus to tell them how to get avoidant browsers to commit, how to cajole quickies into lifelong fidelity or how to transform a 'just one thing' intention into a Roman binge.

Interestingly, many of these big retailers gag the psychologists they hire via non-disclosure agreements. While seeking a consumer psychologist for this chapter, I've consistently happened upon lines like 'department stores we are not allowed to name' upon their websites.

Isn't that interesting? The stores don't want us to know.

I decided to uncover the anthropology of two shops I undertook – both in person and online – by narrating exactly how I felt, reacted and spent, and taking an expert (Patrick Fagan, a behavioural scientist and co-author of *Free Your Mind : The new world of manipulation and how to resist it*) along for the ride – one of the very experts hired by brands to manipulate shoppers like me.

Which shopping decisions are truly ours, and which are nudged from us by clever design, marketing or time-pressure tactics? We'll probably never know, unless we have a behavioural scientist in our ear (as with here). But we *can* know as much as the retailers do, such as what drives us to buy, in order to give ourselves a fighting chance for objectivity.

The physical shops

My nearest city is Brighton, so I head there for the day, intending to buy three things: a gift for a friend, a black knitted hoodie for myself and some new AirPods, given my current set make me sound like I'm making phonecalls from the bottom of the ocean.

The first shop that lures me in is The White Company. It's one of my favourite shops but also one of those I spend the least in – even with my newfound midlife semi-splashy income, it's usually a splash too far for me. The first thing I notice is the smell. It's *unreal*. The lighting is soft, everything is milk or oatmeal, even the shop's fittings feel luxury. Accordingly, I can't see much priced under £50.

I tell the expert what I'm experiencing. 'Smell puts us into a heightened state of physiological arousal, making us more likely to engage with what's in the shop,' says Fagan. 'It can even bait us to visit shops we didn't intend to; this is why bakery items or fresh flowers are often placed near the door.'

He says that 'smell priming' is triggered by retailers deliberately, whereby our behaviour is influenced without us being aware of it. 'Research showed that when a casino sprayed a neutral, nice smell around a certain cluster of slot machines, spends went up significantly.'

Priming even directs us to buy a certain type of item, reveals Fagan. 'When a shop smells of pine trees, people are proven to buy more Christmas-related stuff. Whereas pumping a chocolate smell into a bookshop made sales of romance novels go up.'

My nose leads me to a 'sea salt' product line that smells like a beach day (I'm getting crashing waves, seagrass, cedar trees and coconut sun lotion), and, given the friend I'm buying for is a beach freak, I think it might be perfect. A discreet tag tells me it's £55.

'Expensive items tap into "prestige pricing", whereby we attach more value because it costs more,' Fagan tells me. 'It doesn't make sense that if a brand increases the price they will sell more, yet it happens. The bias behind it is called the "price-quality heuristic" and it happens because we rely on rules of thumb. If something is expensive, we assume it must be better.'

This bias is demonstrated with blind wine tasting, he explains. 'When blindfolded, people can't really discern the differences between the wines. But when they're told a certain wine is expensive, they like it more.'

I pick the gift set up, reflecting upon the fact that I would *never* buy this for myself. I ponder whether I love her enough to spend £55 on the luxury gift set. I decide I do, so I take it to the till.

Many studies show that we spend more when it's a gift, says Fagan. 'Gifts are largely financially ineffective, given we get gifts we don't really want, but we're moved by them because of the offering. It's about someone caring about you enough to spend that money.' The actual item is largely irrelevant, he says.

This is seen in nature too. 'Male fruit flies always give a piece of food to the female before copulation can begin,' he says. In one study, researchers removed the food gift and replaced it with a bit of fluff. 'It still worked,' laughs Fagan. 'After copulation, the male fruit fly picked up the fluff and tried to use it on a different female.'

Back to The White Company. As I'm leaving the shop, I see several items of clothing I want to pick up, to touch – they look like they'd feel soft as a kitten's ear. But I resist, because I'm now aware of the study about us getting attached to items we touch (on page 240).

'Retailers encourage us to touch things because it triggers the endowment effect,' says Fagan. If we touch it, we feel more like we own it. 'And if we own something, we don't want to lose it,' so loss aversion feeds in here. Neuroimaging has shown that it's twice as painful for the brain to lose, say, £50, than it is pleasurable to win £50. The loss is more painful than the gain. 'Brands use lots of marketing tricks to make people feel like they own something before they do; changing rooms so that you can wear the item, or test drives so that you've touched the leather seats.'

I know from previously lustful fondles in here that the clothing costs between £100 and £200 on average, which is too much for me, so I give myself an edge by keeping my hands to myself. I head out of the shop swinging my bag and feeling like I've outwitted *them*. Even though I'm £55 down. Ahem.

Next, I'm drawn to Flying Tiger, because . . . I don't know why, actually. Just because I'm fallible and it's cheap and fun. Nothing in there costs more than £30, so why not, right? I'm already playing into their hands.

Once in the racetrack layout, I'm a mouse in a maze. I can't get out until I've walked past every single item in the store. Much like Ikea, once you're in, you're *in*. There's no such thing as a quick dash to grab one item.

'Research shows we only see a quarter of the average shop we visit,' says Fagan. 'So, retailers try to get us to visit more of it, via devices like racetracks, or putting deals we want to see on end caps (at the end of aisles), or placing essentials such as milk or bread at the back of the store.'

Flying Tiger proudly uses whole pounds in their prices – a cornerstone of its philosophy. This is unique and bragworthy, because they're eschewing the bait of 'charm pricing', which is when a price ends in a 95, 99 or 9. The power of charm pricing is irrefutable; one MIT study found that a dress sold *more* units when priced at $39 rather than $34.

I lose an hour in the racetrack and emerge with a DIY ceramic bowl that I need to decorate myself with teeny tiny paints (I will never do this), a squishy fidget ball filled with coloured beads that will probably take 3,000 years to biodegrade and outlast humankind (legal: I said *probably*), a capybara plushie with an orange on its head (no idea) and a miniature candy shop frontage for my daughter, even though we don't give her sweets. I'm £36 poorer but, hey, I had fun.

It occurs to me, though; I could have bought myself something luxe in the last shop, which I truly wanted, rather than this bunch of essentially meaningless – if beguiling – nonsense.

'Finding a bargain produces a rush of dopamine that's akin to cocaine or porn use,' says Fagan, and I do indeed feel a bit high. 'Finding little trinkets we like also taps into our hardwired need to hoard things.' He adds that shops renowned for bargains (TK Maxx, Poundland, Primark) tend to be confusing, busy, overstimulating and soundtracked by fast music, which makes us more likely to be bamboozled into an impulse buy.

I need to grow the hell up, and I know it, so I go and do a very adult shop that I *know* will not seduce me to spend money I don't intend to spend, as I only buy new tech very rarely, such as when my 12-year-old laptop starts wheezing at the exertion of being on for a whole 10 minutes . . . Enter: the Apple Store.

Everything is so spacious and angular, it feels like a giant exhale. In fact, it's so spacious that I could drive my Mini through the centre of this aisle, but I probably won't, given all the sharp edges and the fact my car already resembles a scratchcard.

'There's research showing that angular shapes are seen as dangerous since they're sharp,' Fagan tells me, 'so this feeds into a brand's desire to be regarded as cutting-edge and efficient. Round or fuzzy shapes are found to be liked by more agreeable people, so if a brand is going for an agreeable consumer, they'll round it, whereas if they want a competitive consumer, they'll sharpen it.'

I pick up an iPad. Do I need a new iPad? I'm reminded of the endowment effect and put it down. This £329 iPad looks downright cheap given the upgrades next to it are priced at £599 and £999. 'Human beings aren't intuitively great at making value judgements in a vacuum,' says Fagan. 'This is because in the big picture of our evolutionary history, we haven't had price tags for all that long.' Homo sapiens have been around for 300,000 years and money was only invented circa 3,000 years ago, ergo it wasn't so long ago in our evolution that we were trading a bag of wool for a bag of wheat. 'But we *are* very good at making relative judgements,' he explains. 'This is why a retailer will place a few similar items together, so that we see an 80p pen alongside two more expensive ones, and can make a judgement call.' Like the cheaper iPad.

The shopping day is nearly at a close, so I dash into Tesco to buy fishcakes for dinner. Despite my knowledge of the end cap effect, I succumb to a two-for-one deal on minty shower gel, remembering at the till that I already have three bottles of half-full shower gel. But it's cheap! I wonder if our stockpiled coffers of BOGOF scores make us actually use more of a product?

'Tesco's branding of white, red and blue is designed to communicate value. It can't charge as much, but more people go there,' says Fagan. 'Whereas Waitrose has opted for dark green and gold to communicate luxury. The footfall is lower, but it commands a higher price.' Colours or fonts are tools with which they control our perceptions. 'Colour can even make us hungry,' adds Fagan. 'Red stimulates the appetite given it's a high-frequency colour, which is why brands such as Pizza Hut, McDonald's, KFC and Nando's all use it.' Whereas blue is a low-frequency colour, which calms.

I get home and realise, while unpacking the Airpods, as well as the miniature sweet shop and other assorted technicolour crap, that I completely forgot to buy the black knitted hoodie I genuinely wanted. Determined to complete my shopping mission, given our bias to complete things, I get online once my daughter is in bed. Thankfully, Fagan is here to help me out.

I browse a number of my favourite shops – COS, Massimo Dutti, AllSaints, Reiss – and notice that almost all of them follow a grid-like pattern, with four items across each scroll width, always worn by a model. We already know that items being touched by a human sell more, so that figures, but I ask Fagan about this quirk: I notice that the more expensive brands have more white space between items. Is this coincidence or design?

'It's absolutely design. In physical luxury boutiques, there's more white space between products, and they do the same online, because it's proven people will pay more.' He compares it to art galleries: the less there is in it, the more expensive it is.

'Another manipulation just in: upscale retailers are now following the lead of gourmet restaurants and dropping the pound sign from the price.' When a designer sweater is listed as '189', as with a main course listed as '35', it weakens our association with it being money, he explains.

Jettisoning the currency sign actually tricks our brain into spending eight per cent more, a study from Cornell University found. 'This only works with experiential, hedonic brands, though,' Fagan warns. 'If the item is functional, dropping the £ sign only puts people off.'

'Hurry, five other people are also viewing this item!' is another tactic online retailers now use, much of which is a fiction. And they've also taken to placing the 'sign up for 15 per cent off' pop-up right at the *beginning* of your browse, rather than after a few minutes, in order to stoke your fear that if you don't take advantage of the pop-up right now, you won't get the discount later.

I order two black hoodies from COS, reasoning that I'll send one back. 'Once they're in your home, though, and you've touched them, you're much more likely to keep them,' says Fagan. 'Many of the buy-now-pay-later services like Klarna leverage this. They encourage people to order three dresses for the same event when they wouldn't ordinarily, given they can opt to pay in 30 days' time. They intend to send two back, but then . . .'

He's too polite to say it, but I will: then we become like mice repeatedly running into the dead ends of a maze, rather than finding our way out.

But now? We're mice with a map. I know I feel empowered by everything I've learned. And if anyone wants to buy a plush capybara with an orange on its head, you know where I am.

ACTIVATING THE PREFRONTAL CORTEX'S POWER

The prefrontal cortex is the grown-up that we all need in a crisis.

The most sensible adult you know.

The one who has three different types of pension, knows how to deal with the gutters and owns packing cubes (which they *use*). The one who you invite to the pub quiz because they know about foreign policy, while your specialist subject is which celebrities have shagged each other. The person who probably isn't that fun to go dancing with . . . but is also the person you would call if your house were on fire.

The prefrontal cortex is the 'adult in the room', neuroscientist Dr Alex Korb told me. Dr Judith Grisel, who's also a neuroscientist, agreed. She called it 'the overbearing adult' of the brain. In the alcohol chapter (pages 34 to 50) you may recall that Dr Sarah Bayless called the prefrontal cortex the controller, 'who makes sure all the systems are running correctly.' It's the source of our ability to make solid decisions, she said.

The personification of this brain region as 'the sensible one' carries across the board, although the metaphors vary. Who cares? We care, because the prefrontal cortex is our secret weapon, when it comes to downregulating addictive urges.

Dr Anna Lembke refers to this brain region, situated behind the forehead, as the 'brakes on overconsumption'.

'We are all now vulnerable to prefrontal cortical atrophy as our reward pathway has become the dominant driver of our lives,' she wrote in *Dopamine Nation*.

Atrophy. Gosh. That sounds melodramatic.

What happens with big addictions?

But it's not. When we're grappling with a big addiction, it's well-documented that the prefrontal cortex loses synaptic density. Or, in regular person terms, it shrinks. 'There's good evidence that the prefrontal cortex is less active in those in active addiction,' Dr Grisel said.

This is a problem, given the role of the prefrontal cortex as the sensible adult. Which is why big addictions are like a devolvement of sorts, Dr Grisel told me. Without the prefrontal cortex steering, the striatum and limbic system lead the charge.

Most experts agree that the striatum specifically – and limbic system at large – are the engines driving addiction. Dr Korb said so back on page 30, calling the striatum the 'seat of addiction', while Dr Grisel calls the limbic system 'the core'.

Once activities become habitual autopilot acts, the prefrontal cortex stops getting involved. 'This is a good thing, evolutionarily speaking,' Dr Grisel says. 'You don't want to really have to think deeply about changing a diaper, or driving home from work. Offloading that stuff to the habit circuits of the brain frees up space for other thoughts. You don't *want* your prefrontal cortex involved.'

But once our little addictions become habitual, that's where we run into trouble. 'Because *then* the prefrontal cortex is no longer regulating – or inhibiting – that behaviour,' she adds.

That little habit can then snowball to become a big addiction, given the prefrontal cortex's lack of intervention. Which is when all hell can break loose. Remember what Dr Korb said, about how our limbic system (the teenager) and the striatum (the dog) would happily lead our lives if we allowed them to? That. That's essentially what occurs with big addictions. The adult of the brain takes a back seat, and the dog and the teen take the wheel. I can confirm that when I had a big addiction, it did indeed feel like a spaniel and an adolescent were driving my life.

However, all is not lost. Like Dr Korb said earlier, there is hope, and lots of it. 'You *can* use your prefrontal cortex to teach your limbic system, and train your striatum, to make better choices,' he said.

The adult of the brain can teach the teen, and train the dog into more desirable choices, whatever those might look like for you.

Blunt tool

These personifications are – of course – crude simplifications of complex neuroscience. Dr Clayton Hickey, a psychology professor who plays a starring role in this chapter, warns me: 'The prefrontal cortex is a huge chunk of cortex, and using oversimplified descriptors for brain regions should be taken with a huge grain of salt.'

Grain of salt added.

'The prefrontal cortex is involved in high-level decision-making, problem-solving and information-organising. It creates cognitive maps,' he explains. 'If there *were* a guy driving the bus, the prefrontal cortex would be that guy. But there isn't.'

All I've heard is that it's the guy driving the bus.

Bus drivers aside, we all know this isn't *real*. We know that there are no teenagers or dogs playing tug of war over a packet of Hobnobs in our heads. Using fun metaphors to denote complex brain regions is a blunt tool, at best, and it's far from elegant.

Yet enough of my experts are into the notion of actionable ways of strengthening the prefrontal cortex ('I love this question,' says Dr Grisel when I ask her) that I feel emboldened to carry on.

If this blunt tool works, then why not use it?

I have a non-magical brain scan

Speaking of blunt tools, I'm at the University of Birmingham to find out more about my brain. I'm here to have an fMRI, or in social media speak, a 'brain scan'. Many of my psychotherapist friends (I collect them, like yoga teachers, because I need their wisdom) bemoan the 'magical brain scans' that get trotted out on social media and have no footing in empirical science.

It's deeply ironic that I'm at this particular university to obtain an image of my brain. I graduated from here in 2002 and this campus is arguably one of the places where I lost the most brain cells. I look for them on the floor outside the student union. All I can see is an avocado skin. Students – *you've changed.*

I applied for this university as a straight-A student (in A Levels as they were called back then), the type who literally handed in extra essays for kicks. But by the time I landed in halls of residence, my alcohol addiction had grown fur and fangs and I'd lost all interest in learning.

I barely attended lectures, showing up to just enough seminars to stop them from kicking me out. Instead of spending those precious years enhancing my grey matter, I systematically destroyed it, spending most of my time downing 99p pints of lager, smoking Marlboro Lights I had to work a bar job to afford, dancing to 'Last Night a DJ Saved My Life' and grabbing a 2am hot dog from a van (not a food truck).

Walking around my old uni campus, I feel a much warmer glow about the library than I do about the Students' Union. I don't even want to go *in* the Students' Union. I had a better time in the library. The Union just reminds me of tears, drama and blurred clinches, its crouching presence a symbol of regret.

I don't believe in 'if only I had' longings, but the one thing I *do* wish I had a do-over for is university.

Kids that are more likely to get addicted

My non-magical brain scan is happening at the Centre for Human Brain Health in the psychology department. When I arranged this fMRI, I wanted to know whether I had a thin prefrontal cortex. Oh, how the professors probably laughed at my ridiculous email.

For context, I wanted to know about my prefrontal cortex for very good reason. We've already covered that a thinner, less synaptically-dense prefrontal cortex can be a *consequence* of a big addiction, but a brand-new study has also found that it might pre-date it.

As an addiction geek, I got very excited when I learned of this finding, making grand statements about it being a 'neurodivergence we have yet to name!' I was then told to calm the F down by every expert I spoke with, so I obediently did. But this finding still breaks new ground and holds exciting future possibilities.

Here's what the study found. They took nearly 10,000 'substance-naive' children aged 9–11, or those who were yet to try any drug, and scanned their brains. The authors then followed up three years later, doing more brain imaging. What they uncovered was remarkable. The kids with a 'thinner prefrontal cortex' and 'greater whole-brain' volume before even picking up an alcoholic drink, vape, cigarette or spliff were *more likely* to pick up an alcoholic drink, vape, cigarette or spliff aged 12–14. These 'neuroanatomical features' predicted early pick-up, essentially, which – as we already know – leads to a greater risk of addiction later in life.

Do you see how important this could be?

'Early pick-up' is just an academic term for starting young. One landmark 1998 US study, looking at a sample of 43,000, found that those who start drinking before the age of 15 are four times more likely to go on to become addicted than those who start drinking at the legal age of 21.

Let's face it, 21 is unlikely as a starting age for drinking, but the study also found that rates of later addiction decreased by 14 per cent with each year of delayed drinking onset, blowing apart the 'teach 'em young at home' theory that many parents have, giving their teenagers glasses of wine with dinner. If kids start drinking before 15, they have a scary 40 per cent chance of later addiction. At 17, you're looking at 24.5 per cent. Those who hold off until 21 only have a 10 per cent chance.

Obviously much of this is beyond parental control, but we can control not giving it to them ourselves. Something I've been guilty of in the past, when I've snuck younger relatives cider at family parties.

Myself, I started drinking aged 12, and I have no doubt that this helped inform how attached my brain became to alcohol as a 'solution' for social anxiety. 'The data is crystal clear on the incidence between early pick-up and higher rates of addiction later,' Dr Grisel told me.

All of this feeds into why this study on brain differences is so fascinating. Because, if brain differences can predict early pick-up, then they can potentially predict later addiction.

I spoke with Professor Alex Miller, who led this exciting study out of

Washington University in St Louis. 'We already know that years of heavy substance use may cause differences in the brain, such as a thinner prefrontal cortex, which can then beget more substance use, making it harder and harder to overcome and abstain.'

'With a thinner prefrontal cortex, you potentially have the reduced capacity to inhibit impulsive behaviour and emotionally regulate,' he says.

'Impulsive behaviour' brings to mind that one time I lay in the road in Soho, in front of a taxi that refused to take me home. I robotically stuffed cheesy chips into my mouth, gravel in my hair, as the black cab beep-beep-beeped. You'll be amazed to hear that the driver still refused to take me.

'This study is the first large-scale effort to find those structural differences in the brain as something that pre-dates the early pick-up,' continues Miller. I ask him, hopefully, whether it's a neurodivergence we have yet to name. 'It's hard to say whether this is a neurodivergence, given there's more about the brain that we don't know, rather than what we do know.'

Bah. I've found myself here many times in the writing of this book: at the crossroads of hyperbolic journalist + cautious academic. I try again, imagining a world in which we can predict which teens are more vulnerable for later addiction . . . I hold my breath and will him to engage in my writerly drama.

'I don't think a future will come to pass where it will be a case of a parent paying for a brain scan of their child,' he says, 'and, based on that alone, receiving a completely accurate print-out of the percentage likelihood they will later grapple with addiction.'

I nod sagely and say, 'Of course, of course' in my most sensible voice.

Genetics and environment obviously play a part in this complex picture too, he points out; it's not just about structural brain differences. 'However, as the technology becomes more accessible, less expensive and less cumbersome, we should be able to form a more complete picture of these risk factors and how they interact.'

I'm asked about secret piercings

Back to my non-magical brain scan. As we touched on, I wanted to discover whether I too have a thinner prefrontal cortex than is the norm, like the kids in this study, and whether that's why I got on the alcohol train so early, riding it for 21 years.

Dr Clayton Hickey, a cognitive neuroscientist at the University of Birmingham, is kind about my utter naivety re: measuring my prefrontal cortex. He emails me ahead of the fMRI, saying that it would take thousands of samples to see any relationship, that this measure provides no predictive power on an individual basis and pointing out that the paper I reference was based on 9,804 scans.

Ahem, OK. I climb back into my box.

They indulge my request for an fMRI anyway, which makes me very happy and fires up *many* jokes among loved ones, such as, 'Cath's so self-involved she even wants a photo of her own cortex.' I'll take it.

Dr Hickey has a warm manner and an easy laugh, but is still authoritative. He's the kind of guy who's elected mayor in the newfound town set up after the zombie apocalypse.

The process is much more involved than I anticipated. I have to remove all metal from my person – jewellery in my case – due to the massive magnetic field of the fMRI machine. Even taking a picture of me next to it has to be done from 20 feet away, as otherwise the phone could go flying, damaging this multi-million-pound machine.

Hickey's pHD student, Thalia, tells me about bobby pins from her hair being whipped into the air. All metal will move, so I'm asked whether I have any secret piercings three times. You would want to remove a nipple piercing, for *sure*.

Then I have to strip completely and wear medical scrubs, which I take really seriously, and snap bathroom selfies of myself in, feeling very *Grey's Anatomy*. I need to be scanned twice for metals, with one of those handheld metal detectors they use in airports, including the soles of my feet. I lie down on what amounts to a big tray for humans, my head secured by pads, and a mask is placed over my face. With slats for eyes, it's not unlike Iron Man's mask, but made of plastic.

'It's important you're completely still for six minutes,' says Dr Hickey. Thankfully I have a toddler, so I am in need of a little lie down. I'm also not claustrophobic in the slightest, and am almost blindly trusting of medical experts. Once I'm raised up and slid into the cylinder, I'm looking forward to a six-minute nap. And I probably would nap, if it were not for the DUNNNG-DUNNNG-DUNNNG noise, much like a giant repeatedly playing a low note on a colossal electronic keyboard, which the foam earplugs muffle, but cannot eradicate.

'That's a nice cerebellum,' says chief radiographer Nina, about the resulting 3D image of my brain. My inner narcissist pops a hip. 'Textbook brain,' agrees Dr Hickey. There's even an image created of how I might look if I didn't have any hair. 'You look serene,' says Nina. She's being generous. I look like an extra on *Star Trek*; the one they don't give any lines to.

I ask Dr Hickey if there's anything he can tell me about my brain. He says I have small ventricles but it's nothing to worry about. Later that day, I will fall into a self-absorbed scrollhole of small ventricles and what they mean, and whether it means I am an inferior or superior human, much like the person who repeatedly Googles their Myers–Briggs personality type (also me).

We're now all talking about our little addictions. Aromatherapy sprays and vaping, says operations manager, Emma. TikTok probably, says Nina. Buying Japanese knives for cooking, says Dr Hickey.

Dr Hickey is equally as circumspect as Professor Miller was when it comes to my vision that we may one day be able to predict future addictions from brain scans. 'The predictive power of a thin prefrontal cortex is very, very low,' he says. 'This has no more implication for your propensity to addiction than it does for your propensity to like anchovies on your pizza.'

But then, Dr Hickey throws me a treat. I jump to catch it.

'Having said that, if you had many, many things you could measure, and you're modelling all of them at the same time, then *maybe* you could then get to the point where you can have the predictive power of saying, "OK, we should be particularly concerned about this 14-year-old kid".'

He points out that the UK is very well positioned for that: 'The NHS is a treasure trove of centralised data.' He tells me there's a lot of discussion in medical circles right now about whether they'll sell this cache of data for AI to use. 'It's worth billions, and they're going to use that data at some point. And they *should* use it because it will save many lives.'

Bigger brains get addicted

The keen-eyed among you may have noticed that the study of the kids also identified another predictive neuroanatomical feature for early pick-up, in the shape of 'greater whole-brain' volumes.

This is exactly what it sounds like – a bigger brain.

Again, this is exciting for geeks like me because, traditionally, addictions have been linked to a *smaller* overall brain volume. Whereas this finding suggests that a larger brain volume than usual exists before the addiction, but the addiction then shrinks the grey matter. How interesting is that?

Talking of big brains, the terms 'highbrow' and 'lowbrow' come from the 19th-century belief that bigger foreheads meant bigger brains (in which case I am a freaking *genius*). This seems simplistic in the extreme, but there is actually some merit to this, because larger brain volume does tend to correlate to a higher IQ, say studies and scientific articles.

'This question is ridiculous,' I say to Dr Hickey, feeling brave due to his generous manner. 'But I'm going to ask it anyway because it's funny . . . I have a big head. Does that mean I have a big brain and, therefore, a higher IQ?'

'Yes, there is a correlation there,' he says. I smile. 'But, we're talking about a relationship observed when you're looking at thousands and thousands of people. Somebody can have a big head but also be dumb as a rock.'

'Not me, though?' I say, my smile fading.

'Not you,' he laughs. Phew.

It's unclear whether the intelligence is a result of the big head, or whether the big head *and* intelligence are a result of genetic and environmental factors. Dr Hickey cites calorific intake as a baby, among many other causal factors in the mix.

The upshot is this – if you too find yourself adjusting baseball caps to the larger settings, you can feel somewhat smug that this probably means you have a higher IQ than your average bear. But – putting all of these puzzle pieces together – it could *also* mean you had/have a higher chance of addiction.

This isn't as much of a leap as it sounds. Many historic studies link higher IQ with higher drug use (this includes alcohol, since it's a drug) and subsequent addiction.

All of this neuro-chat is meaningless, of course, unless we have some actionable tools to take away. So, let's get into that.

NINE WAYS TO ENGAGE THIS SECRET WEAPON

I asked every expert I talked with about specific and practical ways of activating the prefrontal cortex, our foremost neuropower against little addictions. Here's what they said.

1. Reading instead of watching

If you find yourself shovelling *Wotsits* into your mouth mindlessly while watching YouTube, or craving a beer every time you lay down to watch a blockbuster film, you might find that switching to reading of an evening helps downshift your use of [insert thing].

'Watching something is more likely to activate the limbic system,' says Dr Alex Korb. 'Reading may be more effortful, but it brings the prefrontal cortex online, which helps us be more rational.'

2. Naming what's going on

We can activate the prefrontal cortex by naming whatever cognitive distortion is going on. 'It's like Rumpelstiltskin,' Chris Lomas says, an addiction psychotherapist at Delamere residential rehab. 'Once you have the name of the little chap you can control him more.'

For those who don't know, Rumpelstiltskin is the star of a German fairy tale. He's essentially a child-snatcher (19th-century kids' books were *so fun*). He steals the Queen's first-born and the only way she can get him back is by guessing his name.

Because Rumpelstiltskin's name is so weird, he assumes the Queen won't be able to guess it. But she does, and so he has to give the infant back.

It's a masterful simile because that's exactly what naming a cognitive distortion does: gives us the power back. And this works for all little addictions, given they are cognitive distortions in action, whether it's people-pleasing, dating-app fixation or elaborate procrastination.

3. Radical honesty

When I ask Dr Anna Lembke for a specific, actionable way to engage the prefrontal cortex, she's punchy. 'Tell the truth, every day, about things large and small.' I couldn't agree with this point more. When I was writing this book, my partner said, 'Maybe you should write about your weird honesty thing; that feels like a little addiction.'

I am morally resistant to lying now, and have been ever since I quit drinking. I falter sometimes (the average Briton tells two lies a day), but generally I will only lie nowadays if being honest would be cruel.

Radical honesty means eradicating every little lie, even the white ones, wherever possible. Nobody does this perfectly, and the biggest culprits for everyday auto-lies are the tiny self-aggrandisers ('I'm meat-free at home' – you ate some ham on a pizza last week), meeting social scripts to maintain harmony ('you don't look your age' or 'it was nice to see you too') or painting yourself as a victim rather than taking accountability ('I sat in traffic for 20 minutes' – it was more like 10; you left 10 minutes late).

4. Surrounding ourselves with truth-tellers

Lembke tells me that the honesty of those we surround ourselves with has a profound impact. She cites a follow-up to the famous marshmallow test of 1970.

The original Stanford test left kids aged three to six alone in a room with a marshmallow. If they didn't eat the marshmallow, they'd get another in 15 minutes, doubling the treat. It's *the* classic study cited for the ability to delay gratification. There have been many spin-offs, but the most fascinating was carried out by the University of Rochester in New York. We'll call it the 'broken promises' marshmallow test.

Half of the kids in the study experienced broken promises before being asked to wait for the marshmallow, in the shape of promises of better crayons or stickers that failed to materialise. Those kids could only wait three minutes before stuffing the marshmallow in their mouth. When the adult running the experiment made good on their promises beforehand, the kids were able to wait four times longer – an average of 12 minutes. Isn't that wild?

'Surrounding ourselves with truth-tellers cultivates a plenty mindset,' Dr Lembke told me. 'When we can rely on the people around us to do what they said they would do, that gets us out of the scarcity mindset and allows us to delay gratification, which must work through the prefrontal cortex since that's primarily where delayed gratification is strengthened.'

It's one of the reasons why your childhood home environment can be co-creator of your addictive behaviours. As well as why – as an adult – a toxic boss or cheating partner can fuel your overconsumption. It's not your imagination. But, like we said earlier, even when it's not *all* your fault, it is still – inconveniently – all your responsibility.

5. De-centring yourself

Speaking of others, focusing on them can power up the prefrontal cortex, says Dr Grisel. 'Social interactions that elicit theory of mind – so are not about yourself – will work,' she says. (We talked about theory of mind back on page 138 too.) 'Getting out of our own way and not being the centre of all things, essentially.' She adds, 'Of course, with addiction, we and the drug are the centre, and everything else is superfluous.'

She cites volunteer work, or picking up the rubbish in a local park or beach, as good ways to de-centre ourselves. The 12-step structure springs to mind too, where longer-term sober members support newbies. It could also be as simple as supporting a friend through a break-up, or remembering to ask a family member how their job interview went.

6. Meditation

'Meditation clearly works,' Dr Grisel says. I've seen the studies too, about meditation thickening the prefrontal cortex, and they're borderline fantastical. One even suggested that meditation could 'offset age-related cortical thinning', which occurs naturally.

I don't know about you, but it feels like the universe is now repeatedly bopping me over the head with this 'regular meditation is transformative' point.

This transformation takes years, not weeks, experts say. Do swiftly dismiss any outlandish claims from snake-oil salespeople of eight-week courses being able to structurally change your brain. Nope.

7. Exercise

Again, with the exercise. Another tactic repeatedly being bowled to us.

'Exercise works, for sure,' says Dr Grisel, 'because it's healthy for the brain and burns up cortisol, protecting the prefrontal cortex from toxic effects.'

Dr Lembke goes a step further, writing that 'Exercise has a more profound and sustained positive effect on mood, anxiety, cognition, energy and sleep than any pill I can prescribe.' Just a 30-minute walk a day can do the trick, she says.

8. Delay rewards

Delaying a reward lights up the prefrontal cortex, Dr Lembke said. As we covered, relentlessly giving in to rewards of instant gratification – sweets, screen time, another episode, a blast on a vape – is what 'atrophies' the prefrontal cortex. This suggests that when you never delay rewards, the prefrontal cortex can waste away like a muscle during bed rest.

In *Indistractable*, behavioural designer Nir Eyal told me what he and his family use. 'In 10 minutes we can' is their mantra. This even extends to his teenage daughter, whom they've empowered to make her own usage decisions on technology, rather than policing her. He reports that installing this auto-delay means the urge often fades for them as a family, or even disappears altogether.

9. Big-picture judgements

Most of all, the reason the prefrontal cortex is so vital is because it deals in abstracted value judgements, which are bigger-picture choices.

'You like coffee and you like chocolate. But which do you prefer?' asks Dr Hickey (well, *this* feels like a Sophie's choice). 'You need to put them into the same frame of reference, and the prefrontal cortex does a lot of that.'

Here's the interesting part. 'You liked getting high, but you also like being sober,' he says, gesturing to me. 'Getting high had a particular thing about it that you liked, and it was instantly there. Staying sober has a much more complicated, longer-term value structure, which requires cognitive control again and again. It's a back-propagation of that reward signal.'

Long-term sobriety is indeed a massive daisy-chain of delayed gratification, set over many years. It would be far easier to break that chain, capitulate and just have a damn drink already in that first hour of feeling awkward at a party, when we don't know where to put our hands and we can't find the sparkling water. But when we don't, we are activating our prefrontal cortex by zooming out to see the bigger picture, choosing *that* priority over instant relief.

****

I wonder if this last point is why studies show that the prefrontal cortex bounces back in recovery. That the synaptic density lost through big addiction is later regained through abstinence. This is shown over and over again with cocaine, alcohol and nicotine. One study into alcohol found that the lost frontal cortex volume is regained within just 7.5 months of abstaining.

Even more intriguing is this: another study, cited by Dr Marc Lewis in

The Biology of Desire, found that, not only can the volume of the prefrontal cortex be restored, it can even go beyond the baseline of those who were never addicted in the first place.

This makes sense to me, since those in recovery are consistently activating that 'bigger picture' weigh-up of instant vs delay. Which amounts to weekly, daily, hourly sets of reps in resisting. Recovery places our prefrontal cortex in a bootcamp. But this bootcamp isn't exclusive to those in recovery. These resisting reps are available to us all, whatever proportion our addiction is, and whether we opt for abstinence or moderation. On page 126, psychotherapist Hilda Burke brilliantly called it 'wait-training'.

Instead of thinking of it as being tiring, try reframing it as being strengthening. Each time we refrain from that fourth biscuit, it's another arm curl. Each time we delay our TV watching until the allowed slot of 9–10pm, it's another leg press. Every self-bind of 'not right now, darling' whenever we want a weed gummy, vape, or social media bump, is another push-up.

As Hebbian theory says, 'what fires together, wires together'. It'll soon become the new normal for you to refrain, delay, resist, temper. The more you do it, the stronger you – and your prefrontal cortex – will become.

TELEVISION

TV is the dominant artform of the 2020s. It's the one we consume the most; way more than anything else.

But I mean, of course it is. Other than music we're not really listening to, we spend more time watching telly than looking at art, reading and – obviously – attending the theatre given we're not living in Shakespearean England, snacking on pickled herring or talking about who got dunked for being a witch last week.

Your average Brit spends 2 hours and 16 minutes a day watching telly, says the most recent ONS data. The first emotion that slammed into me when I read this was: intense envy. Who are these people?! I'm fortunate if I get an hour. I would *love* to spend over two hours a day. And then I thought: that sounds too low. I was right. It is too low.

That 2 hours and 16 minutes is *self-reported*. And humankind is infamous for rounding down our little addictions, with proven gaps in guesstimating our booze intake or social media use. We need a different source. Enter the industry go-to BARB, which crunches big data from devices and broadcasters themselves, and mines figures from meters in place at 7,000 British households. Turns out the true average is just over three hours a day. That sounds more like it.

Headlines even go so far as to blame TV (specifically, streaming) for the falling levels of shagging across the board, or *even* declining birth rates. It's a reach. Or is it? One scary survey found that 30 per cent of Americans would rather give up sex for a year than Netflix.

Dopamine by design

So, why are we sacrificing almost a fifth of our waking day to the flat-screen altar?

'Streaming services are designed to be addictive,' says neuroscientist Dr Korb. 'It's intentional.' He explains that TV-makers hijack both our natural human curiosity and our reward system, which, as we know, is mostly fuelled by dopamine, 'the molecule of wanting,' as Dr Korb calls it.

Our long-term goals are then shelved, with unwritten novels left in our heads, and start-up businesses becoming start-nots. 'Dopamine is generally just about the short-term,' explains Dr Korb. 'And there's nothing inherently problematic about that, unless it gets in the way of things that are important for your long-term wellbeing.'

'It does! It does get in the way, Dr Korb!' I want to cry. Like how I just watched two episodes of *The Residence* before our interview instead of working on this urgently due chapter. I feel like my reward system has the long-term planning capabilities of a goldfish.

It's fair to say that, left to its own devices, our dopamine doesn't give a rat's ass that we'd intended to paint the hallway this weekend, or read a physical book in the garden, or go for a swim and sauna. It only wants what's right in front of it, and it wants it now, unless we train it to desire differently.

An evolutionary eyeblink

It feels like streaming services, which grant us more TV than we could ever watch in our entire lifetime, have been around forever. But they were only ushered in when Netflix launched in the UK in 2012, followed in 2014 by Amazon acquiring LoveFilm and turning it into Prime. (If you're a Gen Z who's never heard of LoveFilm, I'm about to blow your minds – we used to get sent DVDs through the post. How cute is that?)

The year 2012. Not so long ago, is it? That means we've only had this near-limitless access to telly for just over a decade. Evolutionarily speaking, that amount of time is not even an eyeblink, nor an eyelash; it's the tip of an eyelash. This is one of the reasons why we are hopeless at dealing with it. It's the 'evolutionary mismatch' we talked of on page 27.

Let's go back, before the watershed of streaming. Unless you were able to pay big for Sky (or Tivo in the US) and record and stack episodes, we had this situation: five terrestrial channels in the UK, and a bunch of really fucking weird Freeview channels, with creepy game shows and shopping services selling things nobody wanted. If you did watch a series, you'd have to wait to get your fix as episodes only dropped once a week.

'In the '80s and '90s we would have mimicked our parents' TV-watching habits,' says Dr Korb. 'But the structures we learned were around regular TV, not streaming. This might have looked like, "I'm not going to watch TV, because it's the middle of the day".'

This unwritten playbook was reinforced by the content shown. 'It had an inherent structure inbuilt, because daytime TV was not your favourite thriller or drama,' he says. Think hokey sofa-based chat shows, or treasure-hunting for antiques, rather than *Slow Horses* or *Bridgerton*. 'You had one or two favourite shows per week that only showed during prime time once a week,' he says.

You couldn't binge, even if you wanted to.

They find the bliss point

Have you heard of 'bliss point'? Sadly, it's not a splashy spa set on a peninsula, although it should be. As we covered on page 147, it's a term used by ultra-processed-food designers, which means – 'eureka we've done it!' – they've nailed the exact jive of sugar, salt and fat that make a food irresistibly moreish.

The makers of TV seek to do the same. 'Before streaming, there was less incentive for them to make you want the next episode, because your consumption was limited,' says Dr Korb.

There also weren't dozens of streaming platforms and hundreds of shows fighting for a slice of your pay each month. 'They now design each episode so that it's totally engrossing but, just like with ultra-processed food, it's not fully satisfying and it leaves you wanting more,' he says.

TV also stimulates real emotions in the brain. 'If you like a character and they die, you genuinely feel heartbroken, even though you know they're fictional,' says Dr Korb. The brain knows it's not a live event, of course. 'Thrillers and horrors are only appealing because we know they're not real. Some of the same stress centres *are* stimulated, but if you were really being chased by someone with a gun, you'd be terrified.' It's the same principle as a roller coaster, he says. 'Only fun because you're strapped in.'

We all know that TV use shot up during the lockdowns, with BARB recording the average daily TV set usage in April 2020 as over five hours a day. This happened because TV acts as a 'placeholder for the real human experience', says Dr Korb, and sometimes that's a good thing, like for the housebound elderly or, y'know, the housebound *world*.

TV can also bulk up our empathy muscles, just as reading fiction does. 'It even helps process our own emotions,' he says. 'Sometimes it's tough to move through grief or anxiety, but when you see a character you relate to go through something similar . . .'

I immediately think of watching a gruff father die in a show recently – I won't reveal which show because, *spoiler*. Afterwards, I ugly-cried for a half hour (is there any such thing as a pretty-cry? Discuss), then realised my outsized reaction was because I haven't grieved my own gruff father's death recently. The TV show got me there, un-stoppering emotion I didn't even realise I'd stoppered, with the character's father being a proxy for my own.

'That emotional processing can be even more powerful than therapy or journalling,' says Dr Korb.

So, it's not all bad. Where we get into trouble, however, is when TV becomes a *replacement* rather than a placeholder for real life. 'It allows us to experience these deep feelings,' says Dr Korb. 'But without the same risks of interacting with other humans.'

The dilemma lands. Go to the party vs watch a show depicting a party, therefore experiencing some of the same neuroscientific highs and lows of parties, while using your chest as a popcorn shelf and wearing things made of stretchy jersey. I'll admit, now that I'm 45, the second option often wins.

Storytelling DNA

We've all been storytelling, and story-consuming, since we figured out that certain noises in certain orders could mean specific things, while sitting around fires to do so.

In County Antrim, Northern Ireland – where I'm from and was raised – it's still a thing to sit around flames, often in the 'kitchen' part of a pub (really just a house with some draught stout) and go around the room telling tall tales. I grew up hearing, 'Never let the truth get in the way of a good story, pet.'

We've scratched stories on to the walls of caves, with the charcoal rescued from the fire, colouring these early cartoons in with berry juice and even animal blood. Our drive to reverse-engineer the 'whys' and 'hows' of human existence are arguably as psychologically strong as our biological drives to eat, sleep, drink and procreate.

Hence the irrepressible drive to consume what's being offered to us around the streaming campfires. We want to know: why did the 13-year-old schoolboy of *Adolescence* seemingly commit murder? We want to know: how will the mother and son of *American Primeval* survive their quest across the brutal 19th-century West?

The drive to survive

These two shows – *Adolescence* and *American Primeval* – are a couple of the most watched in 2025 for very good reason. They tap into our urge to protect our family, to be a good parent if we are one and, most of all, to survive. They're tugging on our urge to accrue survival knowledge.

Survival hits different for everyone – for some who equate romantic success with survival (hello, 33-year-old me), a 'will they, won't they' romance will press this button. For others, a whodunnit or action are ways in. For some it's horror but, for most of us, that genre is too much.

Also hardwired within us is a bias to conserve energy in the short-term, because why do something today when you can do it tomorrow, because tomorrow you might need to run from a pack of wolves, so lie down already, would you?

'We are a very "avoid short term pain" oriented species, as are most animals,' says evolutionary psychologist Dr Andrew Thomas.

This *all* coincides with Big Tech luring us into doing just that. There's a mischievous irony here; while lying down conserving energy on our plushy modular sofa, we believe we're also 'learning' how to survive a flooded-world scenario. Pass the seaweed crisps.

I ask Dr Thomas if apocalypse shows like *The Last of Us* or *The Walking Dead* turn us all into doomsday preppers. 'Absolutely,' he says. 'They tap into an ancestral fear. They make us physiologically uncomfortable but also meet a need to understand and plan against such threats.'

In tandem with their ancient heartbeat, the most-watched shows also tend to press into the zeitgeist; the manosphere's disciples in *Adolescence*'s case, the modern Western revival in *American Primeval,* or our fascination with fungi's scary/cool interconnectivity in *The Last of Us*.

The escape-room model

The most addictive shows place the protagonist in a near-impossible predicament. It's 'screenwriting for dummies' lesson one to place the hero in the equivalent of an escape room, even if it's only an emotional one.

In Aaron Sorkin's screenwriting *MasterClass* series, he defines the purpose of each act as:

Act 1: Chase hero up tree
Act 2: Throw rocks at hero
Act 3: Get hero down
(via a way that you introduced in the first act, like a magic rope)

We're then glued to the process of watching the hero think, evolve, fight, therapy or claw their way out of their locked-room conundrum. How will they get off the island, break out of prison, make their doomed relationship work, get justice in a courtroom system rigged against them, or save their child? That's what keeps us gripped.

Any screenwriter worth their salt will make you care about the protagonist. At the most elementary level, there's the 'Save the Cat' principle, which many writers scorn, but which has spawned a whole franchise of 'write by numbers' books and courses, with a 'beat sheet' of notes for writers to hit.

Most importantly, in this formula, the main character needs to do something – and quickly – to show they're decent folk, like save a cat.

But where it gets really interesting, and where screenwriting elevates, is where they have us glued to someone multi-faceted, whom we both like and dislike; think Dexter Morgan of (stating the obvious) *Dexter,* all of the *Girls,* Tom Hardy's character in *MobLand,* the over-privileged *Schitt's Creek* family, *Breaking Bad's* Walter and Jesse, Villanelle from *Killing Eve* and the assassin in *The Day of the Jackal.* They're not inherently likeable, and they're certainly not running around being sweet and saving kittens. They're doing immoral things we actively disagree with, but we root for them anyway. That's when a little bit of genius strikes.

The 'return to the office' part

That's another layer to all this. Many of us are being shepherded reluctantly back into the office, by authoritarian CEOs. David Solomon, the CEO of Goldman Sachs, called working from home an 'aberration', while JP Morgan's CEO, Jamie Dimon, recently ranted about people slacking in Zoom meetings. While this mass move will indubitably cut down on the temptation of 'just one episode' over a WFH lunch, it also brings the social pressure to watch what everyone else is watching.

The streaming designers know this. Which is partly why they're consciously replacing the early 2020s trend of dropping entire seasons wholesale for locked-down workers with the nineties-style weekly drop. (They're *only* doing this with the sexiest new shows. Lukewarm TV is still dropped whole.)

I mean, *bravo*. It's social engineering at its finest, given it means that viewers are placed in holding pens, ensuring many of them watch the latest episode on the same day – ideal for stimulating 'did you see' watercooler chat.

Then, if you're not watching *The Traitors*, or *The Bachelor*, or *Severance*, or *Survivor*, you will feel left out. The latest episode has become a socio-cultural event, just like *Lost* or *Big Brother* were in the 2000s. 'Have you seen?' we ask each other. And when the other person says no, the offered conversation sadly sways to the ground. That's what the streaming services want. That small – 'oh' where the conversation slumps. It's so much more fun to say 'Yes!' and 'It's *so* good right? What about when . . .' and engage.

Fantasies of TV-richness

Like I said earlier, I have this fantasy that the ultimate in a relaxing evening looks like the ability to watch two+ hours of TV. And yet, when I actually had the capacity to do it – thirtysomething, child-free, dog-free, a less demanding work life – I don't recall being extra relaxed.

Think about a similar TV-rich time in your life. You may need to go back to your teens. Do you recall feeling supremely overflowing with relaxation? The fiction of what we *think* will happen is often upended by what actually happens.

This is partly because of hedonic adaptation. For those unfamiliar, this psychological quirk means we always get used to our pleasure-giving thing. It becomes the old normal and, therefore, the glow of it wears off. This means that even self-made oligarchs who once commuted in a beat-up Fiat feel the same way about their helicopter commute as we do about our morning bus.

I wrote a whole book about hedonic adaptation (*The Unexpected Joy of the Ordinary*), so I won't linger on it here, but to summarise, six-figure salaries, holiday homes and Michelin-starred meals don't seal in happiness long-term, because of this collective truth: that which is rare is all the more delicious.

And so, yesterday, when I did have the capacity to watch three back-to-back episodes of *The Diplomat*, and I was dropping chocolate cashews into my mouth like I was Cleopatra, under my heated blanket with my walked dog and no parenting to do all afternoon . . . it felt gorgeous. But the reason it felt gorgeous is because a day like that is now rarefied.

I don't actually want to ***not*** work, or ***not*** see my child, or ***not*** go outside, or ***not*** see my friends and family, or ***not*** walk my dog . . . and nor do you. And yet many of us think that sitting around watching telly – being rich recliners – would be far more satisfying than sitting at our desks or running errands all day.

But, no! There is zero evidence that this is so. Quite the contrary. Take this Brazilian study of 4,607 Brits. The study compared individuals who engaged in sizeable amounts of either mentally-passive sitting down (TV-watching) or mentally-active sitting down (desk work or driving) and tracked their mental health over several years.

They found that the devoted TV-watchers had a 43 per cent higher incidence of depression. And this is far from an isolated finding. Three other studies were also cited which found that mentally-active sitting (work or driving) 'even had a protective relationship' against depression.

That desk job suddenly doesn't look so joy-sucking after all. It's actually more like an anti-depressant.

How much life to sacrifice

This Mary Oliver quote has become an Instagram trope on a par with posting pictures of matcha lattes but, forgive me, I have to: is this *really* what we want to be doing with our 'one wild and precious life'?

Let's take my ideal amount of television time of two hours. Assuming I started this daily watch aged 11 (which is when I first got a TV in my room) and live to the average age of 80.6 years old (the UK ballpark, median across genders) that's just shy of nine years sitting in front of the box, if you whip out eight hours a day to sleep.

Nine years!

Ugh. I don't want to squander nearly a decade of my life watching the entirety of *CSI: NY*, *CSI: Miami* and *CSI: Buttfuck Alaska* (not real, but I would watch it).

We all need to decide how much remaining life we're willing to sacrifice to the altar of TV. Now, while we still have the choice.

Myself, I do love TV, very hard. Nonetheless, now that my eyes are fully open, I've decided that the most I can offer up is two waking years of my theoretical 35 remaining years.

That gives me 54 minutes of TV a day, maximum. I am committing to that here and now, because it's more important to me to live my life, see people, read books, experience things, be in nature and go abroad than it is to sit on my ass and solve ever-more ridiculous fictional crimes.

What about you? Each of us needs to decide.

Dear little TV addict,

Our brains love it when we complete things. It's called 'completion bias'.

'The importance of getting things done is deeply engrained in most people's mindsets,' writes psychologist Eva M. Krockow. She says that completion bias exists because of neurobiological mechanisms that kick in when we complete a task, releasing dopamine. (There goes the dopamine buzzer again.)

Consider this bias for finishing, in an entertainment landscape where TV series are the new movies. Once upon a time, streamers used the hot new movie as bait to lure us into paying for a subscription. Now, it's all about seasons of the sexy new show.

The problem is the time seasons take to complete. Finishing one season – let alone a multi-season epic – takes between five to ten hours. Content that could have been a neat 90-minute film – the Hollywood version of 'this meeting could have been an email' – has been taken and s-t-r-e-t-c-h-e-d.

This is because of – you guessed it – money. Always with the money.

All streamers, save Apple TV+, now feature advertising within the watch (unless you pay a subscription-within-a-subscription. Cheeky monkeys). So, if you spend longer on their platform, they can show more people the adverts and charge advertisers more – cha-ching!

They take iconic movies and create watered-down reboots to colonise another 10 hours of our time – *Fargo* with added supernatural spice, *Training Day* with a reversed racial dynamic, *High Fidelity* with a female lead . . . I could go on and on.

The bias to finish drives us to complete things we're not even enjoying. 'In some cases, completion bias may go as far as driving people to finish futile endeavours that hold no personal benefits,' adds Krockow. I immediately think of almost every lame soap opera I've ever watched.

There's a very easy fix for this. We can decide to pick up a shorter completion bias tugline by going old-school and watching films instead.

For a start, scarcity is on our side; it's harder to find a hot new film than a show, given less of them are being made now. Hollywood studios made 40 per cent fewer movies between 2022 and 2024.

Second, starting a film is more daunting than a season broken into more bitesize chunks, even though we should logically be *more* fearful of starting a whole new show. 'It's 9pm, we can't start a film now,' is heard in households up and down the land. But watching one episode? It's disarmingly small but, before we know it, we're three episodes and two hours deep, because we were tricked into seeing the show as a 40-minute task, rather than what it really is: a six-hour one.

We can outthink completion bias – by recognising the true size of the thing we're taking on when we click on episode one of eight.

Love,
Cath x

TELEVISION MICRO TACTICS

Build your own structure

Modern life took a sledgehammer to the structures we inherited around TV and so, we need to build our own, whether as a pledge to ourselves or a pact with family or housemates. What do you want it to look like?

Science says it takes an average of 66 days to form a new habit so, while the habit is bedding down, using physical reminders – such as a Post-it on the TV detailing your intentions, or throwing a blanket over it until evening time – will be immensely helpful.

The more radical option

If you're a late-nighter who regularly stays up until 1am, then this one is for you. Just as you can set parental controls on your WiFi, you can also use it to set time limits for yourself. Log into your provider's web interface and look for 'time limits', 'scheduled pauses' or similar. It'll then automatically cut you off at whatever time you choose. Re-activating it will be such a ball-ache that you probably won't bother.

Focus on the long-term want

Remember the 'guilt paradox': telling yourself off for wanting something only makes your cravings intensify. 'If you focus on "It would be *so bad* if I watched another episode", that'll only get your dopamine system all riled up, and then it's going to take over and want it even more,' explains Dr Korb. 'The secret is to redirect and focus on the longer-term want – like getting a good night's sleep – rather than the thing you don't want.' This re-angles your dopamine – which loves to complete a goal, remember – towards that healthier 'want' instead.

Then, step away

Directly after this, Dr Korb says you need to take a physical action towards the longer-term want. 'Don't just sit there in front of the TV. Go brush your teeth and put your pyjamas on. Or, if you need to work, go to the office and sit at your desk.'

If it helps get you off the sofa, tell yourself, 'I can always come back' (this helps me).

Identify your addictive genre

Mine is whodunnits. And so, after writing this chapter, I banned them altogether until I've finished this book. I know that I can easily sit and watch four straight hours of red herrings, hooked by the urgency of unmasking the true killer. I have to know who it is! Tell me! And so I restricted myself to comedies and dramas instead. I don't struggle to stop *Hacks* or *The Buccaneers,* probably because there's no life-or-death imperative caffeinating the plot.

You're self-aware too. You already know what your most addictive telly is. If you don't press play during a particularly busy phase of life, it can't suck you in.

USE THIS LIFE-SACRIFICE CALCULATOR

You may well be canny enough with maths to figure these workings out by yourself, without my help. But, if not, I've provided the workings for you here, in order to calculate how much life you're willing to lose to watching telly.

We're going to assume you live until the average age of 80.6 (non gender-specific), to get Figure B.

Step one

Figure B: Minus your current age from 80.6. So, I'm 45, which means my calculations are 80.6 – 45 = 35.6

Figure A: Then, decide how many of those waking years you are willing to spend watching telly.

Write both figures in the boxes below and then do the calculations to get figures C and D.

Figure A x 365 days x 16 waking hours = Figure C

Figure B x 365 days = Figure D

Step two

Figure C ÷ Figure D =

Figure E

Figure E is how many hours per waking day that you can spend watching TV. This will be a decimal number (like mine; 0.9, or 1.2, say).

Step three

You can then figure out how many minutes that is exactly, by using the below:

Figure E x 0.6 = Figure F

The number after the decimal point is how many minutes you get. For instance, my calculation is 0.9 x 0.6 = 0.54, so that's 54 minutes of TV per day.

Your figure may well be less than an entire film. Incidentally, the easiest time to pause a film is at the mid-point, because there are almost always tantalising turning points deliberately placed 20 minutes in and 20 minutes from the end. The middle always sags a little, in comparison.

Set a timer on your phone, or oven, and stick to it. This helps me. Or gorge the whole film and take the next day off telly.

CAFFEINE

Dr Judith Grisel is wearing a floral kimono and sitting in an office that looks like it smells like leather-bound books. She is poised, but in a *real* way. I bet her students at Bucknell University say things like, 'When I grow up, I want to be like Professor Grisel.'

We both confess that we're knackered. She because she hosted 30 people last night. Me because it took four hours to put my three-year-old to sleep, which meant I had to work until 1am.

We turn our cameras off after saying our hellos, so that we can really concentrate, and I can type as she talks. All Zooms should be more like this. Maybe if we didn't all have to *pretend* not to be knackered, then feel we must make eye contact for 60 minutes (nobody would do that in person), we would all be a little less knackered.

I'm almost scared to ask her this next question. Because, if you could track what words tickertape across people's brains the moment they wake, mine would be: **COFFEE.**

Brewing coffee is the very first thing I do after attending to my basic bodily needs. I only have one a day (when I have two, I regret it). I enjoy it immensely, preferring single-origin, Ethiopian ideally, sourced from a local roastery. I even grind my own beans.

I feel mildly disgusted when I think of my twenties, when I drank instant. The smell now turns my stomach. Yep, I'm that person. A coffee ~~knob~~ snob. (I'm not quite as bad as my partner. When we visit a new city, we can't leave until he has befriended all the premium coffee shop owners and talked to them about 'extraction' and the altitude their beans were grown at.)

And so, I'm scared that Dr Grisel, a world-class expert in the neuroscience of addiction, will run roughshod over my ritual, my lovely morning coffee. My *precious*.

But she's a fan too. 'I drink it every morning as well,' she says. 'I go to the coffee pot almost comatose. Then I feel normal.' Are we hooked, I wonder?

'Coffee wakes me up, so I don't wake up until I get coffee, which is really a simple sign of dependence. It's like when people say, "Alcohol relaxes me, so I don't relax until I have alcohol." Or "Cannabis makes things interesting, so nothing's interesting unless I'm stoned." But the one justification we both have is that caffeine is actually good for you.' I mentally punch the air. Tell me more, Dr Grisel.

'Caffeine is good for your brain. It's good for your heart. It protects against Parkinson's, maybe Alzheimer's too. So, I don't think coffee is so bad.'

I check into all of this about caffeine. It all holds up.

One study found that, when participants had the Parkinson's gene, caffeine reduced their risk of onset by four to eight times. However the claim of reduced dementia risk is only shown in some caffeine studies, not all, which is why Dr Grisel prefaced this one with 'maybe'. Many studies I read called caffeine 'neuroprotective'.

Let's get into the heart-protecting too. The British Heart Foundation recently reported on a study that found this fascinating nuance with regards to coffee: the heart-protective element only appears to work if you're a *morning* drinker of it.

I need to tell Judith. I mean Dr Grisel. (We're friends now, in my head. She doesn't know yet.)

This coffee study took 40,000 American adults, dividing them into those who didn't drink coffee, morning drinkers of coffee or those who drank it all day long. They revisited all of these people a decade later and found that the morning drinkers were 31 per cent *less* likely than non-coffee drinkers to have died from heart/circulatory disease, as well as 16 per cent less likely to have died full stop.

'In comparison, people who drank coffee throughout the day did not have a significantly lower risk of dying over the following decade,' the British Heart Foundation wrote.

If you're a tea-lover, I also have good news for you. A similar UK study about black and green tea took in data from half a million people aged 40 to 69, then followed up with them 11 years later. 'Compared with non-tea drinkers, people who reported drinking two or more cups of tea a day had a 9–13 per cent lower risk of dying from any cause,' the British Heart Foundation wrote. The very best results came from those who drank their tea black, with no milk or sugar, but there wasn't much in it, and it was generally consistent across the board.

Great, so we've now enabled our tea and coffee habits, especially if it's coffee in the morning, or two+ cups of tea. Which, very handily, overlays with my habit of one coffee + two breakfast teas. I am delighted.

Cortisol's role

Caffeine tells the central nervous system to make cortisol. Cortisol gets a rough time in the press and on socials, I keep getting served ads for supplements that claim to lower cortisol. Everyone be hating on cortisol, and it's not warranted.

A bit like Meghan née Markle, when all she's done is be successful in her own right, marry a sexy prince and become entirely cottagecore by keeping bees. 'I find it astonishing, the vitriol levelled at Meghan,' said Bryony Gordon, on *Lorraine*. 'It's entirely disproportionate . . . She's not Vladimir Putin, she's just a mum from California who quite likes making her own bath salts.' *Yes*, Bryony.

Let's jump to cortisol's defence too. Cortisol is oft cited as the 'stress hormone' and everyone just wants to get rid of it. But Professor Murphy makes a point of calling it the 'stress *and* arousal hormone'. It's just not as snappy. Dr Grisel has strong thoughts in its favour too: 'There's no living without cortisol,' she says. 'They tried to blunt cortisol in depressed people, thinking it might help and, *no*, it didn't work at all.' There's a sweet spot we need to find, she says. 'Too little or too much are bad. If you look at the circadian or diurnal rhythm [the daytime version of circadian] of cortisol, it's up and down in healthy people throughout the day.'

Let's get into something even more contentious; I want to delve into the truly disturbing craze sweeping the West (or is it just my friends?) for people to now say you oughtn't drink coffee for the first 90 minutes of the day, because Dr Andrew Huberman said so.

If you've been living beneath a rock, or just have better things to do than 'pull to refresh' on socials, Dr Huberman is like the George Clooney of neuroscience. He has an impressive beard, arms the size of babies and nine million followers on socials. His podcast is considered required listening for most Millennials.

****

The professor is wearing enormous bright blue gloves to open the fridge full of human tissues. They look like the gloves an oversized Smurf might wear. Lab Smurf.

'Normally it's -80 centrigade. But at present it's -56,' says Professor Philip

Murphy, a psychobiologist from Edge Hill University. 'Your domestic freezer is about -20 so, as you can imagine, you want to get in and out as quickly as possible.'

Jsssh goes the massive fridge. I'm hit by an icy blast, even standing six feet away. As swiftly as possible, like somebody doing a task in *The Crystal Maze*, he opens the drawer to whip out the human tissue samples. Impressive.

'These are saliva samples, for an ongoing study on cortisol levels,' he says. 'We have something called the cortisol awakening response [CAR],' he tells me. 'When you wake up in the morning, for the first 45 minutes to an hour, your cortisol levels increase sharply – and then decline gradually for the rest of the day. Unless something stressful occurs.'

Cortisol is a 'biological measure of arousal', he says, which can be measured by taking a series of staggered saliva samples over the day.

We start talking about the Dr Huberman method of delaying caffeine in order to allow our cortisol to rise slowly and naturally. Professor Murphy has no opinion on this trend. But he drinks a coffee himself within 30 minutes.

I say that making a coffee is the very first thing I do in the morning. The professor looks more worried than I think he should be.

****

'Cortisol itself is not bad. Cortisol is wonderful,' Dr Huberman says. It is one of the things that wakes us up in the morning, it enhances the immune system, stimulates our metabolism and makes us alert and focused, he says. Most of all, cortisol clears out adenosine, the molecule that makes us sleepy.

You would think that caffeine – which creates even *more* cortisol than CAR – would, therefore, be a good thing. But no, says Dr Huberman. And here's why he recommends delaying your first cup of the day.

For mystical reasons only known to geniuses, the cortisol produced by caffeine fails to help that usual adenosine clearance, which usually happens via CAR. Instead, the caffeine blocks the clearance of the sleep molecule. The adenosine is placed in a holding bay of sorts. Think of it as a vault full of yawns. The sleepiness sits in the vault until the caffeine wears off, then it is released, usually after lunchtime. And – *yawn*. Which means we reach for more caffeine because we literally can't cope with the slump. This is what we call the 'afternoon crash'.

I am so convinced by Dr Huberman's argument and logic that when I listen to the podcast myself, I decide to try it out. The next morning, instead of waking up and brewing coffee immediately, I force myself to take my dog out for a run. I do this most mornings anyway, but usually *after* the lovely *jjjjhhhh* of pressing down my AeroPress. I don't manage 90 minutes until the coffee, but I do manage 60 quite easily.

I kind of hate that I'm doing it, because it means I've become one of *those* people. The 90-minute caffeine people. Except I'm a 60-minute caffeine person, because I'm counterculture, and don't tell me what to do, OK?

Turns out that delaying my coffee just means that I'm really grumpy for the first hour of the day. When I see people on my run who smile and say 'hello!' I want to hiss at them like an angry cat. It doesn't make any discernible difference to my energy levels in the afternoon, or to my sleep at night so, sod it, I tossed it after three days.

Dr Grisel is not convinced, either. 'If you really want your cortisol to be all natural, then don't drink coffee,' she says. I flinch. 'Drinking coffee when you first wake up *is* working with our natural rhythms, however,' she says. I smile.

Maybe you will find that a caffeine delay changes your life, eradicating your afternoon crash and persistent insomnia. The science is robust, and it makes sense, which is why I've included it, but, for me, the difference would have needed to be dramatic to make it worthwhile. And it wasn't.

Dr Huberman himself admits that, when he's doing strength-training or similar in the morning, he will ditch the 90-minute delay, grabbing coffee within 10 or 20.

If you don't want to delay your coffee, Dr Huberman also says there *are* some natural ways to help clear your adenosine so that less of it goes into this holding bay. He recommends getting outside into sunlight (or in Britain, cloudlight) as soon as possible, even if it's just to sit in the garden. And try to do a spot of exercise too; if you don't have the energy for a proper mat workout first thing, even just five minutes of star jumps would help. Or skipping, if you're mysteriously co-ordinated first thing. I would almost certainly end up falling over.

You can help this adenosine-clearance along some more by having half of your usual morning caffeine upon waking, and half of it an hour later, he suggests. I start doing this, and after my run with the dog, I genuinely don't want the other half. I'm perky enough, and I also haven't hissed at any friendly strangers.

So, to be fair to Dr Huberman, this tack means I effortlessly cut out 40mg of caffeine. I'll forgive him the grumpy mornings, then.

What about the afternoon slump?

We've pretty much established that caffeine is a great idea in the morning, and given even Dr Huberman – the bad-news bear of caffeine – says an 8- to 12-hour gap between a cuppa and bedtime is sufficient, it won't affect your sleep.

After lunchtime is when we tend to get into trouble. It's the afternoon caffeine that we regret most, that we wish we hadn't partaken of, when we're lying there at 1am, eyeballs stinging, wondering whatever happened to the *Karate Kid* or having an existential crisis and turning over conversations that happened ten years ago, scripting better responses.

It's normal to experience an afternoon dip in energy, which is when our body's diurnal rhythm naturally chimes in, says Dr Grisel. 'There's a dip in cortisol at that time,' she says. 'So, if you're drinking caffeine as an antidote to that 4 o'clock dip then, yeah, that's not the best.' She used to do this herself, but she quit.

So, what can we do when we can't have a cuppa but need to push through? Dr Grisel now takes an afternoon walk instead of re-firing the coffee pot. 'It stimulates a little,' she says. 'There are some very famous scientists who did this – went for an hour-long walk every day at 3 or 4pm, then back for a couple more hours on the second wind.'

She's right; Charles Darwin reportedly did this and, inspired by him, so did Albert Einstein. Marie Curie, Caroline Herschel and Steve Jobs apparently did this too.

Dr Huberman agrees on going with the flow, rather than spiking a slump into submission with caffeine: 'Many people, including myself, do need a short nap or non-sleep deep rest* or other form of relaxation, for 10–30 minutes in the afternoon. That is natural.'

* Not sure what a 'non-sleep deep rest' is, but it sounds well naughty.

A note on Diet Coke

Three of my very good friends have told me of savage Diet Coke addictions. We're talking hiding crushed cans, having a secret stash and, when people started to comment on the frequency, drinking it furtively in the loos or downing it in the car.

It's probably the only time I've agreed with Donald Trump. He once tweeted: 'Let's face it – this stuff just doesn't work. It makes you hungry.' He accidentally appears to have hit on something real, which is that Diet Coke seems to create a gap, which you then feel the urge to fill. Sometimes with more Diet Coke, sometimes with food.

Why the gap? Artificial sweeteners promise the brain a sweet reward that never comes, which can induce fierce craving. This is relevant for energy drinks, too.

'Sweet taste in the mouth prepares the body for sugar,' wrote Dr Chris van Tulleken in *Ultra-Processed People*. 'If that never arrives, it's a problem.' He writes about studies showing it increases the cravings for sugary foods.

In fact, Dr van Tulleken himself developed a Diet Coke habit, putting away six cans a day. 'I have no way of explaining how addictive these felt . . . I never craved real Coke as much as Diet Coke.'*

One compelling study showed that even when a rat is clinically addicted to cocaine, if you introduce an artificial sweetener (in this case, saccharin) into its bevy of substance choices, it chooses to hit the sweetener instead, 94 per cent of the time. The study's authors concluded that intense sweetness can override the importance of drug addiction because of an 'inborn sensitivity to sweet tastants'. As we've covered, we evolved in a sugar-scarce environment, where we were lucky if a forager found a honeycomb for the whole settlement once in a while. The rat study said that sweetness – even if it's not from sugar – provokes a supernormal reward signal in the brain. We find it *very* difficult to override that, which is why addictions abound.

Sidenote: if you're hooked on sugar-free chewing gum (like me), this phenomenon could be why. It's not the gum itself making it sticky; it's probably

* My legal team want me to add: 'Coca-Cola say their products are "perfectly safe" and can be enjoyed as part of a balanced lifestyle.'

the artificial sweetener. That realisation just relocated my spearmint Extra habit in my brain; from the innocuous suburbs, into living next door to mainlining Diet Coke.

Where's the line, please?

I'm intrigued as to where the line sits, where the risks of caffeine kick in.

Most experts, including the US Food and Drug Administration (FDA), agree on where the line is.

THE LINE: 400mg of caffeine.

This equates to: four cups of percolated (from bean) coffee; five cups of instant coffee; eight cups of black tea; twelve cans of cola; twelve cups of green tea; or five 80mg energy drinks.

If you slide over that 400mg line, you're starting to play health roulette with nasties including high blood pressure or heart disease.

It's worth emphasising that different people metabolise caffeine differently. This is influenced by weight, activity levels, age (older people metabolise it more slowly) and genes (linked to liver enzymes). For some, just a little can cause palpitations or anxiety. Others can put away a lot without really feeling it.

Personally, if I drank 400mg of caffeine a day, I'd be a nervous wreck, with a bell in my hand and a 'The end is nigh' sign round my neck.

You're an adult, and you probably already know what amount is OK for you. Sticking to it is the challenge. We'll get into that.

Dear little caffeine addict,

I'm going to cheat here by telling you how I downsized my medium addiction to another hot drink, which doesn't contain caffeine. But the way I used it? It may as well have come laced with caffeine, sugar, MDMA, rainbow sprinkles and eternal youth.

I had a medium addiction to peppermint tea. I *still* had it when I started writing this book, putting away an average of two teapots a day – about eight cups. I was also taking a flask of it when I left the house.

(Speaking of which, I once announced, 'I've got my flask, anyone want some?' at a recovery get-together in America. Turns out, in America, a 'flask' means a hip flask. So, to clarify for any Americans reading, I mean what you might call a 'Thermos' for a hot drink, *not* a flask full of bourbon.)

I would love to stay cosy in denial and claim that my medium peppermint tea addiction has never harmed me, but it has. I once dumped half a boiling hot flask over my thigh in a moving car (I was the passenger, you'll be relieved to hear), while trying to pour some into my keep-cup.

It was agony, and I still have a palm-print-sized patch on my thigh that never tans.

Friends would always make sure they had a box of peppermint tea in their cupboards, lest I go into narked withdrawal. They needn't have bothered; I always had some in my wheelie-case or handbag as a contingency plan for their abject failings.

A friend and I once wound up another friend who'd said, 'Cath is addicted to mint tea!' We told her I'd started chewing mint leaves in the toilets to get my fix. She believed it.

The way I downsized this addiction to a non-addiction was ridiculously basic. I now have a very pedestrian two cups of peppermint tea a day. And the key-turn was so simple.

I reasoned that I was getting most of my hydration from this herbal tea. And so I started doing this one tiny thing. Every time I boiled the kettle to make a coffee or tea, I drank a glass of water.

That's it. And because I was soon sufficiently hydrated, I no longer craved an unreasonable amount of herbal tea.

This trick, of pairing a thing you *already* do with a thing you want to do, is called various things depending on who you're reading.

The forefather of habit-formation, BJ Fogg, called it 'anchoring'. Then, his ardent student James Clear called it 'habit stacking' in his book *Atomic Habits*. But, before both of them, let's give it up for Professor Katy Milkman, a behavioural scientist.

In 2015, Professor Milkman published a genius paper called 'Holding the *Hunger Games* Hostage at the Gym' (and compared to most academic paper titles, this name is jalapeño-level spicy). This was back when iPods existed and Milkman's big idea was that if people could only listen to a moreish audiobook on an iPod at the gym, which was being 'held hostage' in a monitored locker there, maybe they would go to the gym more.

On the iPods were four audiobooks the participant had picked. The choices were ultra-addictive stories, such as *The Hunger Games*, the *Bourne* trilogy, *His Dark Materials*, some John Grisham classics and *Twilight* (mock the sparkly vampire saga all you like, and I will too, but I stayed up until 4am to finish the final book).The results were remarkable. That 'temptation-bundling' group, as Milkman called them, visited the gym 51 per cent more than the control group. Yep, 51 per cent!

'Temptation-bundling' is one to keep in your back pocket for all little addictions. And maybe try the water hack. Now that we know caffeinated drinks do indeed hydrate us (wisdom of yore said they didn't, because caffeine is a diuretic), it's entirely possible that if you make sure you drink a bunch of water instead, you'll want less tea, coffee, energy drink or similar.

I also slept better after the water hack, given I was no longer waking in the night wanting water (and then waking again to pee). I woke each morning to a nearly full glass of water beside my bed and an infinitely more rested head.

Sometimes the simplest things really are the most life-enhancing. What will you put into your temptation bundle?

Love,
Cath x

CAFFEINE MICRO TACTICS

Full-life calculator

There's a weird quirk with caffeine literature where they report on the 'half-life', like 'it takes five hours for half of the caffeine to leave your system'. I don't know why this is, so I will report the *full* life.

It takes up to 10 hours for caffeine to leave your system, depending on how you metabolise it. Studies have shown that having your last caffeine at 4pm will 'significantly disrupt' a 10pm bedtime, cleaving off more than an hour from your sleep. (That shocked me. I love you, single-origin beans, but I love sleep more.)

For pregnant women, because the liver enzyme that metabolises caffeine recedes, particularly in the final trimester, it can take up to *30 hours* for caffeine to clear the body.

Mushroom coffee could dampen anxiety

I had a beautifully scathing passage about mushroom coffee (aka adaptogenic) prepared for this chapter. It withered:

'The ex-reality TV stars who are smart enough to now slay on Instagram say it has changed their life #ad. It has quietly expensive black and white packaging, matt of course, and features 'activated' mushrooms (whatever that means) and monk-blessed matcha, and is shade-grown. But it's still coffee. It just costs more. You can roll a cake in bee pollen but it's *still a cake.*'

But then I found out that lion's mane or cordyceps (mushrooms that are often found in these coffees) have been shown to lower anxiety. Although, more research is needed to determine whether the amounts present in coffee blends *actually* work.

Also on the plus side, mushroom coffees do usually contain less caffeine than your usual ground cuppa, so are handy if you want to cut down.

Doll-sized cups

Do you remember that bonkers doll-sized diet that was hot for a minute in the noughties? I remember because I had to write an absurd piece about it, and try to find serious experts to endorse it, which was just embarrassing. It recommended using children's plates (and utensils!) to cut down on your portion sizes. Quelle loadabollocks.

Or so I thought. Actually, because of 'unit bias', shrinking the receptacle makes sense and is a beverage version of 'self-binding': if you drink out of smaller cups, you will probably drink less tea or coffee. Try switching your veritable vat for a cute clay mug. See what happens. You could also try brewing per cup, via an AeroPress or similar, rather than making a pot or cafetière. The faff of doing another cup is a friction-filled 'obstacle', which famously works with any size of addiction.

Switch to energy drinks with less kick

Cans of Monster Energy or Relentless can contain up to 160mg of caffeine – the equivalent of two filter coffees. Red Bull gets a bad rep (probably because of all the thumping hangovers it co-sponsored via 'VodBull' nights), but it's pretty tame, at only 80mg. A bottle of Lucozade has 46mg (Lucozade Alert is almost threefold).

Energy drinks can contain up to seven teaspoons of sugar, just so you're aware. Sugar-free versions seem like the solution but, given they use artificial sweeteners, which we covered earlier, this sets up a craving cycle for a reward that never comes.

It's only a week

Most people clear the withdrawal of caffeine within a week, so if you're only reducing, you most certainly will. Keep some painkillers handy for the potential headaches, and hydrate like crazy.

PROCRASTINATION

Bill Gates was a chronic procrastinator at Harvard. 'People thought it was funny,' he said. 'That was my positioning. The guy who did nothing until the last minute.' He cites it as the number one behavioural drag he had to tackle when he got into business.

'I'm still working on it,' he admitted in 2005, 30 years after founding Microsoft and becoming one of the most successful entrepreneurs in history.

Margaret Atwood, too, is another walking contradiction; both a compulsive procrastinator and a work machine (56 books for the adult market, eight for children; more besides). She's described herself as a world-class procrastinator ('I'd hate to be a *failed* procrastinator,' she laughed), watching films like *Captain Underpants* on airplanes when she should be working.

Atwood describes routinely spending the morning 'procrastinating and worrying', before eventually knuckling down at about 3pm, and inching herself into the deep work.

'It's like going into a very cold lake,' she told psychologist Adam Grant on his podcast. 'You put your foot in, you take it out . . . It's still too cold. You think, "Am I gonna do this or not? No? Yes. No. Yes." That goes on for a while. And then . . . if you're going to do it, you run in screaming.'

You run in screaming. Yes. I relate. You may do, too.

Gates and Atwood are far from alone. Many gifted and productive icons delay the inevitable, causing themselves stress. White House staff reportedly used to give Bill Clinton – another chronic procrastinator – a full six-week runway to write his State of the Union address, only for it to always be a harried last-minute affair.

Steve Jobs took eight years to pick a sofa, his wife revealed. 'Madam Speaker' Nancy Pelosi is one too, it seems. And the author of *Moby Dick*, Herman Melville, apparently had his wife chain him to his writing desk.

It's commonly cited that one in five of us do it chronically, while over half of Brits are more casual procrastinators, saying that it has 'affected their lives'. Even pigeons procrastinate, according to another study.

But it's not all bad. In fact, there's a proven link between procrastination and creative originality (an enabling lever if ever I saw one). A 2018 study found that those who were allowed to procrastinate by playing Minesweeper or Solitaire (*downloads both immediately*) came up with new business ideas that were rated as 28 per cent more creative by independent adjudicators, than those who were forced to start working instantly.

Adam Grant said that, 'When you procrastinate, you're more likely to let your mind wander. That gives you a better chance of stumbling on to the unusual and spotting unexpected patterns.'

It seems that our brains need a little free-range roaming time to come up with something beautifully original. 'You call it procrastination. I call it thinking,' Aaron Sorkin told one interviewer, who challenged him on his last-minute screenwriting antics.

It's not laziness

Putting the eleventh-hour creative surge aside, procrastination is ultimately self-sabotage. It's allowing our short-term self to call the shots, while our long-term self looks on in horror.

Almost all procrastinators believe this is caused by a deep character flaw. If you ask them, 'Why do you do this?' they'll usually say that laziness is the root of it (this includes Atwood, Gates and other self-confessed procrastinators, including the Dalai Lama). I know I feel wretchedly lazy when I do it.

Yet it's not about indolence, any more than it's about IQ or overall productivity. You'll be hard pressed to find any psychologist who says that procrastination is about laziness.

Right on cue: 'It's not laziness,' says psychotherapist Anna Mathur, author of *The Uncomfortable Truth*. 'It's a form of emotional self-regulation.' A mis-regulation, as some experts call it.

'We do it to avoid the negative emotions that come with the task we're putting off,' adds Mathur. She points to overwhelm or fear of failure as the main ones, but also sometimes boredom, if the task is a grind, such as a tax return.

Procrastinators are often the opposite of lazy. 'Classic, chronic procrastinators will have the neatest houses, all the dishes will be done, everything will be clean,' psychologist Professor Fuschia Sirois told the *Granted* podcast, 'but the big looming task that they're supposed to be doing isn't being done.'

Procrastination is funny – but also isn't

We crack jokes about doing it. 'I love deadlines. I love the whooshing noise they make as they go by,' said Douglas Adams, author of *The Hitchhiker's Guide to the Galaxy*.

But it also isn't funny. The one in five of us who do it consistently truly suffer. I'm sure Douglas Adams has had some dark nights as a result of the whoosh. It's the stress of the constant self-beration during the procrastinate, followed by staring down the barrel of the impending deadline, and then the physical ordeal of having to work intensely to meet it.

It leaves a mark.

I was originally planning to open this chapter with a cute list of things I had done instead of write this chapter (meta!), a few of which are preserved below:

- Mopped the kitchen floor, because I couldn't stop thinking about it.
- Told myself I had to feel perfect before I started, so went for a 6km run, then a bracing dip in the sea, then had to wash my hair. Two hours later . . .
- Prepped food, reasoning that it would mean I wouldn't have to break later to cook. Then it was 'too late' to start, so I ate the food, while watching *Smoke* on Apple TV+.

I also tend to learn an unnecessary amount about the thing rather than do the thing – telling myself I have to read all the articles, listen to all the podcasts, read all the books. As Mark Manson quips, 'Learning more is a smart person's favourite form of procrastination.' I'll take the inherent compliment; you should too.

I razed this cute list and started afresh on a brand-new empty document; a procrastinator's worst nightmare. Because what this meta list didn't communicate is the pain that chronic procrastination has caused me.

The pain of procrastination

Indeed, a study of 2,500 adults assessed on the General Procrastination Scale (pretty sure I'd ace that test) concluded that procrastinators experience more stress, distress and fatigue than their counterparts.

Let's get into the fatigue. I've had to pull all-nighters to meet book deadlines more than once. On one memorable occasion, I showed up to my co-working space on a sunny Friday wearing a summer dress and open-toed sandals, planning to finish my final draft of a book and file that same day.

On the Saturday, 27 hours after entering the office, I had to do a 'walk of procrastinator shame', wearing the same clothes, in a thunderstorm. We all know what the people I walked past *thought* had happened.

All-nighters are almost exclusively the reserve of procrastinators, but many of us also deprive ourselves of sleep on a regular basis. Sleep scientists coined the term 'bedtime procrastination' around a decade ago, which then extended to become 'revenge bedtime procrastination' (acronymed to RBP). The 'revenge' was added in when it was discovered that many of us do this as a misdirected 'fuck you'. Revenge against the day, for feeling we haven't had enough 'me' time.

A follow-up 2023 study found that 'self-love therapy' decreased RBP 'significantly'. The paper was annoyingly vague as to what this 'self-love therapy' comprised of, but it makes sense that it would act as a foil. RBP may feel like delicious revenge against the mean day, but it only harms ourselves.

I write gratitude lists before bed, and find they help enormously in mitigating RBP. So, learning about this study just made me realise why my nightly gratitudes work.

Not only does this nightly act insist that my negatively biased brain (which most of us have, naturally) seeks out the positives, but it also taps into some self-love. Over the past 12 years of gratitude-ing, I've learnt to insert an element of congratulating myself, for all I've achieved that day, even if it was only 'kept daughter, dog and self alive and fed'. I should probably call these 'congratitudes'.

These congratitudes aren't written to puff myself up; it's to find my healthy size of ego, something many of us in recovery call becoming 'right sized'. Unless I find the things I've done right during that day, I will tend to lie and stare at the inside of my eyelids – or at the ceiling – reproaching myself for everything I did wrong.

The self-love of congratitudes helps me feel sleepy, but also deserving of sleep. I believe my toddler deserves enough sleep, so why not myself? Self-parenting is a therapy-speak cliché now, which can be deemed the reserve of snowflake Millennials, but whatever. *So melt me*; it works.

The procrastination gene

A tendency to procrastinate is genetic around half of the time, according to a study of 347 sets of twins. The procrastinating phenotype overlaps significantly with impulsivity, another heritable trait. It's thought that procrastination is actually an evolutionary by-product of this impulsivity ('Sod it! I'll do something else instead of the scary/boring task'), which makes sense.

We very rarely procrastinate by doing nothing. We usually choose itty bitty tasks, such as cleaning, exercising, social media updating, laundry, messaging, cooking, tidying or email-replying. Only, these small tasks refill each day. So, day after day, they consistently get in the way.

'I'll play an instrument, read my Substacks, clean things that are already clean,' says psychotherapist Josh Fletcher. 'It's about creating the illusion of doing something.'

It seems like our brain is misbehaving, but our brain is actually doing something that makes sense to it. Overwhelmed by the much bigger, longer-term, heavier task that looms before it, it's choosing a much smaller, short-term, spicier task. Why does it feel spicier? Because: dopamine. (I *am* going to put it on a T-shirt.)

This bias evolved for good reason. 'Evolutionarily speaking, our brains prioritise short-term regulation over long-term reward,' says Mathur. 'We're built to hunt in the minute, live in the moment and reach for the immediate reward. Because the *moment* we switch from the task we're supposed to be doing to one we're not, we get that dopamine release. It's the reward of rebellion, of escape from the overfacing or boring.'

We're a very 'avoid-short-term-pain-oriented species,' Dr Thomas said earlier, 'as most animals are'. This inbuilt short-term bias works against our long-term requirements and desires. 'It's a battle of wills,' he adds. 'Something that is perhaps unique to humans.'

Delayed gratification works against our 'minimise pain, maximise pleasure' operating system. 'Pursuing short-term needs is our default setting, while meeting long-term needs is the effortful deviation.'

Procrastinators have different brains

There's even a neuroanatomical difference in those who procrastinate. We tend to have larger amygdalas, said a study that scanned the brains of 264 people.

Remember the amygdala? Our expert described it as the oldest, dumbest, most fearful part of the brain, back on page 221. It seems that the fear of failing at the task immobilises us. 'Over-analysis leads to paralysis,' as my father used to say.

'This [greater amygdala volume] means they will also be more sensitive to the potential negative consequences of their actions,' explained Professor Sirois, 'leading to more negative emotions and procrastination.'

But a larger amygdala is not a lifelong affliction. We can change our brains. In response to the study, Professor Tim Pychyl told *BBC News* that meditation is the best counterbalance to this brain quirk, given meditation has been proven to shrink the amygdala's volume and, in turn, expand the prefrontal cortex. (*God*, why does everyone keep telling us that meditation is the answer to everything? OK, OK, we hear you, meditation-thumpers.)

There's also more good news in that most of us tend to grow out of chronic procrastination, with a 2016 study finding that it's most rife in our twenties. Maybe you're thinking 'Not me, I'm still doing it at 53!' Well, I don't fit neatly into this wellbeing box either. I was 39 when I did that 'walk of procrastinator shame'. I guess some of us are so good at procrastination that we even manage to delay growing out of it.

Procrastination lifts stress from the shoulders of today's us, for sure. But only to heap it on to the shoulders of future us. One meme turned an important cog in my head. It said: 'Procrastination is like masturbation. Fun for a while, but in the end, you're only screwing yourself.'

Dear little procrastination addict,

We can outwit our urge to procrastinate over the big stuff by throwing our brain a few smaller tasks to begin with. This is because of the 'urgency effect', whereby we prefer tasks with smaller completion windows.

As President Eisenhower once said: 'I have two kinds of problems: the urgent and the important. The urgent are not important, and the important are never urgent.'

Ain't that the truth.

Smaller tasks tug on our sleeves as 'urgent' – that WhatsApp your friend now knows you've read, that email from your boss, the basket of washing bleeping in your mind-map – but they're not truly important. We all know that. They can usually wait.

Your friend isn't going to un-friend you (unless they're a knob), your boss doesn't expect an instant reply (ditto) and the washing isn't going to grow legs and run from the house.

The reason we favour these seemingly urgent tasks over the profoundly life-changing deep *important* work is because they're small and snappy and will give us a burst of dopamine once we attend to them, just like Dr Korb told us.

So, attend to them. Do it. Why not? Let your brain indulge in the 'urgency effect'. Do that tiny task gnawing at you right now. Your brain likes it – wants it – because it's accomplishable within five-to-ten minutes.

'Finishing immediate, mundane tasks actually improves your ability to tackle tougher, important things,' said a piece in *Harvard Business Review*. 'Achieving a small goal can result in a positive feedback loop that makes you more motivated to work harder going forward.'

This was confirmed by a study of 500 workers, half of whom were asked to use this method of 'a few small first, big later' in each working day. They were also asked to keep lists of tasks, checking them off as they went.

The results were compelling. 'Those who completed a couple of short tasks first and then checked off others as they completed them were the most satisfied with their job, felt the highest level of motivation and, based on their records, had accomplished the most throughout the week,' wrote the lead researchers, Francesca Gino and Bradley Staats.

You can leverage this – and simultaneously limit the impact of procrastination – by deliberately choosing a few quick tasks for the beginning of your day. This will place you on a fun roll, like starting your day on a waterslide, rather than needing to launch yourself into the icy water of the deep task; or running in screaming, Atwood-style.

Ding, ding, ding, the dopamine will go. And, as long as you make sure to switch tack after three maximum, you'll be better positioned for the big picture.

Love,
Cath x

PROCRASTINATION MICRO TACTICS

Forgive yourself for procrastinating – right now
A fascinating 2010 study found that if we can forgive ourselves for *past* procrastination, we make future procrastination less likely. Finding empathy for ourselves unlocks it. 'This is about standing beside that "naughty" kid who's tired of doing what they're supposed to – or the scared kid who doesn't want to do the exam because they're scared of failure – and telling them they *can* do it,' says Mathur. 'Hand-holding the part of you that wants to procrastinate and encouraging it into doing the boring or scary thing anyway.'

Let an auto-reply do the talking
Unattended-to emails chirp in a procrastinator's brain, asking to be attended to, even when they're entirely optional. It's a fiction of our own creation that they're urgent.

An auto-reply can really help undo that imagined time pressure. Even if it's something as simple as 'I'm travelling/doing deep work today, so I will be slow to reply/will reply tomorrow.' It could help dis-enable your procrastination, because you will already know that the sender doesn't expect an instant reply, or a reply at all.

Make it so small that you can't say no
You can hack an overfacing task into teeny, tiny slices. That's what I had to do with this book. I carved it up into 'print this', 'email them', mostly turning it into tasks achievable in five to ten minutes.

As the proverb goes, you eat an elephant a bite at a time, which is why annoyingly successful people, such as Instagram's former CEO Kevin Systrom, swear by setting a timer for five minutes, to get them going. The pomodoro method is an extension of this, where you work in 25-minute chunks. But, frankly, I find that too overwhelming.

Twenty-five minutes?! Err, I want to *flirt* with the work, not *marry* the work.

Double the time you allow for chunky tasks

The 'planning fallacy' is a psychological quirk whereby we consistently underestimate how long things will take. One classic study on this tendency found that mid-thesis students, on average, guesstimated it would take them 34 days to complete the body of work, but it actually took them 56 days. Nearly *double* the amount of time.

Define a 'learning' cut-off

If you're like me and you get obsessed with listening to, reading and absorbing everything about something, before you start *doing the thing*, you're going to need to self-bind. Think about what a reasonable amount of learning time is, write it down someplace, tell someone else if you like and then stick to it. Hopefully that way you won't watch five hours of YouTube tutorials and have no time to actually enact what you've learned.

Schedule appointments for first or last thing

Experts in time management have found that we're much less productive in the hours leading up to an appointment. This is why appointments in the middle of the day make us feel like our day is shorter. We literally do less that day.

The secret is creating as many sequential free hours as you can, of what the experts called 'unbounded' work time, by scheduling that Zoom for first thing, and that dentist appointment for last.

Find your rebellion elsewhere

'If you've historically been a people-pleaser, it can feel really good to rebel by doing the "wrong" thing c/o procrastination,' says Mathur. But you can find that elsewhere. 'I get this recipe delivery service, and never follow the instructions,' she laughs. 'I have to turn the mash into chips, or cut the vegetables in a different way to how they tell me. If you've worn that "good girl" or "good boy" hat your entire life, those tiny acts of rebellion give you an important buzz.'

Get yourself a Peggy
Margaret Atwood has an alter ego, just as Beyoncé has Sasha Fierce for stage shows, or David Bowie had Ziggy Stardust. Only, Atwood's alter ego is the opposite of fun – 'Peggy' tells Atwood to log off social media and do the laundry. I feel like we could all use a Peggy.

WHY WE NEED TO MAKE VISION BOARDS (YES, REALLY)

I've always thought vision boards were the act of a teenult with access to too much stationery.

But my British cynicism has been squelched, as I discovered while writing this book that there is some science behind cutting out pictures of holiday destinations, dream homes and chilled-looking people from magazines, then gluing them on to a big bit of card.

And that science is this: long-term goal-setting brings the prefrontal cortex online, says addiction psychotherapist Chris Lomas. Who you're envious of is an unexpected – and great – place to start when it comes to a vision board. Why? You're envious because they have something *you* want.

'Our egos get bad press but they have to be involved to some degree,' Lomas says of becoming our best selves. 'Because it's about looking at people you feel a pull towards, who activate that "want" in you. What is it about them that you want to replicate?'

Strong emotions are clues denoting things we want ourselves. So, seeing your ex-colleague host networking dinners might make you want to throw your phone across the room in disgust. *Clue.*

Myself, I find people who brag about batch-cooking on Sundays, or make big jam jars of miso-soy dressing . . . triggery. *Clue.*

Therefore, networking dinners or jam jars of homemade dressing should go straight on that board. Get them on there.

'Once you identify where you want to go and what kind of person you want to become, the prefrontal cortex is fully engaged,' says Lomas. 'This means that things in the way no longer feel like stop points. They're now obstacles to navigate instead.'

Indeed, since I became the kind of person who batch-cooks buddha bowls on Sundays, replete with miso-soy dressing from nine ingredients, I no longer find those people annoyingly smug. Because the reason those people triggered me was not because they're annoyingly smug. It's because I wanted what they had. A sense of order, advance prep, healthy food, a full fridge, the creation of ease in the working week.

If you really can't be arsed to get covered in glue and glitter – and, besides, you haven't bought a physical magazine in forever – you could try doing what I do to activate the same self-knowledge with less collaging.

Write an 'In five years' time, I want . . .' letter to the universe. Just try sending it out there.

I also write a 'This year, I want . . .' letter every January. Usually, by the end of the year, I've made most of it occur.

The universe isn't going to grant your wishes. It isn't a genie from a bottle. But knowing what your wishes are is profoundly key and, as we've already covered, is a way of getting our prefrontal cortex going. We need to give this powerful part of the brain a target to aim towards.

Otherwise, how will it know where to go?

CONCLUSION

The Cabin

While in the thick of writing this book, I went to a cabin.

One of those unplugged places in forests, where you forsake your phone while you're there. The type that rich stressed Londoners pay £150 a night to stay at in order to grind their own coffee beans using a spinny thing and live in what is essentially a caravan for Millennials.

My cabin is made out of wood, has a matt black bathroom with a rainfall showerhead, 100 per cent linen sheets and shower gel that smells like freshly squeezed grapefruit. The cabin-goers then take photos (to share on socials) of the Polaroids they took over the weekend, showing them dancing to the Madonna tape that's been provided with a cassette player, next to the fire pit that was super-easy to build given the ultra-flammable firelighter balls.

I mean, I sound superior, but I've been to these cabins myself four times as a paying guest, always for writing retreats. Frankly, I go to get away from my toddler who is only in childcare three days a week. The rest of the time she stands at the bottom of the stairs shouting 'MUMMY! MUMMY! MUM-MMMY!' We've tried pretending I'm out. She's not fooled; she can smell me. 'Mummy upstairs, hmmph,' she says, folding her chubby forearms like a '90s boyband member at the close of a song.

And so, I *am* the cabin-going cliché. If you're aware of it, does that make it better or worse? I'm not sure, but I will go again, more please, forever.

We now pay through the nose for this kind of experience. We go through the theatrics of locking our smartphones in a box and firing up a dumbphone, even though we have the tiny key for the phone prison in our pocket. We will talk for months after about how we felt like we had all the time in the world; how delicious it was to be unreachable; how we read a whole book in a day.

In my childhood, all of that was just called 'going to the caravan'. My father and stepmother had a caravan in Donegal next to a beach that wasn't just pebbly, it had massive rocks on it. But we had a Swingball set so everything was grand.

And when we went to the caravan, my father and stepmother were utterly, totally unplugged. For a tenth of what an unplugged retreat now costs us.

They only had a landline at home, so that was that dealt with. Leave your home = unreachable. And a TV never would have got coverage there, even if it had had an aerial the size of the caravan itself, so they read books. They didn't grind their own single-origin coffee, they just drank instant coffee that smelt a little like bin juice and gravy granules. Still, they really got that wholesale break from their lives that a holiday is meant to be.

They weren't still enmeshed in the drama blowing up on WhatsApp about the stag do, nor were they still hooked into the snafu at work, having turned on a fierce 'I will not be reading emails' OOO and then still reading emails (*me*). Nor were they keeping up with their binge-watching via their iPad, or browsing the seasonal sales at Urban Outfitters or Tu.

It's easy to fall back on 'weren't the good old days grand' but, no, sometimes they weren't. If you wanted to pay a bill, order food, access some entertainment, quickly organise something with a friend, or find something out, it was a clunky long-arsed nightmare.

I have been thinking about 'non-attachment' a lot while writing this book. The opposite to having things and processes and substances that we are far too stuck on. I've been thinking about it because I've finally started meditating (without the easy button of a guided meditation – I knew I needed to graduate), given the universe kept repeatedly bopping me over the head with that particular lesson (such as on pages 260 and 269). For just ten minutes a day, I put on a sound bath (see page 86) and try not to hook myself onto the thoughts that flicker through my mind, like coloured feathers hiding a barb.

It's difficult, really bloody difficult, but it's the deeper work I've known I needed to do for a long time. I can already feel my psychological core building into that thing that will stabilise me when I'm stood in the eye of the storm. Is meditation like plank for the mind, I wonder?

Despite this, when I set off on my 'unplugged' retreat, which was all about detaching from worldly attachments and getting back to nature, I packed my work backpack, a suitcase so big your average eight-year-old could hide inside, a tote bag and a huge bag of UPF, plus a few tokenistic pieces of fruit. I'd brought so much that the wheelbarrow they provide to house the belongings of two guests was overcome. This was all for three days.

It got me thinking about how many things – as well as thoughts – I can't unhook from and, therefore, in my view, am overly attached to. Lip balm, pocket tissues, an eye mask, antacids, my bluetooth speaker, tiger balm, sleepy tea, my slippers, body lotion, earplugs, unsalted nuts, hand cream, a hot-water bottle, noise-cancelling headphones, chocolate, running gear, my pregnancy pillow even though I'm not pregnant . . . the list goes on and on. This was all as well as the little addictions already outlined: nicotine lozenges, chewing gum, coffee.

Most of these extraneous items orbit comfort, and for good reason. I was frequently so uncomfortable (cold, hungry, tired, scared) and cared so little for myself in active alcohol addiction that, now, I want life to be *soft*. Cashmere soft if you can, please, even though that sounds like an overly floral fabric conditioner that probably kills fish.

After I spent an hour unpacking the frankly unhinged amount of stuff I had brought to this cabin, I was so disgusted with myself that I went for a 90-minute walk without any of it – even lip balm and chewing gum, and if you know me, you'll know that's big. I had my keys, one tissue (because hayfever) and the dumbphone they'd provided for emergencies.

Within a half hour of walking through woodland, I felt my chattering monkey mind slow and my mental core switch on. The dense trees broke into a clearing, which opened into a valley and – *oh my word*. It looked like some of the artwork you might see on a Jehovah's Witness leaflet; this is what heaven looks like, people.

Bucolic was the word that kept wanting to come out of my mouth. And, given I've only ever used this word in English essays about fictional settings, that's unusual. I tramped off down the valley feeling like an Austen character, making a beeline for some sort of gorgeous monument thing on the hill yonder, which looked like a stone birdcage. Once I'd crested that hill, I saw – I shit you not – lambs gambolling in a field just below. If this were a kid's book, this valley is definitely where the unicorns would base their HQ.

I stood on that hillside and burst into tears. But it went so much deeper than how beautiful it all was. I was crying because of this: modern life is disconnecting us from this exact feeling. The wonder. The quiet joy. Not the shallow, loud, nervous, hit-me-again buzz.

This is the good stuff – the deep-down shift, the slow dopamine – that can only be achieved by tramping up a hill. This is what it's all about, and we're missing it, *I'm missing it*, because we've all got our faces in our screens repeatedly pressing on the fast-dopamine button.

I wanted to get a closer look at the lambs, so I approached the field slowly, attracting the attention of a couple of grizzly older members of the herd, who probably served in Vietnam as marines, and are called Jed and Bruce, and definitely own a set of throwing knives. They eyeballed me, grunting, pawing slightly at the dirt. The lambs in the background stopped their cavorting.

I read a long time ago that animals intimate human intention via tone of voice and body language. Anyone who works with traumatised animals will likely tell you that this is true. So, I sat myself on the ground and, for the next 10 minutes, I murmured gently and continuously to Jed and Bruce. After five minutes, they softened from death stares to head cocks. Ten minutes in they came closer, ears flicked forward, posture relaxed, rubbing their noses on their knees, curious to see what I'd do.

I'm still not even sure why the next thing happened. Maybe because I'd run out of things to say about how I thanked them for their service, wished them no harm and that all I wanted was to just sit here for a while to watch their grandkids gambol, because I live in a place called the 'suburbs' and, instead of watching lambs, I spend my time watching things about funghi zombies eating people.

And so, I started to sing to them: 'Twinkle Twinkle Little Star', which is my daughter's favourite jam. And half of the herd looked up, stopped what they were doing and listened. I swear to you, they were rapt. The ex-marines came closer and closer; they were now six feet from me. Dozens of others came too. Mothers brought their newborn lambs within 20 feet.

I was now on 'Star Light, Star Bright', which they didn't like as much, so I switched to 'Hush Little Baby', which they were more in to. Bruce lay down. A lamb poked his sooty nose through the fence to breathe me in. He was so close I could have touched him (I didn't).

I know that this sounds like I'm propping myself up as some sort of 'mothers bring their baby animals to me' guru, especially given my previous anecdote about the horses when I was suicidal (page 82), but I am far from that. I don't have golden 'bring all your baby animals to my yard' energy. Anyone who knows me will tell you that I'm sometimes kind, sometimes irritable, sometimes thoughtful, sometimes thoughtless, sometimes lovely, sometimes impatient, sometimes gentle, sometimes intolerant, sometimes funny, sometimes boring.

But I can also tell you this. If you spend the time to make yourself soft and talk to random animals in fields, genuinely convincing them that you mean them no harm, you'll find that remarkable things happen. When I got up to leave, many of the herd came to follow me, weaving along the edge of the field, and there was a big chorus of baas like they were saying goodbye.

You could argue the herd just wanted feeding, or that they were telling me to bugger off – and to not audition for *Farm Idol* again – with those baas, but given they'd been wary and watchful when I first arrived, and half an hour later the difference was so dramatic, I took it as a sign that my non-attachment had improved my energy. Probably to monastic levels. Had I hacked the system and become like the Dalai Lama within 30 minutes of being lip balm-, phone- and chewing-gum-free?

It moved me so much that, over the next three days, I decided to forsake not only my phone, but lots of other dopamine cheat codes too, and use the nature around me for feelgood vibes instead. To use *doing my work* for satisfaction. I know! To dangle my feet in a lake with lily pads, build fires with the flammable balls and dance around a forest shouting the lyrics to Lola Young's 'Messy' even though I didn't have it blasting out of my AirPods.

I'd taken three pieces of leftover birthday cake to the cabin. I didn't eat any of it. I'd taken nine nicotine lozenges – 3mg for each day. Didn't have 'em. I'd taken valerian over-the-counter sleeping pills, which I often take, for fear the 3am wake-up's gonna get me (hiiii, perimenopause). Left those alone too. I'd downloaded three episodes of *MobLand*, intending to watch one a night, but it felt like it would be a desecration of my surroundings to watch gangsters kill each other in ever-more imaginative ways.

I used many of my comforts – the essential oils, one coffee a day, music from the ancient iPhone that I turned into an iPod (page 125), lip balm beside the bed, the sleepy tea, body lotion . . . but I was judicious about what I used. I only used it if I *knew* it wasn't too sticky a thing for me.

You know your sticky things too. They're the chapters you read in this book. They're the things you might feel nervous about doing without for three days if you went to a cabin. Or, if they're less frequent, for a week or a month.

Proving to yourself that you don't need them as much as you thought you did, that there is still pleasure and joy everywhere – better still, it's organically grown and free – might do something unexpected. Flexing the element of choice we still enjoy over these little addictions helps us detach from them.

We find out that the lower-case wants, the slow sources of dopamine (see page 182) don't carve out a hole – they actually fill it. We still want them, just not as urgently, and we find that we don't *need* them. They're what our bodies and brains were designed for, rather than the artificially supersized stickies that overpower us because of the evolutionary mismatch we've talked about throughout.

Once you step into your untapped power, the *not doing the thing* can become more of a rush than the sugar/alcohol/nicotine/gaming/porn whatever it was, ever was. Because we pick it.

You feel that small push of pride in your chest, that pulse of slow dopamine from what you choose to do instead, which sustains you for much longer than instant gratification ever did. It's a home-cooked protein breakfast rather than a shop-bought sugary pastry.

Our rebelliousness, our mischief, our kicks start to come from the *not doing.* And we don't find ourselves as darkened as we expected to by the deprivation. We've reframed the refrain as the bigger, better choice for us. The reward from it isn't the flicking on of spotlights – it is a steady, flickering oil lamp.

A fascinating thing I gained from researching this book was this: nature is our brain's neutral. Professor Murphy told me that, when he and his fellow researchers are trying to establish a neurophysiological 'cognitive baseline' to measure against during experiments, they show people a nature video. Corny though it may sound, science says that hilltops, waves, the chirp of birds and the shadows of a forest are our brain's big sigh. We unwind into this baseline.

The cogs we place into our reward system *can* change, like we talked about on page 88. We can be sustained by slow dopamine as the main, with the odd consciously chosen flash of fast. We don't have to be powered by fructose and thriller bingeing and Crunchy Nut Cornflakes and 'everything is content'. We don't have to be pacified by weed or booze at the end of the day just to feel OK.

Instead of iPhone neck, I choose sky neck. I want 'content enough not to create content', chutney and cheese rather than MSG, cuddles with my dog instead of staring at someone typing… This can be my new operating system, should I allow it to be.

I also, let's be real, want my one coffee a day, my ice cream cones, my flop in front of the TV, my daily two hours of screen time, the odd almond croissant from a bakery, my posh peppermint tea, that 'new dress' feeling, a takeaway once a month. Although I will quit nicotine, I'm not going to give up these other little addictions altogether. Now that I've tamed, bound and boxed them, I feel like they're the right size.

Personally, the ways that I've downsized my little addictions have been as follows. With ice cream, I've harnessed unit bias (by encasing it in a cone, see page 157) and identity change 'I'm not the kind of person who eats ice cream most nights', (page 157). Whereas peppermint tea was moderated down to two per day thanks to temptation bundling (page 287) and I now swerve all online shopping, now that I know of the endowment effect once the items are in my home (page 243) and the power of touch (page 240).

My screen time has almost halved due to the use of a symbolic storehold (mine's a rainbow seal, see page 127) and with Instagram, I simply post much less, and therefore obsess much less (page 125).

Elsewhere, I reclaimed my untapped power over biscuits (page 153), and even though I can host them, I choose not to (page 154). Television is now timeboxed within 9–10pm a day (page 189), but if I want a binge of a Sunday, I don't flog myself over it (because of the guilt paradox from page 27), I merely rebalance by taking a couple of days off. Learning about artificial sweeteners naturally downregulated my chewing gum habit, meaning I'm now on a pedestrian two tabs a day, while with caffeine, I really haven't changed anything, given everything I found out (page 285).

What will you keep, what will you seek to shrink and what will you discard? You're an intelligent adult who can decide the path from here. The only thing you must do is *something*. Which is why I've given you 130 specific, grabbable tips in this book. The lessons you take away and run with will be entirely personal to you. But of all the recovery sayings, this one is most true: 'Nothing changes if nothing changes.'

While trying to shrink a little addiction from this book, you may find you can't. That it was larger than you thought and had more of a grip on you than you'd realised. If that's the case, there may be a sense of mourning as you contemplate quitting that thing, rather than allowing its sway over you to enlarge, whether it's porn, UPF, gambling or gaming. I'm here to tell you that what feels like an ending could be the beginning of something lovelier than you could have imagined.

People who quit things don't quit because they can't do it any more. They quit because they see the path ahead and don't like what they see. They could continue on the path of not-moderating. Instead, they decide to prioritise their marriage over YouTube, or their job over alcohol . . . and, most of all, *themselves* over the *thing*.

Everyone can do anything they damn well please, if it's legal and they can afford to. The secret rarely shared is that these people choose to quit. They have to choose it, to quit effectively. Daily, if needs be, but they do.

But this book isn't about quitting. That's just a sidebar.

The final thing I want to leave you with is this. As the saying goes, whether you think you can, or you think you can't, you're right. Your self-belief is a coat hanger that will determine the shape of how your future hangs. That's why we've gone deep on items such as mindset, knowing our behavioural biases backwards and choosing empowering language.

You're no marionette. I *know* you can change your life. After all, you're already examining what so many leave unexamined by virtue of buying this book. Plus, you've endured my thousand or so mentions of my dog to get to the robust science underlying him. The question now is: *will* you change your life?

We don't need to waste another second being the chess piece. We're the chess players. Person uses thing, rather than thing uses person.

Love,
Cath x

PS: I've enjoyed every second of writing this book. Thank you for coming on this ride with me. Please, do stay in touch. I can't reply to everything, although I do reply to as much as I can. But I do read and love it all.

Instagram: @unexpectedjoyof
Web: catherine-gray.co.uk

RESOURCES FOR BIG ADDICTIONS

If you discovered back on page 16, that your addiction is a medium or big one, then here are some resources that are proportionately appropriate for you. I gained so much help from outside sources when I was recovering from my intense alcohol addiction, and would not have been able to do it alone. So, I greatly recommend seeking out external support.

None of these resources are affiliated with industry actors or funded by the industries themselves (see page 39 on how industries sometimes fund resources, which compromises the impartiality of these resources).

SMART Recovery
This covers alcohol and other drugs, plus gambling, nicotine, food, shopping, phone and internet-based addictions. Secular and advocating self-efficacy, it is particularly prevalent in the USA, Canada and Australia, but it operates globally too.

You can find meetings near you, or access free online meetings via **www.smartrecovery.org.uk** or **www.smartrecoveryglobal.org**

Alcoholics Anonymous and incarnations thereof (including Narcotics/Cocaine/Sex and Love Addicts/Gamblers/Overeaters/Gaming Addicts/Marijuana Anonymous)
Based on the 12 steps, this is a spiritual program involving a 'Power greater than ourselves', although some secular meetings are available. Find in-person meetings, or access free online meetings via the following:

www.alcoholics-anonymous.org.uk or **www.aa.org**
www.ukna.org or **www.na.org**
www.cocaineanonymous.org.uk or **www.ca.org**
www.slaauk.org or **www.slaafws.org**
www.gamblersanonymous.org.uk or **www.gamblersanonymous.org**
www.oagb.org.uk or **www.oa.org**
www.gamingaddictsanonymous.org
www.ma-uk.org or **www.marijuana-anonymous.org**

For secular versions geared towards atheists or agnostics , try the following:

www.aaagnostica.org
www.aasecular.org
www.secularna.org
www.secularovereaters.org

Refuge Recovery
A program based on the core principles of Buddhism, this can be used for any sort of addiction.

In-person meetings are all in the USA and Canada, but there are plenty of online meetings to join, plus free meditations, via **www.refugerecovery.org**

LifeRing Secular Recovery
For those seeking self-empowered and secular abstinence from alcohol and other drugs. Global, accessed online and running specialised meetings on co-occuring conditions, such as ADHD, Visit **www.lifering.org** for more details.

Women for Sobriety
Based on 13 acceptance statements, and geared towards emotional growth and lasting happiness. Visit **www.womenforsobriety.org** for more details.

Smoking/nicotine cessation
The NHS offers a range of support, which varies regionally, and can be found at **www.nhs.uk/live-well/quit-smoking**

Gaming addiction
The NHS offers free support from London-based The National Centre for Gaming Disorders. Self-referral is available at **www.cnwl.nhs.uk/national-centre-gaming-disorders**

SOURCES

INTRODUCTION

Sample paper title: Boolani A, Fuller DT, Mondal S, Wilkinson T, Darie CC, Gumpricht E, 'Caffeine-Containing, Adaptogenic-Rich Drink Modulates the Effects of Caffeine on Mental Performance and Cognitive Parameters: A Double-Blinded, Placebo-Controlled, Randomized Trial', *Nutrients,* 29 June 2020 (doi:10.3390/nu12071922).

NO GENERATIONAL PRECEDENT

Fish and chips escapes WWII rationing to boost morale: Caitlin Zaino, 'Chipping away at the history of fish and chips', *BBC Travel Online,* 19 April 2013.

82 per cent of Brits had mobile phones in 2005: Alexandra Bourgeaud, 'Share of mobile phone users in the United Kingdom (UK) from 2005 to 2024', *Statista,* 10 March 2025.

92 per cent of Brits still had landlines in 2006: Thomas Alsop, 'Percentage of households with landline telephones in the United Kingdom (UK) from 1970 to 2018', *Statista,* 6 August 2023.

We spend an average of four hours and twenty minutes on our phone in the UK overall. Gen Z spend an average of six hours: Ofcom, 'Online Nation 2024 Report', 28 November 2024.

Gen Z's social media time has decreased since 2021: Celeste Huang, 'Gen Z daily social media consumption falls, while boomers increase usage', *WARC,* n.d.

Gen Z's attitudes to social media: National Education Union, The New Britain Project and More in Common, 'Public attitudes to smartphones, social media, and online safety', *More in Common* website, 6 March 2025.

Headline asking 'What's wrong with young people today? They don't get drunk any more': Richard Goodwin, writing in *The Guardian,* 11 October 2018.

43 per cent of Gen Z don't drink: 'Almost half of young people no longer drink alcohol', *The Times,* 27 January 2025.

'Boring phone' launched: James Tapper, Aneesa Ahmed, 'The "boring phone": stressed out gen Z ditch smartphones for dumbphones', *The Guardian,* 27 April 2024.

OUR BRAINS EXPLAIN EVERYTHING

Hunter gatherers operating today: Jeff Leach, 'Trying the Hadza hunter-gatherer berry and porcupine diet', *BBC News Online,* 23 July 2017.

ALCOHOL

One in four Brits drinks over 14 units: 'Alcohol Statistics', *Alcohol Change UK* website, n.d.

NHS definition of one unit: 'Alcohol units', *NHS* website, n.d.

NHS defines a binge as six units: Royal Cornwall Hospitals, 'Alcohol: How much is too much?', V2, 2015.

World Health Organization states even one alcoholic drink a week carries risks: 'No level of alcohol consumption is safe for our health', *World Health Organization* website, 4 January 2023.

Meta-analysis of 107 alcohol studies questions health benefits of low-volume drinking: Tim Stockwell, Jinhui Zhao, Jim Clay, Ashley Levesque, Nathan Sanger, Adam Sherk, Timothy Naimi, 'Why do only some cohort studies find health benefits from low-volume alcohol use?', *Journal of Studies on Alcohol and Drugs*, July 2024 (doi:10.15288/jsad.23-00283).

Alcohol industry funding into alcohol research: University of York, 'Increase in alcohol-industry-funded research is a cause for concern, study suggests', *University of York News*, 17 September 2020.

Alcohol increases stress levels rather than relaxing you: Andrew Huberman, 'How alcohol actually increases stress levels, rather than relaxing you', *YouTube*, 2 January 2023.

Study identifies 500 neurons linked to binge drinking inhibition: P Gimenez-Gomez, T Le, M Zinter, P M'Angale, V Duran-Laforet, T G Freels, R Pavchinskiy, S Molas, D P Schafer, A R Tapper, T Thomson, G E Martin, 'An orbitocortical-thalamic circuit suppresses binge alcohol-drinking', *bioRxiv*, 5 July 2024 (doi:10.1101/2024.07.03.601895).

29 per cent of the brain's neurons are in the prefrontal cortex: Richard Levy, 'The prefrontal cortex: from monkey to man', *Brain*, Vol. 147, Issue 3, March 2024 (doi:10.193/brain/awad389).

Ozempic shown to dampen alcohol cravings: Michaeleen Doucleff, 'Ozempic seems to curb cravings for alcohol. Here's what scientists think is going on', *NPR Health Shots*, 28 August 2023.

GLP-1 spin-off semaglutide studied in patients with Alcohol Use Disorder: C S Hendershot, M P Bremmer, M B Paladino, et al, 'Once-Weekly Semaglutide in Adults With Alcohol Use Disorder: A Randomized Clinical Trial', *JAMA Psychiatry*, 2025 (doi:10.1001/jamapsychiatry.2024.4789).

Private cost of weekly Ozempic injections: 'Ozempic UK', *Medicspot UK*, n.d. (www.medicspot.co.uk/weight-loss/injections/ozempic-uk).

Institute of Alcohol Studies warns on 'dark apps' backed by alcohol industry: 'Dark apps uncovered: popular alcohol-tracking apps backed by the alcohol industry mislead users', *Institute of Alcohol Studies* website, 25 February 2025.

Drinkaware's funding comes predominantly from alcohol producers: 'About us', *Drinkaware* website, n.d. (www.drinkaware.co.uk/about-us).

Identity change and habit formation: James Clear, *Atomic Habits: Tiny changes, remarkable results*, 2018.

Study shows CBD (800mg) reduces alcohol cravings: S Zimmermann, A Teetzmann, J Baeßler, et al, 'Acute cannabidiol administration reduces alcohol craving and cue-induced nucleus accumbens activation in individuals with alcohol use disorder: the double-blind randomized controlled ICONIC trial', *Mol Psychiatry 30*, 2025 (doi:10.1038/s41380-024-02869-y).

GAMING

SnowWorld study demonstrates VR pain relief: H G Hoffman, G T Chambers, W J Meyer III, L L Arceneaux, W J Russell, E J Seibel, T L Richards, S R Sharar, D R Patterson, 'Virtual reality as an adjunctive non-pharmacologic analgesic for acute burn pain during medical procedures', *Annals of Behavioral Medicine*, April 2011 (doi:10.1007/s12160-010-9248-7).

Hunter Hoffman on SnowWorld's immersive distraction effect: 'Soldiers Get Virtual Reality Therapy for Burn Pain', *Sciencentral YouTube*, 10 November 2008 (www.youtube.com/watch?time_continue=128&v=jNIqyyypojg).

MRI scans show SnowWorld reduced pain-related brain activity by 50–97%: 'Virtual reality significantly reduces pain-related brain activity', *University of Washington News*, 21 June 2004.

SpiderWorld game used to distract adolescents undergoing burns procedures: University of Washington Seattle and UW Harborview Burn Center, 'Virtual Reality Pain Reduction', *HITLab*, n.d, (www.hitl.washington.edu/projects/vrpain).

Candy Crush still played by 200 million users in 2024: Keza MacDonald, 'Crushing it: why millions of people still can't stop playing Candy Crush', *The Guardian*, 1 August 2024.

Candy Crush motto 'Swipe the stress away': 'Candy Crush Saga—TV Commercial', *YouTube*, 2013 (www.youtube.com/watch?v=-KXGC4O3UL4&t=29s).

Reddit threads reveal users spending £1,000s on open-world games: 'How much have you spent on D&D in the past year?', *Reddit (r/DnD)*, 2024. 'How much have you spent on WoW over the years?', *Reddit (r/wow)*, 2022.

Runescape hat sells for $4,500; Amsterdam item sells for $50,000: 'The 10 most expensive in-game items ever sold', *1v9.gg*, 10 January 2025.

Meta-analysis of 116 gaming studies on cognition: Marc Palaus, Roser Viejo-Sobera, et al, 'Neural Basis of Video Gaming: A Systematic Review', *Frontiers in Human Neuroscience*, 2017 (doi:10.3389/fnhum.2017.00248).

Marc Palaus discusses gaming's brain effects: Thom James Carter, 'What gaming does to your brain–and how you might benefit', *Wired*, 26 June 2021.

Study on 33 surgeons shows video gaming improves surgical skills: James C. Rosser Jr., Paul J. Lynch, et al, 'The impact of video games on training surgeons in the 21st century', *Archives of Surgery*, February 2007 (doi:10.1001/archsurg.142.2.181).

Fortnite faces lawsuit in Canada: Isaac Olson, 'Addicted to Fortnite? Montreal law firm says video game company should pay up', *CBC News*, 4 October 2019.

Top 5 games linked to addiction support searches: 'World's most addictive video games revealed', *Rehabs UK* blog, 14 December 2022.

Expert compares Fortnite to heroin: Jef Feeley and Christopher Palmeri, 'Parents losing battle with Fortnite as children forced into rehab for video game addiciton', *The Independent*, 3 December 2018.

Gaming addiction associated with loneliness: Haohao Dong, Ming Wang, Hui Zheng, Jialin Zhang and Guang-Heng Dong, 'The functional connectivity between the prefrontal cortex and supplementary motor area moderates the relationship between internet gaming disorder and loneliness', *Prog Neuropsychopharmacol Biol Psychiatry*, 8 June 2021 (doi:10.1016/j.pnpbp.2020.110154)

NICOTINE

Over one in 10 of us vape, almost half of those are not ex-smokers: ASH Factsheet, 'Use of vapes (e-cigarettes) among adults in Great Britain', *ASH*, August 2024.

Nicotine was used as a pesticide: Joanna Dowle, 'How safe are natural insecticides?' *Environmental Protection Authority (New Zealand)*, 2 August 2024.

The USA banned use of nicotine as an insecticide in 2014: A Mishra, P Chaturvedi, S Datta, S Sinukumar, P Joshi, A Garg, 'Harmful effects of nicotine', *Indian Journal of Medical and Paediatric Oncology*, January–March 2015 (doi:10.4103/0971-5851.151771).

Unregulated vapes contain nickel, lead and chromium: Hugh Pym and Lucy Watkinson, 'Vaping: High lead and nickel found in illegal vapes', *BBC News*, 23 May 2023.

A quarter of school kids aged 11–15 have tried vaping; nearly one in 10 do it regularly: 'Almost 1 in 10 secondary school pupils currently vape, new NHS survey shows', *NHS England*, 17 October 2024.

Example of 'disposable alternatives' marketing and a £4.99 vape unit: www.vapeuk.co.uk/pod-vape-kits/disposable-vape-alternatives

Average mg of nicotine in a cigarette vs how much we actually ingest: Sarah Marsh, 'How much nicotine is in a cigarette compared to a vape', *The Guardian*, 23 June 2023.

Northerner.com answer to average consumption of nicotine pouches: 'Nicotine pouch use: How many per day', *The Northerner*, 6 May 2025.

The 'bioavailability' of nicotine in pouches is around 44 per cent, and can increase the heart rate by 22.5bpm: Hauke Reimann, Matthias Berger, Elisabeth Eckert, Katja Merches, Frederik Börnke, 'Beyond smoking: Risk assessment of nicotine in pouches', *Toxicology Reports*, Vol.13, 2024 (doi:10.1016/j.toxrep.2024.101779).

2015 meta analysis into nicotine's harmful effects, 90 studies in all: A Mishra, P Chaturvedi, S Datta, S Sinukumar, P Joshi, A Garg, 'Harmful effects of nicotine', *Indian Journal of Medical and Paediatric Oncology*, January–March 2015 (doi:10.4103/0971-5851.151771).

2018 study shows nicotine has cognitive-enhancing effects: G Valentine, M Sofuoglu, 'Cognitive Effects of Nicotine: Recent Progress', *Current Neuropharmacology*, May 2018 (doi:10.2174/1570159X15666171103152136).

Goop recommended 'vagus nerve oil': '4 Stress-Reduction Strategies to Keep in Your Pocket', *Goop*, n.d.

Gadgets that claim to biohack a vagus nerve reset: Emilie Lavinia, 'Why experts are urging caution on the "vagus nerve reset" trend', *The Independent*, 23 April 2025.

Study of 53 people shows iced water creates more of a 'vagal enhancement': CT Chiang, TW Chiu, YS Jong, GY Chen, CD Kuo, 'The effect of ice water ingestion on autonomic modulation in healthy subjects', *Clinical Automatic Research*, December 2010 (doi:10.1007/s10286-010-0077-3).

Rituals help relax us: Alison Wood Brooks, Juliana Schroeder, Jane L Risen, Francesca Gino, Adam D Galinsky, Michael I Norton, Maurice E Schweitzer, 'Don't stop believing: Rituals improve performance by decreasing anxiety', *Organizational Behavior and Human Decision Processes*, 2016 (doi:10.1016/j.obhdp.2016.07.004).

Financial incentives shown to bring about smoking/nicotine cessation: J Hartmann-Boyce, J Livingstone-Banks, JM Ordóñez-Mena, TR Fanshawe, N Lindson, SC Freeman, AJ Sutton, A Theodoulou, P Aveyard, 'Behavioural interventions for smoking cessation: an overview and network meta-analysis', *Cochrane Database of Systematic Reviews*, 4 January 2021 (doi:10.1002/14651858.CD013229.pub2).

FIVE-STAR REHAB

2022 meta-analysis of residential rehabs: Scottish Government, 'Residential rehabilitation: literature review', 30 May 2022.

Autism expert discussing lack of interoception skills leading to meltdowns: Dr Emma Goodall, 'Interoception and mental wellbeing in autistic people', *National Autistic Society*, 16 March 2022.

Sound bath 2023 Korean study into brainwaves: SC Kim, MJ Choi, 'Does the Sound of a Singing Bowl Synchronize Meditational Brainwaves in the Listeners?' *International Journal of Environmental Research and Public Health*, June 2023 (doi:10.3390/ijerph20126180).

Harvard Medical School says several studies show blood pressure decreases when you pet a dog: 'Having a dog can help your heart – literally', *Harvard Health Publishing*, 1 September 2015.

2006 study by Dr Qing Li and 12 others into phytoncides aromatherapy, and how it can mimic the effects of forest bathing in person: Qing Li, A Nakadai, H Matsushima, Y Miyazaki, AM Krensky, T Kawada, K Morimoto, 'Phytoncides (wood essential oils) induce human natural killer cell activity', *Immunopharmacology and Immunotoxicology*, 2006 (doi:10.1080/08923970600809439).

Dr Qing Li tells Goop that phytoncides have the 'greatest effect' of all the aspects of forest bathing: 'The Science—and Magic—of Forest Bathing', *Goop*, n.d.

GAMBLING

Most popular forms of gambling in the UK: Gambling Commission, 'Statistics on gambling participation – Year 2 (2024), wave 4: Official statistics', *Gambling Commission* website, 22 May 2025.

Swedish study on lottery winners' happiness: Erik Lindqvist, Robert Östling, David Cesarini, 'Long-Run Effects of Lottery Wealth on Psychological Well-Being', *The Review of Economic Studies*, November 2020 (doi:10.1093/restud/rdaa006).

Previous Omaze prize winners: Nic North, 'The truth about winning the Omaze "dream" ', *MailOnline*, 28 August 2023.

Coastal erosion beliefs leave Omaze North Devon home empty: Alice Giddings, 'A £1,000,000 mistake? The "Omaze curse" plaguing these stunning dream homes', *Metro*, 22 March 2025.

Omaze as a 'charity raffle': Louise Parry, 'Omaze house winner overjoyed despite planning issue', *BBC News*, 28 March 2025.

One per cent of National Lottery's revenue is profit: John Woodhouse, 'The National Lottery: Research briefing', *House of Commons Library,* 8 February 2024.

National Lottery took in £7.8bn in sales 2023–24: 'Annual sales of the National Lottery in the United Kingdom from April 2008 to March 2024', *Statista*, 9 July 2025.

Omaze investigation: Will Sibley, 'Omaze: How does it work and what are your chances of winning?', *The Telegraph,* 15 March 2025.

'Let me dream on' effect: Martin G Kocher, Michal Krawczyk, Frans van Winden, '"Let me dream on!" Anticipatory emotions and preference for timing in lotteries', *Journal of Economic Behavior & Organization,* Vol.98, February 2014 (doi:10.1016/j.jebo.2013.12.006).

The reason people use gambling apps or gamble online: Gambling Commission, 'Investigating the relationship between reasons for gambling and different gambling activities', *Gambling Commission* website, 30 January 2025.

Best lotteries to play, odds wise: Emma Lake, 'POT LUCK: The lottery games you have the highest chance of winning and those with the biggest jackpots', *The Sun,* 4 January 2025.

OUR PHONES

Stanford's Persuasive Technology Lab alumni: Yasmin Samrai, 'How Stanford Profits Off Addiction', *The Stanford Review,* 4 February 2020.

Center for Humane Technology: 'About us: Impact and Story', *Center for Humane Technology* website.

BJ Fogg founds the Peace Innovation Lab at Stanford: BJ Fogg, 'The Facts: BJ Fogg & Persuasive Technology', *Medium,* 18 March 2018.

Dr Timnit Gebru's dispute with Google: Karen Hao, 'We read the paper that forced Timnit Gebru out of Google. Here's what it says', *MIT Technology Review,* 4 December 2020.

Sarah Wynn-Williams' claims about Facebook: Katie Razzall and Sarah Bell, 'Facebook was "hand in glove" with China, BBC told', *BBC News,* 10 March 2025.

Sarah Wynn-Williams' testimony to the US Senate: U.S. Senate Committee on the Judiciary Subcommittee on Crime and Counterterrorism, 'A Time for Truth: Oversight of Meta's Foreign Relations and Representations to the United States Congress. Questions for the Record for Sarah Wynn-Williams', *U.S. Senate Committee on the Judiciary,* 16 April 2025.

Meta on *Careless People*: Steven Poole, '*Careless People* by Sarah Wynn-Williams review – Zuckerberg and me', *The Guardian,* 13 March 2025.

55 per cent of Brits check their phones during dinner: Matthew Smith, 'YouGov reveals the extent of Britain's addiction to our phones', *YouGov,* 18 October 2018.

Three quarters of us sleep in the same room as our phone: Milan Dinic, 'The YouGov Sleep Study: Part Four – The impact of screens, lights, and noise on sleep', *YouGov,* 29 June 2022.

A third of us check our phones in the night: Fiona Simpson, 'One in three Brits check their smartphones in the middle of the night', *The Standard,* 26 September 2016.

A quarter of teens check their phones more than ten times during the night: 'Teenage use of mobile devices during the night', *BASW: The professional association for social work and social workers,* n.d.

Tristan Harris BBC interview: 'One to One: Is social media ruining our lives?', *BBC Radio 4,* 4 May 2021.

Tristan Harris and Jaron Lanier quotes from *The Social Dilemma*: '*The Social Dilemma* (2022) – Transcript', *Scraps from the Loft,* 3 October 2020.

Harris on our phone being 'the slot machine in your pocket': Von Tristan Harris, 'The slot machine in your pocket', *Spiegel International,* 27 July 2016.

Gmail stopped scanning contents of our emails to serve ads in 2017: Alex Hern, 'Google will stop scanning content of personal emails', *The Guardian,* 26 June 2017.

67.5 per cent opt in to push notifications: Andrew Buck, '50+ push notification statistics for 2025', *MobiLoud,* 3 July 2025.

'Brain drain' experiments from University of Texas: Adrian F Ward, Kristen Duke, Ayelet Gneezy, and Maarten W Bos, 'Brain Drain: The Mere Presence of One's Own Smartphone Reduces Available Cognitive Capacity', *Journal of the Association for Consumer Research*, April 2017 (doi:10.1086/691462).

University of Texas press release: 'The Mere Presence of Your Smartphone Reduces Brain Power, Study Shows', *UT News*, 26 June 2017.

2023 meta-analysis of 22 studies to investigate 'brain drain' effect: T Böttger, M Poschik, K Zierer, 'Does the Brain Drain Effect Really Exist? A Meta-Analysis', *Behavioral Sciences*, 11 September 2023 (doi:10.3390/bs13090751).

Kids with phones in the room score 15 points lower on tests: Paige MacPherson, 'Quality testing data shows why smartphones have no place in classrooms', *Fraser Institute*, 9 February 2024.

It takes 23 minutes after interruption to resume: Gloria Mark, Shamsi Iqbal, Mary Czerwinski, Paul Johns, 'Focused, Aroused, but so Distractible: A Temporal Perspective on Multitasking and Communications', *Cooperative Work & Social Computing*, 14 March 2015.

Those who are interrupted complete work in the same time frame, but with more stress, frustration and time pressure: Gloria Mark, Daniela Gudith and Ulrich Klocke, 'The Cost of Interrupted Work: More Speed and Stress', *Conference on Human Factors in Computing Systems*, 2008.

Dr Anna Lembke berries/wheat quote: Dr Anna Lembke, *Dopamine Nation: Finding balance in the age of indulgence*, 19 January 2023 (152).

Typical British adult now spends 3 hours, 21 minutes on their phones: Mark Sweney, 'Adults in Great Britain now spending more time on mobiles than watching TV', *The Guardian*, 25 June 2025.

Google agree to settle $5 billion class action lawsuit: Reuters reporters, 'Google agrees to settle $5bn lawsuit claiming it secretly tracked users', *The Guardian*, 29 December 2023.

Daily news consumption calamitous for mental health; a few of hundreds of studies: J K Kellerman, J L Hamilton, E A Selby, E M Kleiman, 'The Mental Health Impact of Daily News Exposure During the COVID-19 Pandemic: Ecological Momentary Assessment Study', *JMIR Mental Health*, 25 May 2022 (doi:10.2196/36966). B McLaughlin, M R Gotlieb, D J Mills, 'Problematic News Consumption and Its Relationship to Mental and Physical Health: A Replication Study', *Health Communication*, 2 December 2024 (doi:10.1080/10410236.2024.2434955). Çağrı Güneç, 'Frequent News Consumption Might Negatively Impact Mental Health', 11 September 2022 (doi:10.13140/RG.2.2.17519.71843).

Survey of therapists on news consumption and mental health: Alan Deibel, 'The negative effects of news and how to protect your mental health', *Growtherapy*, 11 March 2025.

Press release on 2015 study on 5,000 Facebook users: Louis DiPietro, 'Addicted to Facebook: why we keep returning', *Cornell Chronicle*, 10 December 2015.

Aza Raskin quote on infinite scroll, plus Tristan Harris on 'vibrate': 'What happened in Vegas with Natasha Dow Schüll', *Your Undivided Attention* podcast from Center for Humane Technology, 11 June 2019.

Brian Wansink's bottomless bowls study: Susan S. Lang, '"Bottomless" bowls of soup win CU's Wansink an "Ig Nobel"', *Cornell Chronicle*, 9 October 2007.

Brick: getbrick.app [accessed 2 October 2025].

CANNABIS

Where cannabis is legal or has lower penalties: Sarah Sinclair, 'Where Is Cannabis Legal In Europe? A Guide To The Latest Policy Changes', *Forbes*, 28 March 2024.

UK is the highest exporter of medicinal cannabis: Reality Check team, 'Is the UK the world's biggest exporter of legal cannabis?', *BBC News*, 23 May 2018.

Fine for smoking on the streets in Amsterdam: Senay Boztas, '"Potheads, go giggle elsewhere": public weed ban begins in Amsterdam', *The Guardian*, 25 May 2023.

Dabs or oils can be as high as 90 per cent: Isabella Backman, 'Marijuana: Rising THC Concentrations in Cannabis Can Pose Health Risks', *Yale School of Medicine*, 30 August 2023.

THC: CBD ratio: David J Potter, Kathy Hammond, Shaun Tuffnell, Christopher Walker, Marta Di Forti, 'Potency of Δ9–tetrahydrocannabinol and other cannabinoids in cannabis in England in 2016: Implications for public health and pharmacology', *Drug Testing and Analysis*, vol.10, iss.4, April 2018 (doi:10.1002/dta.2368).
The 'entourage effect' in popular media: Raj Chander, 'What is the interaction between CBD and THC?', *Healthline*, 24 January 2024.
The 'entourage effect' challenged: SD Pennypacker, K Cunnane, MC Cash, E A Romero-Sandoval, 'Potency and Therapeutic THC and CBD Ratios: U.S. Cannabis Markets Overshoot', *Frontiers in Pharmacology*, 6 June 2022 (doi:10.3389/fphar.2022.921493).
Indica vs sativa strains: Kimberly Holland, 'What to Know About the Differences Between Sativa, Indica, and Hybrid Strains of Weed', *Healthline*, 26 February 2025.
Edible with high CBD enhanced the negatives of THC: 'CBD May Increase the Adverse Effects of THC in Edible Cannabis Products, Study Shows', *John Hopkins Medicine Newsroom*, 13 February 2023.
One in ten who try cannabis become addicted: Fact sheet, 'Cannabis/Marijuana Use Disorder', *Yale Medicine*, n.d.
Cannabis is not a gateway drug: Elizabeth Hlavinka, 'Massive study of adolescent brains puts "gateway drug" theory into question', *Salon*, 6 January 2025.
US study of 500,000 finds cannabis use risen among high-earners and college graduates: DT Mattingly, MK Richardson, JL Hart, 'Prevalence of and trends in current cannabis use among US youth and adults, 2013–2022', *Drug & Alcohol Dependence Reports*, 28 June 2024 (doi:10.1016/j.dadr.2024.100253).
Teen use of marijuana falling between 2013 and 2023: Centers for Disease Control and Prevention, 'Youth Risk Behavior Survey Data Summary & Trends Report: 2013–2023', *US Department of Health and Human Services*, 2024.
Joe Biden walks back his stance that marijuana is a gateway drug: Jason Silverstein, 'Joe Biden rolls back his stance on marijuana being a "gateway drug"', *CBS News*, 26 November 2019.
Dr Peter Grinspoon quote: Peter Grinspoon, 'The endocannabinoid system: Essential and mysterious', *Harvard Health Publishing*, 11 August 2021.
Study on 1,000 teens, cannabis use and IQ: Harold S Koplewicz, 'Does Teenage Marijuana Use Affect IQ?', *Child Mind Institute*, 5 June 2024.
2014 Study on rats, resistance exercise and endocannabinoid activation: G Galdino, T Romero, J F Pinho da Silva, D Aguiar, A M de Paula, J Cruz, C Parrella, F Piscitelli, I Duarte, V Di Marzo, A Perez, 'Acute resistance exercise induces antinociception by activation of the endocannabinoid system in rats', *Journal of Anesthesia, Analgesia and Critical Care*, September 2014 (doi:10.1213/ANE.0000000000000340).
Runner's high thought to be endocannabinoids: Christopher Bergland, '"Runner's High" Depends on Endocannabinoids (Not Endorphins)', *Psychology Today*, 26 February 2021. Prakash Nagarkatti and Mitzi Nagarkatti, 'People produce endocannabinoids – similar to compounds found in marijuana – that are critical to many bodily functions', *University of South Carolina*, 22 February 2023.
15 minutes of weightlifting is enough to increase endocannabinoids: Christopher Bergland, 'Endocannabinoids and the Anti-inflammatory Power of Exercise', *Psychology Today*, 18 November 2021.
Kitchen Safe KSafe: www.thekitchensafe.com [accessed 4 October 2025].

ULTRA-PROCESSED FOOD

All Dr David A Kessler quotes: David Kessler, *Food or Fiction: the truth about the ultraprocessed foods making America sick*, 7 May 2024. Previous relationship with food (8), rat studies (79), reward response in gut (78), 'calorific torpedo' (38), unprocessed vs ultra-processed food study (84–5), bread basket heuristic (98), overeating guilt trap (180).
All Dr Chris van Tulleken quotes: Chris van Tulleken, *Ultra-Processed People: Why do we all eat stuff that isn't food... and why can't we stop?*, 2 May 2024. He and brother Xand were addicted to UPF (303), bingeing and purging cheap takeaways (163, 165), rule of thumb (160), food isn't addictive, but UPF is (165), scientists' conflicts of interest (305–6), sandwich (303).

Shahroo Izadi quotes: 'Behaviour Change Scientist: How I Lost 120lbs With Kindness: Shahroo Izadi', *The Diary of a CEO with Steven Bartlett* podcast, 16 February 2023.

A few of many sources confirming that Coca-Cola Inc funds clinical studies: P Serodio, G Ruskin, M McKee, Stuckler, 'Evaluating Coca-Cola's attempts to influence public health "in their own words": analysis of Coca-Cola emails with public health academics leading the Global Energy Balance Network', *Public Health Nutrition*, 3 August 2020 (doi:10.1017/S1368980020002098). David Stuckler, Gary Ruskin and Martin McKee, 'Complexity and conflicts of interest statements: a case-study of emails exchanged between Coca-Cola and the principal investigators of the International Study of Childhood Obesity, Lifestyle and the Environment (ISCOLE)', *Journal of Public Health Policy*, vol.39, 27 November 2017 (doi:10.1057/s41271-017-0095-7).

Coca-Cola can quash clinical studies if they don't find the data favourable: Elisabeth Mahase, 'Coca-Cola contracts could allow it to "quash" unfavourable research findings', *BMJ*, 8 May 2019.

British Nutrition Foundation funding: 'About the British Nutrition Foundation', *British Nutrition Foundation*, British Nutrition Foundation 'Healthy Eating Week', 2023.

Coca-Cola has donated over $1 million to the BNF: I M Del Giudice, K A Tsai, J Arshonsky, S Bond, M A Bragg, 'Food industry donations to patient advocacy organisations focussed on non-communicable diseases', *Public Health Nutrition*, March 2023 (doi:10.1017/S1368980022001859).

PORN

Seven in 10 teens have watched porn, up from four in 10 in 2005: 'New Report Reveals Truths About How Teens Engage with Pornography', *Common Sense*, 10 January 2023.

Three per cent of 8–9-year-olds in the UK accessed a porn site in the past month: 'Age checks for online safety – what you need to know as a user', *Ofcom*, 26 June 2025.

22 per cent of women watch porn; males are threefold: 'We asked men how they feel about dating, sex, and porn in 2023. The answers are not simple', *GQ*, 29 March 2023.

Survey of younger women finds 47 per cent use porn: 'BBC Three releases survey findings for new porn documentary', *Daily Nightly*, 14 March 2019.

Filipino women watch more porn than Filipino men: Jemy Gatdula, 'Porn and the damage to Philippine society', *Business World*, 12 January 2024.

Women under-report porn use, men over-report: Aikaterini-Maria (Katerina) Litsou, 'Women's Reported Motivations for, and Outcomes from, their Pornography Use', *University of Southampton* PhD thesis, January 2024.

Celebrity porn use: Iris Goldsztajn, '19 Celebrities Share Their Thoughts on Porn', *Cosmopolitan*, 19 July 2016.

Billie Eilish: Reuters reporters, 'Billie Eilish says watching porn as a child "destroyed my brain"', *The Guardian*, 15 December 2021.

Study into the porn use of 217 couples: Alice Bourne and Grace Schwenck, 'How does using porn alone affect relationship quality?', *Couples & Sexual Health Research*, 13 May 2024.

Couples who use porn together report higher relationship satisfaction: T Kohut, K A Dobson, R N Balzarini, R D Rogge, A M Shaw, J K McNulty, V M Russell, W A Fisher, L Campbell, 'But What's Your Partner Up to? Associations Between Relationship Quality and Pornography Use Depend on Contextual Patterns of Use Within the Couple', *Frontiers in Psychology*, 30 July 2021 (doi:10.3389/fpsyg.2021.661347).

THE DOPAMINE-HUNTERS

Dopamine discovered to be a neurotransmitter in 1957: V K Yeragani, M Tancer, P Chokka, G B Baker, 'Arvid Carlsson, and the story of dopamine', *Indian J Psychiatry*, January 2010 (doi:10.4103/0019-5545.58907).

'Liking and wanting' experiment: KC Berridge, T E Robinson, 'Liking, wanting, and the incentive-sensitization theory of addiction', *American Psychologist*, 1 November 2017 (doi:10.1037/amp0000059).

Dopamine-fasting: Peter Grinspoon, 'Dopamine fasting: Misunderstanding science spawns a maladaptive fad', *Harvard Health Publishing,* 26 February 2020.

Dr Cameron Sepah backpedals: Nellie Bowles, 'How to feel nothing now in order to feel more later', *Irish Times,* 5 December 2019.

Dr Stephanie Borgland quote: Celia Ford, 'Dopamine, explained', *Vox,* 22 May 2024.

All Dr Anna Lembke quotes: *Dopamine Nation: Finding balance in the age of indulgence,* 19 January 2023. Measures addictive potential (49), rat in a box (50), anhedonia (57), rats cocaine study (101–2). *The Official Dopamine Nation Workbook: A practical guide to overcoming addiction in the age of indulgence,* 1 October 2024. Human brains survival (62), hormesis and baseline quote (101), 'slow dopamine' activities (105).

All Dr TJ Power quotes: *The Dose Effect: Small habits to boost your brain chemistry,* 16 January 2025. Sources of 'quick dopamine' (27), homeostasis (29).

Changes in tonic rate of dopamine: Park Jeongrak, Kang Seongtak, Lee Yaebin, Choi Ji-Woong, Oh Yong-Seok, 'Continuous long-range measurement of tonic dopamine with advanced FSCV for pharmacodynamic analysis of levodopa-induced dyskinesia in Parkinson's disease', *Frontiers in Bioengineering and Biotechnology,* vol.12, 24 January 2024 (doi:10.3389/fbioe.2024.1335474).

Low dopamine linked to restless leg, depression and Parkinson's: 'Dopamine Deficiency', *Cleveland Clinic,* 23 March 2022.

Some of many clinical papers linking ADHD with dopamine dysfunction: K Blum, AL Chen, ER Braverman, DE Comings, TJ Chen, V Arcuri, SH Blum, BW Downs, RL Waite, A Notaro, J Lubar, L Williams, TJ Prihoda, T Palomo, M Oscar-Berman, 'Attention-deficit-hyperactivity disorder and reward deficiency syndrome', *Neuropsychiatric Disease and Treatment,* October 2008 (doi:10.2147/ndt.s2627). Hayley J MacDonald, Rune Kleppe, Peter D Szigetvari, Jan Haavik, 'The dopamine hypothesis for ADHD: An evaluation of evidence accumulated from human studies and animal models', *Frontiers in Psychiatry,* vol.15, 15 November 2024 (doi:10.3389/fpsyt.2024.1492126).

Some of many clinical papers linking autism with dopamine dysfunction: Denis Pavăl, 'Chapter One – The dopamine hypothesis of autism spectrum disorder: A comprehensive analysis of the evidence', *International Review of Neurobiology,* vol.173, 2023 (doi:10.1016/bs.irn.2023.08.009). GE DiCarlo, MT Wallace, 'Modeling dopamine dysfunction in autism spectrum disorder: From invertebrates to vertebrates', *Neuroscience & Biobehavioral Reviews,* February 2022 (doi:10.1016/j.neubiorev.2021.12.017). 'New study links dopamine to autism symptoms', *Karolinska Institutet,* 22 January 2025.

Those with ADHD three times more likely to experience addiction (15.2 per cent vs 5.6 per cent): 'ADHD and Co-occurring Conditions', *CHADD,* n.d. www.chadd.org/about-adhd/co-occuring-conditions.

University of Cambridge study finds autistic adults less likely to use drugs, but nine times more likely to self-medicate: E Weir, C Allison and S Baron-Cohen, 'Understanding the substance use of autistic adolescents and adults: a mixed methods approach', *The Lancet Psychiatry,* 1 July 2021.

JUDGEMENT & GOSSIP

Women and men gossip equally: Chris Matyszczyk, Howard Raucous, 'Men gossip just as much as women, says just published study (and, boy, do we spend a lot of time gossiping)', *Inc.,* 17 May 2019.

Lainey articles and nicknames: Jessica Biel (https://www.laineygossip.com/Jessica-Biels-publicist-explains-why-one-of-her-pit-bulls-died/7514), Tom Cruise (https://www.laineygossip.com/Tom-Cruise-and-John-Travolta-at-Scientology-Super-Power-Centre-opening-in-Florida/28668), Katie Holmes (https://www.laineygossip.com/Tom-Cruise-walks-Katie-Holmes-to-work-in-NYC/10588), Ryan Phillippe (https://www.laineygossip.com/Ryan-Phillippes-Carb-Face-and-loser-pants-leaves-Villa-with-Abbie-Cornish/10327), Ryan Reynolds (https://www.laineygossip.com/Ryan-Reynolds-to-host-Saturday-Night-Live-and-Scarlett-Johansson-in-Paris-to-promote-album-with-Pete/14530).

DATING, FLIRTING & SEX

Lawsuit filed against dating apps: Rachel Hall, 'Are dating apps fuelling addiction? Lawsuit against Tinder, Hinge and Match claims so', *The Guardian*, 17 February 2024.

Tinder use a 'desirability rating': Matt Burgess, 'Tinder knows how desirable you are (but it won't tell you)', *Wired*, 12 January 2016.

Dating app use down: Daniel Roman, 'The Incredible Shrinking Dating App', *Wired*, 13 February 2025.

11 per cent of Brits met their long-term partner through a dating app: Shahed Ezaydi, 'In an era of dating apps, a new study shows that 53% of Brits met their partners in person', *Stylist*, 2023.

Two-thirds of Tinder users are in a relationship: 'Almost two-thirds of Tinder's users are already in a relationship – and half don't even want a date', *Sky News*, 14 July 2023.

Skin hunger: Denise Renye, 'What is Skin Hunger?', *Good Therapy Blog*, 13 December 2022. Claire Postl, 'What is skin hunger?', *The Ohio State University Wexner Medical Center*, 16 March 2020.

Expert endorsements of weighted blankets and skin hunger or 'touch starvation': Suzanne Degges-White, 'Skin Hunger, Touch Starvation, and Hug Deprivation', *Psychology Today*, 20 November 2020. Sarah Barkley, 'What Does It Mean to Be Touch Starved?', *Psych Central*, 2 August 2022. 'Weighted blankets guide for occupational therapists', *Royal College of Occupational Therapists*, 1 February 2023.

PEOPLE-PLEASING

Brits apologising: Xantha Leatham, 'The number of times Brits say sorry per day revealed – so, are you guilty of over-apologising?', *MailOnline*, 8 May 2025.

SHOPPING

Gabor Maté addicted to classical music: Leslie Garrett, 'Gabor Maté: Why We're a Culture of Addicts', *Spirituality & Health*, n.d.

Anna Lembke addicted to romantasy: Joel Stein, 'Book Review: All You Can Read', *Stanford Mag*, July 2022.

Ecological overshoot: JJ Merz, P Barnard, W E Rees, et al, 'World scientists' warning: The behavioural crisis driving ecological overshoot', *Science Progress*, 20 September 2023 (doi:10.1177/00368504231201).

Satin bowerbirds collect blue things to attract mates: Emma Siossian, 'Satin bowerbirds fall victim to plastic waste, wildlife experts urge mindfulness', *ABC.NET.AU*, 6 October 2018.

Study into the hunter/gatherer assignment: Daniel Kruger, Dreyson Byker, 'Evolved foraging psychology underlies sex differences in shopping experiences and behaviors', *Journal of Social, Evolutionary, and Cultural Psychology*, December 2009 (doi:10.1037/h0099312).

'Neural predictors of purchases': B Knutson, S Rick, G E Wimmer, D Prelec, G Loewenstein, 'Neural predictors of purchases', *Neuron*, 4 January 2007 (doi:10.1016/j.neuron.2006.11.010).

Temu investigation finds 'extremely high risk' of child labour: Sam Gruet, 'Temu shoppers risk buying items made by forced labour, M P warns', *BBC News*, 21 December 2023.

Illegal deforestation: Dimitri Selibas, 'Report links H&M and Zara to major environmental damage in biodiverse Cerrado', *Mongabay*, 17 April 2024.

Shein lawyer refused to answer committee about region associated with forced labour: Michael Race, 'M Ps urge checks as Shein refuses to answer questions', 10 January 2025.

Brian Knutson on the insula: Nikhil Swaminathan, 'This Is Your Brain on Shopping', *SCI AM*, 5 January 2007.

When using credit cards, costs are 'out of mind': S Banker, D Dunfield, A Huang, et al, 'Neural mechanisms of credit card spending', *Scientific Reports*, Vol.11, 18 February 2021 (doi:10.1038/s41598-021-83488-3).

Exposure to 'age-progressed' versions of ourselves: H E Hershfield, D G Goldstein, W F Sharpe, J Fox, L Yeykelis, L L Carstensen, J N Bailenson, 'Increasing saving behavior through age-progressed renderings of the future self', *Journal of Marketing Research,* November 2011 (doi:10.1509/jmkr.48.SPL.S23).

Denis Diderot: 'Regrets for my old dressing gown', *Oeuvres Complètes,* Vol IV, translated by Mitchell Abidor, 1769 (translated 2005).

Insula activation via interoceptive sensations: W K Simmons, J A Avery, J C Barcalow, J Bodurka, W C Drevets, P Bellgowan, 'Keeping the body in mind: insula functional organization and functional connectivity integrate interoceptive, exteroceptive, and emotional awareness', *Human Brain Mapping,* 13 June 2012 (doi:10.1002/hbm.22113).

Butt brush effect: Bill Page, 'Shoppers' movements might come down to fears of caves and the "butt brush"', *Ehrenberg-Bass Institute for Marketing Science,* 12 June 2018.

Touching study: Joann Peck and Suzanne B Shu, 'The effect of mere touch on perceived ownership', *Journal of Consumer Research,* vol. 36, October 2009 (doi:10.1086/598614).

We prefer items being touched online too: Andrea Luangrath, 'Consumers value a product viewed online more if they see it being virtually touched', *Canadian Manufacturing,* 7 December 2021.

THE SECRETS RETAILERS DON'T WANT YOU TO KNOW

All prices cited in this chapter correct at time of shopping in February 2025.

Consumer psychologist's website example: www.humanising-brands.com/about/

Flying Tiger store example bio: www.experienceguildford.com/directory/home/flying-tiger/

Charm pricing study: Eric T Anderson; Duncan I Simester, 'Effects of $9 Price Endings on Retail Sales: Evidence from Field Experiments', *Quantitative Marketing and Economics,* March 2003 (doi:10.1023/A:1023581927405).

Dollar (or pound) sign dropping: Susan S Lang, 'Diners spend more when menus don't use dollar signs', *Cornell Chronicle,* 9 December 2009.

ACTIVATING THE PREFRONTAL CORTEX'S POWER

The prefrontal cortex as the 'brakes on overconsumption': Dr Anna Lembke, *The Official Dopamine Nation Workbook: A practical guide to overcoming addiction in the age of indulgence,* 1 October 2024.

One of many studies showing the prefrontal cortex loses synaptic density in addiction: H Garavan, K L Brennan, R Hester, R Whelan, 'The neurobiology of successful abstinence', *Current Opinion in Neurobiology,* 16 March 2013 (doi:10.1016/j.conb.2013.01.029).

Those who drink under 15 are more likely to develop addiction: 'Age of Drinking Onset Predicts Future Alcohol Abuse and Dependence', *National Institute on Alcohol Abuse and Alcoholism,* 14 January 1998.

Addiction routinely linked to lower overall brain volume; two studies of many: Scott Mackey et al, 'Mega-Analysis of Gray Matter Volume in Substance Dependence: General and Substance-Specific Regional Effects', *American Journal of Psychiatry,* vol.176, 2019 (doi:10.1176/appi.ajp.2018.17040415). X Liu, J Matochik, J L Cadet, et al, 'Smaller Volume of Prefrontal Lobe in Polysubstance Abusers: A Magnetic Resonance Imaging Study', *Neuropsychopharmacology* 18, 1 April 1998 (doi:10.1016/S0893-133X(97)00143-7).

Brain size opinion: Christof Koch, 'Does Brain Size Matter?', *SCI AM,* 1 January 2016.

Greater brain volume and higher IQ: J Pietschnig, D Gerdesmann, M Zeiler, M Voracek, 'Of differing methods, disputed estimates and discordant interpretations: the meta-analytical multiverse of brain volume and IQ associations', Royal Society Open Science, 11 May 2022 (doi:10.1098/rsos.211621). J J Lee, M McGue, W G Iacono, A M Michael, C F Chabris, 'The causal influence of brain size on human intelligence: Evidence from within-family phenotypic associations and GWAS modeling', *Intelligence,* 7 May 2019 (doi:10.1016/j.intell.2019.01.011).

Higher IQ linked with higher chance of addiction: W Johnson, BM Hicks, M McGue, WG Iacono, 'How Intelligence and Education Contribute to Substance Use: Hints from the Minnesota Twin Family Study', *Intelligence*, 1 November 2009 (doi:10.1016/j.intell.2008.12.003). Adam Clark Estes, 'Science Is Sure: Smart People Love Drugs', *The Atlantic*, 15 November 2011.

Dr Anna Lembke quote: *Dopamine Nation: Finding balance in the age of indulgence*, 19 January 2023 (105).

Dr Anna Lembke quote on delayed rewards: *Freedom Matters & Anna Lembke: Digital Dopamine 24/7* podcast, 20 January 2022.

The original, marshmallow test: Sofia Deleniv, 'A new take on the marshmallow test', *The British Psychological Society*, 15 October 2020. W Mischel and EB Ebbesen, 'Attention in delay of gratification', *Journal of Personality and Social Psychology*, 1970 (doi:10.1037/h0029815).

'Broken promises' marshmallow test, press release and study: 'The Marshmallow Study Revisited', *University of Rochester*, 11 October 2012. Celeste Kidd, Holly Palmeri, Richard N. Aslin, 'Rational snacking: Young children's decision-making on the marshmallow task is moderated by beliefs about environmental reliability', *Cognition* vol.126, iss.1 (doi:10.1016/j.cognition.2012.08.004).

Studies on meditation thickening the prefrontal cortex: Caroline Williams, 'Different meditation types train distinct parts of your brain', *New Scientist*, 4 October 2017. SW Lazar, CE Kerr, RH Wasserman, JR Gray, DN Greve, MT Treadway, M McGarvey, BT Quinn, JA Dusek, H Benson, SL Rauch, CI Moore, B Fischl, 'Meditation experience is associated with increased cortical thickness', *NeuroReport*, 28 November 2005 (doi:10.1097/01.wnr.0000186598.66243.19).

Debunking claims an eight-week course of meditation can change your brain: Natalia Mesa, 'How Meditation Changes the Brain: New Study Challenges Popular Beliefs', *The Scientist*, 19 June 2025.

Dr Anna Lembke exercise quote: *Dopamine Nation: Finding balance in the age of indulgence*, 19 January 2023 (152).

Lost cortical volume is reversible with abstinence: TC Durazzo, A Mon, S Gazdzinski, P-H Yeh, DJ Meyerhoff, 'Serial longitudinal magnetic resonance imaging data indicate non-linear regional gray matter volume recovery in abstinent alcohol-dependent individuals', *Addiction Biology*, 29 August 2014 (doi:10.1111/adb.12180).

Prefrontal volume can increase above baseline with abstinence: Marc Kewis, *The Biology of Desire: Why addiction is not a disease*, 23 August 2016 (137).

TELEVISION

Average British adult self-reports two hours 16 minutes TV a day: Census, 'Time Use in the UK: March 2023', *Office for National Statistics*, 4 July 2023.

BARB data on average TV use per day (TV figure isolated), and BARD data during first UK lockdown month (April 2020): 'Total Identified Viewing summary. All aged 4+', *Barb*, August 2025. 'What People Watch: April viewing summary', *Barb*, 11 May 2020.

30 per cent of Americans would rather give up sex for a year than Netflix: Dana Feldman, 'Netflix Or Sex?', *Forbes*, 12 February 2019.

Declining sex lives and the falling fertility rate linked with the rise of streaming: Shalini Ramachandran, 'Let's Watch Netflix: Three Words Guaranteed to Kill a Romantic Mood', *The Wall Street Journal*, 21 April 2019. Louise Atkinson, 'The Great British SEX drought: 30 years ago, we carried out a landmark survey that revealed what really goes on in the nation's bedrooms. Now we've asked a new generation the same questions – with startling results . . .', *MailOnline*, 8 July 2022.

Aaron Sorkin's MasterClass series: 'Film Story Arc', *MasterClass* (www.masterclass.com/classes/aaron-sorkin-teaches-screenwriting/chapters/film-story-arc).

***Adolescence* most-watched UK TV show:** '*Adolescence* Grips Viewers for Second Week at No. 1', *Tudum by Netflix*, 25 March 2025.

***American Primeval* most-watched US TV show on Netflix:** Ernesto Valenzuela, '"American Primeval" Brings Brutal Western to Top of Netflix Chart', *Movieweb*, 12 January 2025.

Jamie Dimon's leaked town hall rant: Nic White, 'Hear full audio of JPMorgan employee's work-from-home challenge that triggered CEO Jamie Dimon's foul-mouthed meltdown', *MailOnline*, 18 February 2025.

TV-watching linked with higher incidence of depression: 'Watching TV, Passive Sitting, Linked to a 43% Higher Risk of Depression', *Psychiatrist.com*, 28 November 2023.

Study comparing mentally-passive and mentally-active activities and mental health outcomes: André O Werneck, Neville Owen, Raphael HO Araujo, Danilo R Silva, Mats Hallgren, 'Mentally-passive sedentary behavior and incident depression: Mediation by inflammatory markers', *Journal of Affective Disorders*, vol. 339, 2023 (doi:10.1016/j.jad.2023.07.053).

40 per cent decline in Hollywood film productions: Regan Morris, 'Hollywood's big boom has gone bust', *BBC News*, 29 September 2024.

66 days to form a new habit: 'How long does it take to form a habit?', *UCL News*, 4 August 2009.

Average age of death in the UK, median of gender averages: 'National life tables – life expectancy in the UK: 2020 to 2022', *Office for National Statistics*, 11 January 2024.

CAFFEINE

Research on Parkinson's and caffeine: Corrie Pelc, 'Coffee may help lower Parkinson's risk in genetically predisposed ethnic groups', *Medical News Today*, 13 October 2023. Yujia Zhao et al, 'Association of Coffee Consumption and Prediagnostic Caffeine Metabolites With Incident Parkinson Disease in a Population-Based Cohort', *Neurology*, 21 March 2024 (doi:10.1212/WNL.000000000020920). Tim Newman, 'Parkinson's: Caffeine may lower risk but doesn't slow progression', *Medical News Today*, 31 May 2024.

Mixed results on caffeine lowering the risk of dementia: 'Caffeine and the risk of dementia', *Alzheimer's Society*, December 2023.

Drinking coffee in the morning: 'Is coffee in the morning good for you?', *British Heart Foundation*, 17 January 2025.

Study of 40,000 adults: Xuan Wang, Hao Ma, Qi Sun, Jun Li, Yoriko Heianza, Rob M Van Dam, Frank B Hu, Eric Rimm, JoAnn E Manson, Lu Qi, 'Coffee drinking timing and mortality in US adults', *European Heart Journal*, Vol.46, Iss.8, 21 February 2025 (doi:10.1093/eurheartj/ehae871).

Tea comments and study: 'Can drinking tea help you to live longer?', *British Heart Foundation*, 7 September 2022. Maki Inoue-Choi et al, 'Tea Consumption and All-Cause and Cause-Specific Mortality in the UK Biobank', *Annals of Internal Medicine* vol.175, 30 August 2022 (doi:10.7326/M22-0041).

Bryony Gordon defending Meghan Markle on *Lorraine*: 'Bryony Gordon CLAPS BACK on Lorraine & SHUTS DOWN Meghan Lies with FACTS!', *Glam Star Report YouTube*, 7 March 2025 (www.youtube.com/watch?v=qsl0df7uHAU).

Dr Andrew Huberman quotes: Andrew Huberman, 'Using Caffeine to Optimize Mental & Physical Performance', *Huberman Lab Podcast 101*, 5 December 2022.

Donald Trump tweet on Diet Coke: x.com/realDonaldTrump/status/260392425552482307.

Dr Chris van Tulleken quotes: *Ultra-Processed People: Why do we all eat stuff that isn't food... and why can't we stop?*, 2 May 2024 (158, 203).

Artificial sweeteners are thought to be addictive and rat study: Holly Strawbridge, 'Artificial sweeteners: sugar-free, but at what cost?', *Harvard Health Publishing*, 29 January 2020. M Lenoir, F Serre, L Cantin, SH Ahmed, 'Intense sweetness surpasses cocaine reward', *PLOS One*, 1 August 2007 (doi:10.1371/journal.pone.0000698).

400mg maximum of caffeine: 'New Study Finds Chronic High Caffeine Consumption May Heighten Risk for Cardiovascular Disease', *American College of Cardiology*, 15 August 2024. 'Spilling the Beans: How Much Caffeine is Too Much?', *U.S. Food & Drug Administration*, 28 August 2024.

Ballparks for what mg of caffeine is in each drink: 'Caffeine content for coffee, tea, soda and more', *Mayo Clinic*, 6 February 2025. Dr Nish Manek, 'Here's what a high-caffeine drink like PRIME Energy actually does to your body', *BBC Science Focus*, 18 September 2023.

Temptation-bundling: KL Milkman, JA Minson, KG Volpp, 'Holding the Hunger Games Hostage at the Gym: An Evaluation of Temptation Bundling', *Management Science*, February 2014 (doi:10.1287/mnsc.2013.1784).

Coffee and tea count as water intake: 'Water, drinks and hydration', *NHS*, 17 May 2023.
Pregnant women caffeine half-life 15 hours: H Lakin, P Sheehan, V Soti, 'Maternal Caffeine Consumption and Its Impact on the Fetus: A Review', *The Cureus Journal of Medical Science*, 4 November 2023 (doi:10.7759/cureus.48266).
Caffeine six hours before bed leads to a loss of more than one hour's sleep: C Drake, T Roehrs, J Shambroom, T Roth, 'Caffeine effects on sleep taken 0, 3, or 6 hours before going to bed', *Journal of Clinical Sleep Medicine*, 15 November 2013 (doi:10.5664/jcsm.3170).
Lion's mane reduces anxiety: Megan Giec Perry, 'Mushroom Coffee: An Evidence-Based Review', *Rupa Health*, 14 August 2024.
Cordyceps makes us better able to deal with stress: Dr Chinta Sidharthan, 'The Truth About Mushroom Coffee: Benefits vs. Hype', *Life Sciences Medical News*, 20 February 2025.

PROCRASTINATION

Bill Gates quote: 'Procrastination is not a good habit', *Motivation and Affirmations YouTube*, 2 February 2024 (www.youtube.com/watch?v=bBHQ9iOjJx4).
Margaret Atwood quote: 'The real reason you procrastinate', *TED WorkLife with Adam Grant*, 18 March 2020.
Bill Clinton given six weeks for State Address: Michael Duffy, 'The State of Bill Clinton', *Time*, 7 February 1994.
Steve Jobs took eight years to choose a sofa: John Brownlee, 'Steve Jobs's Quest For Perfection Could Make Even Buying A Sofa Into A Decade-Long Ordeal', *Cult of Mac*, 25 October 2011.
Nancy Pelosi is reportedly a procrastinator: Brittany Brolley, 'The Real Reasons You Procrastinate', *The List*, 21 August 2023.
Herman Melville chained to his desk: Caroline Gold, 'Confessions of a procrastinator', *The Spectator*, 24 September 2024.
Those allowed to procrastinate being more creative: Jihae Shin and Adam M Grant, 'When Putting Work Off Pays Off: The Curvilinear Relationship Between Procrastination and Creativity', *Academy of Management Journal*, 15 June 2021 (doi:10.5465/amj.2018.1471).
Over half of UK adults say procrastination has affected them: 'Worry about it later', *Legal & General*, n.d.
Pigeons procrastinate: J E Mazur, 'Procrastination by pigeons: preference for larger, more delayed work requirements', *Journal of the Experimental Analysis of Behavior*, January 1996 (doi:10.1901/jeab.1996.65-159).
Aaron Sorkin quote: Katie Couric, '*The Today Show* interview with Aaron Sorkin', *Bartlet4America News Archive*, 22 May 2022.
Douglas Adams quote: '42 Douglas Adams quotes to live by', *BBC Radio 4 in Four*, n.d.
Dalai Lama quote: Pico Iyer, 'The Heart of the Dalai Lama', *Small Giants Academy*, n.d.
A 'mis-regulation' of emotion: Chris Weller, 'A leading expert says procrastination has almost nothing to do with willpower', *Yahoo! Finance*, 26 November 2016.
Bedtime procrastination: F M Kroese, D T De Ridder, C Evers, M A Adriaanse, 'Bedtime procrastination: introducing a new area of procrastination', *Frontiers in Psychology*, June 2014 (doi:10.3389/fpsyg.2014.00611). R Herzog-Krzywoszanska, L Krzywoszanski, 'Bedtime Procrastination, Sleep-Related Behaviors, and Demographic Factors in an Online Survey on a Polish Sample', *Frontiers in Neuroscience*, 18 September 2019 (doi:10.3389/fnins.2019.00963).
Self-love therapy decreases RBP significantly: Wardah Alqo'idah, Tsania Nabila, Muhammad Ar-raza, Ratna Supradewi, 'Revenge Bedtime Procrastination: A Self-Love Phenomenon or Revenge Against Yourself?', *Jurnal Psikologi Perseptual*, December 2023 (doi:10.24176/perseptual.v8i2.10229).
Procrastination as heritable: D E Gustavson, A Miyake, J K Hewitt, N P Friedman, 'Genetic relations among procrastination, impulsivity, and goal-management ability: implications for the evolutionary origin of procrastination', *Psychological Science*, 4 April 2014 (doi:10.1177/0956797614526260).
Procrastinators have larger amygdalas: Caroline Schlüter, Christoph Fraenz, Marlies Pinnow, Patrick Friedrich, Onur Güntürkün, and Erhan Genç, 'The Structural and Functional Signature of Action Control', *Association for Psychological Science*, 4 May 2018 (doi:10.1177/0956797618779380).

Professor Sirois quote: Thomas Ling, 'How to finally break your procrastination habit, explained by a psychologist', *BBC Science Focus Magazine*, 7 January 2025.

Professor Timothy Pychyl quote: Nazima Pathan, 'Procrastination: It's pretty much all in the mind', *BBC News*, 26 August 2018.

Meditation proven to shrink amygdala volume: R A Gotink, M W Vernooij, M A Ikram, W J Niessen, G P Krestin, A Hofman, H Tiemeier, M G M Hunink, 'Meditation and yoga practice are associated with smaller right amygdala volume: the Rotterdam study', *Brain Imaging and Behavior*, February 2018 (doi:10.1007/s11682-018-9826-z).

Procrastination most rife in people in their twenties: M E Beutel, E M Klein, S Aufenanger, E Brähler, M Dreier, K W Müller, O Quiring, L Reinecke, G Schmutzer, B Stark, K Wölfling, 'Procrastination, Distress and Life Satisfaction across the Age Range – A German Representative Community Study', *PLoS One*, 12 February 2016 (doi:10.1371/journal.pone.0148054).

The urgency effect: Meng Zhu, Yang Yang, Christopher K Hsee, 'The Mere Urgency Effect', *Journal of Consumer Research*, Vol.45, Iss.3, 9 February 2018 (doi:10.1093/jcr/ucy008).

'Small first, big later' method: Francesca Gino and Bradley R Staats, 'Your Desire to Get Things Done Can Undermine Your Effectiveness', *Harvard Business Review*, 22 March 2016.

Forgiving ourselves for past procrastination: Michael J A Wohl, Timothy A Pychyl, Shannon H Bennett, 'I forgive myself, now I can study: How self-forgiveness for procrastinating can reduce future procrastination', *Personality and Individual Differences*, Vol.48, Iss.7, May 2010 (doi:10.1016/j.paid.2010.01.029).

Kevin Systrom's five-minute hack: Betsy Mikel, 'Instagram's billionaire CEO does this for 60 minutes every single morning', *Inc.*, 10 June 2017.

Students' mid-thesis expectations: Roger Buehler, Dale Griffin and Michael Ross, 'Exploring the "Planning Fallacy": Why People Underestimate Their Task Completion Times', *Journal of Personality and Social Psychology*, Vol.67, 1994.

We're less productive before appointments: Gabriela N Tonietto, Selin A Malkoc, Stephen M Nowlis, 'When an Hour Feels Shorter: Future Boundary Tasks Alter Consumption by Contracting Time', *Journal of Consumer Research*, Vol.45, Iss.5, February 2019 (doi:10.1093/jcr/ucy043).

Margaret Atwood's alter ego, 'Peggy': Jessica Stillman, '*Handmaid's Tale* Author and Self-Described Lazy Person Margaret Atwood Explains How She Beats Procrastination', *Inc.*, 24 May 2020.

ACKNOWLEDGEMENTS

Caitlin Moran quote: Caitlin Moran, 'After 25 Years, Here's What I've Leant About A "Good Marriage"', *Grazia*, 28 September 2020.

ACKNOWLEDGEMENTS

I wrote this book – my most challenging book yet – in just eight months. That would not have happened, were it not for the tireless patience and support of my partner, George.

He looked after our three year-old Mia – and our highly anxious dog, who can never be left alone, ever – while I travelled the country talking to experts, pulled late nights and worked weekends, and went on writing retreats when the panic set in.

A long time ago, I read a quote from Caitlin Moran saying that 'All too often, women marry their glass ceiling' and I never forgot it. Thank you for being the opposite of that, George.

I am wildly grateful to all of my 24 experts, who shared their insights so generously, but special thanks goes out to those institutions who hosted me physically: Delamere residential rehab, which I spent two full days at and left very impressed by; the University of Birmingham's CHBH (Centre for Human Brain Health), where I had an fMRI and unexpectedly, a lot of fun while also learning; Edge Hill University, which provided me access to many fascinating aspects; and the University of Winchester, where I saw not only Wendy's 'bar lab', but much more besides. I was inspired by everyone I met and interviewed along the way, and only hope to match their vigour for the cause. Thank you for having me.

I am lucky enough to have the best team behind me, from my indefatigable agent Rachel Mills, to the kind and highly skilled team at Octopus: Jo Morrell, Pauline Bache, Karen Baker, Katie Forsythe, Matt Grindon and Mel Four, who all went over and beyond. I'm also delighted that Michaela Twite, who I've known for many years, has been able to come on board as a freelancer for the copy edit too.

My first readers, Kate Faithfull and Laurie McAllister, for both telling me when I've got it right, and when they think I've gotten it wrong. You need the hearts as well as the constructive criticism, they're both equally important, and I hugely appreciate the many hours you both spent reading my early drafts.

I'm grateful to the welcoming gang at St Julian's Hall co-working space, particularly Aimee, for allowing me to work late nights and weekends in order to get this done. I also spent many happy days on writing retreats at Starcroft Farm Cabins, in East Sussex, where Hannah's flawless taste and attention to detail really elevated my experience. You deserve those 70 five-star reviews. I'll be back.

Last but far from least, I want to extend the hugest thanks to my readers, many of whom have stuck around for the past nine years, supporting me ever since *The Unexpected Joy of Being Sober*. Thank you for sending me the most beautiful messages over the years. I hope you like this one too.

INDEX

ABOUT THE AUTHOR

Catherine Gray is the author of six books, including *The Unexpected Joy of Being Sober*. *Little Addictions* is her seventh. She's sold well over half a million books in English-speaking territories alone, and her books have been translated into fourteen languages.

With a background in journalism, she has written for *The Guardian*, *Grazia*, *Stylist*, *The Telegraph* and many more. Her books have received acclaim from the likes of *The New York Times*, *BBC Breakfast*, *Good Morning America* and BBC Radio 2.

In 2018, Catherine founded the charitable campaign Sober Spring – a three-month sabbatical from alcohol – with Alcohol Change UK, for whom she is an ambassador. She's been sober since 2013.

Catherine lives in a little house by the sea with a high-maintenance dog, a medium-maintenance partner and a low-maintenance toddler.

You can follow Catherine on Instagram @unexpectedjoyof or sign up for (very infrequent) emails from her on www.catherine-gray.co.uk

Dear Reader,

We'd love your attention for one more page to tell you about the crisis in children's reading, and what we can all do.

Studies have shown that reading for fun is the **single biggest predictor of a child's future life chances** – more than family circumstance, parents' educational background or income. It improves academic results, mental health, wealth, communication skills, ambition and happiness.[1]

The number of children reading for fun is in rapid decline. Young people have a lot of competition for their time. In 2024, 1 in 10 children and young people in the UK aged 5 to 18 did not own a single book at home.[2]

Hachette works extensively with schools, libraries and literacy charities, but here are some ways we can all raise more readers:

- Reading to children for just 10 minutes a day makes a difference
- Don't give up if children aren't regular readers – there will be books for them!
- Visit bookshops and libraries to get recommendations
- Encourage them to listen to audiobooks
- Support school libraries
- Give books as gifts

There's a lot more information about how to encourage children to read on our website: **www.RaisingReaders.co.uk**

Thank you for reading.

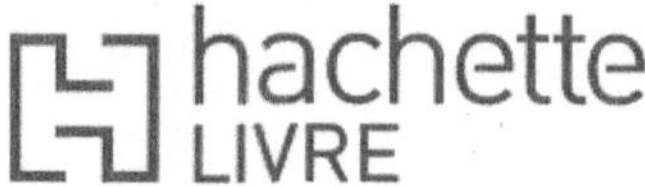

---

[1] OECD, '21st-Century Readers: Developing Literacy Skills in a Digital World', 2021, https://www.oecd.org/en/publications/21st-century-readers_a83d84cb-en.html

[2] National Literacy Trust, 'Book Ownership in 2024', November 2024. https://literacytrust.org.uk/research-services/research-reports/book-ownership-in-2024